When Treatment Fails

David J. Bearison

When Treatment Fails

How Medicine Cares for Dying Children

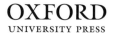

OXFORD
UNIVERSITY PRESS

2006

OXFORD
UNIVERSITY PRESS

Oxford University Press, Inc., publishes works that further
Oxford University's objective of excellence
in research, scholarship, and education.

Oxford   New York
Auckland   Cape Town   Dar es Salaam   Hong Kong   Karachi
Kuala Lumpur   Madrid   Melbourne   Mexico City   Nairobi
New Delhi   Shanghai   Taipei   Toronto

With offices in
Argentina   Austria   Brazil   Chile   Czech Republic   France   Greece
Guatemala   Hungary   Italy   Japan   Poland   Portugal   Singapore
South Korea   Switzerland   Thailand   Turkey   Ukraine   Vietnam

Copyright © 2006 by David J. Bearison

Published by Oxford University Press, Inc.
198 Madison Avenue, New York, New York 10016
www.oup.com

Oxford is a registered trademark of Oxford University Press

Library of Congress Cataloging-in-Publication Data
Bearison, David J.
When treatment fails : how medicine cares for dying children /
David J. Bearison.
p.   cm.
Includes bibliographical references and index.
ISBN–10: 0–19–515612–9
ISBN–13: 978–0–19–515612–6
1. Terminally ill children—Care.   2. Terminally ill children—Medical care.   3. Terminally ill
children—Care—Psychological aspects.   I. Title.
RJ249.B43 2005
362.17'5'083—dc22   2005005898
1 3 5 7 9 8 6 4 2
Printed in the United States of America
on acid-free paper

Foreword

Twenty years ago, as a fellow in pediatric oncology, I sat with Audrey Evans, an eminent pediatric oncologist, while she told the parents of a 2-year-old child with Stage IV neuroblastoma that their child had an invariably fatal disease. Taken out of the context, and away from her inimitable presentation and presence, those words seem to reverberate with cruelty. However, her words were in fact suffused with kindness, and she employed the intensity of the moment to invite the stricken parents to join her in a journey of clinical investigation exploring new methods of therapy and reaching for cure. Once engaged in the struggle, the parents and physician became allies in the fight against the disease and the care of the child. Her honesty enabled the parents to begin to prepare themselves for the cruel loss, but her activity and endeavor continuously signaled to them that there was some hope. The child experienced a brief partial remission from the disease, but within the year, the child's disease progressed. The progression of the disease signaled to both parents and physician that the time for more "clinical research" had passed, and the goal was now to render comfort to the child and to provide time for the parents and child to be together without technical interventions. When the child died, this extraordinary senior physician joined mother and nurses by the bedside to bathe the dead child and help shroud the body.

Stage IV neuroblastoma remains a difficult disease to cure. Enormous advances have been made in understanding the varieties of the disease, allowing us to categorize prognosis finely and to tailor treatment to the biological parameters. An enormous leap forward has been made in understanding the molecular basis of the disease, and some incremental progress has also been made in achieving long-term survival for some of the children. It is, unfortunately, one of the diseases in pediatric oncology that has been relatively resistant to cure.

What has changed dramatically from those days, it seems to me, is the way physicians and parents alike approach this and other potentially fatal diseases.

Using the Internet and the conversational net woven among the parents themselves, parents often see themselves as pivotal in the search for cure. Information about investigational agents that appear to be "the cure" is frequently televised, and a seemingly endless variety of complementary cures are publicized. Thus, many parents have the unshakable belief that a child's death is not just the failure of medicine, but the failure to find the correct practitioner and the correct drug in the correct hospital. Physicians themselves seem less and less inclined to view death as an acceptable end for a child. Although a partnership between parent, patient, and physician and other medical caregivers is the ideal and seemingly could positively fuel the dissemination of medical knowledge, too often the incomplete or inaccurate barrage of information the parents find creates a profound lack of trust in medical staff. The parents often see themselves as the guardians of their child against the physician's or the hospital's lack of knowledge, disinterest, or even ineptitude. Parents and physicians seem to have increasingly disparate ways of experiencing the progression of an illness. Despite this gulf between professionals and parents, they are often united in inadvertently allowing the quest for cure to interfere with the provision of comfort and relief of suffering for the patient. The shared acceptance of a child's coming death, and collaboration in providing comforting care for a dying child, seems to be an ever less likely occurrence.

A great challenge of pediatric medicine today is to reconcile the quest for cure, including the clinical investigation of new agents and methods of cure, with the reality of loss. Without pushing the borders of clinical investigation, treatment advances cannot be achieved. However, in advancing new therapies, we must not ever lose sight of the need to accept loss. Each practitioner must know how to guide parents toward such acceptance when, for their child, the end of life approaches. Above all we must work to minimize the suffering of parents and children. These words, though so easy to say, are profoundly challenging to enact at the bedside.

In these stories of children's deaths as seen through the eyes of the hospital staff who cared for them, the complexities of the child's end of life are sharply etched. There is a paucity of research in this area, and whatever has been done is approached mainly from the patients' and parents' perspective. Through the iteration of the professional caregivers' stories, one can see the inevitable conflict between the quest for cure and the acceptance of death in sharpest relief. In seeing the trajectory toward death through the professionals' eyes, we can begin to formulate better ways to care for the families we serve and also find ways to care for the caretakers. Caring for the caretakers results in better care for parents and children alike. I hope that this book will provide ways of bringing together medical caregivers and parents in the journey toward cure of children when possible and toward death when inevitable.

Linda Granowetter, M.D.
Bellagio, Lago di Como, Italy

Preface

I'm not afraid of death, I am afraid of dying.
— DEREK JARMAN
At Your Own Risk

In the unconscious, each of us is
convinced of his own immortality.
— SIGMUND FREUD

I began spending time with children who had cancer 20 years ago as a way of understanding how they struggled to adjust and make sense of what was, for them, a bewildering and frightening experience that involved many hospitalizations, and invasive, painful medical procedures, sometimes lasting 3 or more years. As I became more familiar with the culture of childhood cancer, I was concerned by the efforts parents and caregivers made to blindly and falsely reassure children that having cancer was "no big deal" and certainly nothing for them to be scared about. Of course, this was done with good intentions—as a way of trying to "protect" children. But time and time again, I saw that it didn't help children at all and that, furthermore, it led them to a frantic, and often lonely, search to find meaning and make sense of their having cancer in spite of efforts to deny them as much. So I wrote a book about what it is like to talk openly and honestly to children about having cancer, *"They Never Want to Tell You": Children Talk About Cancer.*[1] I relied on the children's narratives about having cancer in order to give unrestrained voice to how they dealt with cancer and how they chose to talk about their fears, hopes, and aspirations. I hoped that hearing the candor in their voices would help adults overcome their fear of talking to children about life-threatening situations.

In the decade and some since I wrote "*They Never Want to Tell You*," attitudes about talking to children about cancer have changed dramatically. Today, pediatric oncologists, at least in the United States, consistently appreciate the value of open and honest discourse with children of all ages about what it means to have cancer and the nature of their treatment protocols. They also see the value in encouraging parents to follow suit and to recognize that they do not comfort or protect their children when they falsely reassure them. Hence, we have increasingly come to find the means of talking honestly about a frightening and life-threatening illness while providing hope and promise.

This has not been the case, however, in discourse about end of life. Because dying is no longer linear or progressive and makes no sense in our attempts to reconcile our ways of living, it is particularly difficult for us to talk openly about it. Our lack of honesty with dying patients (who today face a greater likelihood of dying in a hospital than at home because of the growing medicalization of dying) and our reluctance to allow public display of emotions contribute to making death and dying a hidden, even forbidden, subject.[2] Yet, it is during end-of-life care that medical staff come to appreciate how much each organ and tissue ultimately serves as "palpable testimony that we are material and mortal."[3]

Dying as Metaphor

Most children who die in hospitals have cancer, and despite remarkable medical advances, cancer survival, in individual cases, remains frustratingly uncertain and increasingly complicated. I am drawn to this inquiry about what it is like to care for children at the end of their lives because it remains a topic that has not been adequately addressed either professionally or publicly and, when it is finally broached, it is shrouded in metaphors and euphemisms that obscure its realities. Given our ambivalence about death and our unwillingness to face it directly, we try to "protect" child patients and families—which represents the most grueling, heart-wrenching, and frustrating aspect of pediatric practice. Like Susan Sontag in her essays *Illness as Metaphor* and *AIDS and Its Metaphors*,[4] I find that we can achieve better ways of caring for children at end of life by stripping the discourse about death and dying of some of its tenacious and insidious metaphors. These kinds of metaphors make it more difficult for medical staff to come to grips with what they are doing to provide family-centered care at the end of a child's life. It also makes it more difficult for families to know what to do, and it denies children their autonomy.

The language we use to describe the conditions of death and dying has been culturally and historically constructed over time. Our stories about death and dying are sustained less by biological determinants than by sociohistorical and cultural metaphors that reflect our collective fears and torments. Metaphors are phrases ordinarily used to designate one thing that are then applied to implicitly convey beliefs and values about other things.[5] They often are couched in comparative terms. For example, in the case of death and dying: living is dynamic, dying is moribund; living has a cause and purpose, dying is senseless; living is progressive, dying is regressive; living might be a triumph, dying always is a failure. We resort to metaphors about death and dying to hide our fears and protect ourselves. What stronger evidence could there be of this practice than the range of euphemisms we use to avoid speaking of death in ordinary discourse.[6] In some countries, even common euphemisms of death and dying are intolerable because they are too threatening. Death has replaced sex as the most forbidden topic of discourse.[7,8]

For me, the inspiration to elicit the narratives that form the core of this book lay in the mystery of it all: I never knew what stories I was going to hear, what they might be like, and where they might lead me in thinking about children dying in hospitals. I remember that when I began approaching medical staff about telling me what it is like for them to care for a dying child, one senior attending physician said, "Yeah, great idea. I'll give you 10 minutes" and then we met and he talked for more than an hour and a half. At the end of our meeting, he realized that he had never spoken to anyone (including himself) about these kinds of end-of-life issues about any of his patients. He thanked me for giving him the space to talk about it, and said how much it helped him. As I continued eliciting narratives, I was pleased to find that his reaction was the norm rather than the exception.

As a pediatric psychologist who worked and studied with medical staff long before I began the present study, I thought I knew most of the participants pretty well. But when I sat down with them—one-on-one and in confidence—and listened to them tell what it was like to care for a dying child, I began to know them in different and quite remarkable ways. They spoke compassionately in ways that reflected their own particular sense of who they were in the context of what happens when a child is dying. Although, for many of them, caring for a dying child happened repeatedly, it was never a routine matter for any of them. Each child and family brought forth particular medical issues and a varying range of emotions. From their trenchant stories, I came to realize that abstract principles and universal guidelines about how to care for children at the end of their lives don't fit the clinical demands, uncertainties, and increasingly complex parameters of any given family's situation.[9]

Often, when people heard that I was preparing this book, they asked me how I could do it—why was I such a glutton for such anguish? Such questions reminded me of a nurse who told me, "What keeps me going is knowing that, for some reason, I'm somehow making a difference in these kids' lives and in their parents' lives." I found that talking to staff about end-of-life care in pediatrics was inspiring. Their concern for children and families was paramount in everything they did, and, for me, it was contagious.

When reading the standard texts in the field of pediatric end-of-life palliative care, I am discouraged by how remote they are from the critical and compelling issues that constitute the day-by-day uncertainties and complications involved in end-of-life care for children and their families. These texts typically begin with a history of the topic without ever acknowledging how it authorizes a certain privileged position about the topic. They convey a false sense that we have historically arrived on secure ground through systematic accumulative advances in theory and scientific research. However, this kind of rhetoric is challenged the moment we try to apply it in practice. The practical decisions that staff confront about end-of-life care of children profoundly capture the fundamental differences between abstract principles and clinical practices in medicine. Standard texts fail to recognize or adequately acknowledge essential differences between the logical coherence of formal, abstract, theoretical ideas and the immediacy of the clinical press of day-to-day practice. In practice, issues frequently arise that are neither logical nor coherent in any systematic way. They are messy, complex, and frustratingly uncertain. In place of science, we often have to rely on our beliefs and values about the quality of life. We like to think that science informs practice, but that is not necessarily the case in medicine when treatment for curative intent is failing. Such times provide the means for practice to inform theory and to challenge it in ways that are profoundly disturbing; in other words, the science of medicine is always grounded in clinical practice.

In my dual roles of academic and practitioner (in medicine, law, and clinical psychology), I have always been drawn to these kinds of challenges and provocations. I don't particularly like the cloistered atmosphere of the "ivory tower," and, unlike most of my colleagues there, I often venture out to explore scenes of drama, chaos, trauma, and tumult. Maybe I find it exciting, in the sense of ambulance-chasing, but, in the spirit of the psychologist and philosopher William James, I always find that what I learn on the edge can be brought to better understand the center of life.[10]

Acknowledgments

For many years, I have benefited from discussions, ideological disputes, and heated debates with friends, students, and colleagues about the issues considered in this book. Our fervent dialogues led the way for me to advance my ideas in doctoral seminars, colloquia, professional meetings, plenary speeches, and medical rounds. As I came to appreciate how the trajectory of care for children dying in hospitals is not so rational and linear, I grew to realize how my own thoughts about this topic are not so constrained. I have wavered between seemingly contradictory perspectives while always trying to avoid any kind of orthodoxies about how to care for children dying in hospitals. In the end, I learned to appreciate that it is enough to raise the issues that address essential questions about this, even when I don't have decisive answers.

Those who know me understand what a struggle this might have been for me and how it complicated my sense of mission when preparing this book. So many of them were there to help me in this struggle. Among my institutional benefactors, I thank the Faculty Research Awards Program of the City University of New York. On two occasions, they provided seed money for this project. I thank Robert Granger, President of the W. T. Grant Foundation, who arranged substantial financial support for me to do this work. I am grateful to the Rockefeller Foundation for providing me with the ideal place and comforts to write major sections of this book—the Villa Serbelloni, Lago di Como, Bellagio, Italy. The Graduate Center of the City University of New York gave me a fellowship leave and, the following year, a Scholar Incentive Award in order first to gather data and then to write this book. I thank Anna Stetsenko, Head of the Ph.D. Program in Developmental Psychology, Judith Kubran, Administrative Assistant of the Program, and Joseph Glick, Executive Officer of the Ph.D. Programs in Psychology, for assisting me during these leaves.

I was fortunate to initiate my study of end-of-life care, in a systematic way, when I was a Visiting Professor at Mount Sinai School of Medicine in 1995 when Diane Meier invited me to participate in its Open Society Institute's Death in America project and to continue that affiliation as an Adjunct Professor of Pediatrics at Mount Sinai School of Medicine. My participation in the Pediatric Oncology Group (POG) and later in its reincarnation as the Children's Oncology Group (COG) brought me into productive collaborations with an amazing group of pediatric psychologists, nurses, and oncologists who recognize the contributions of psycho-social issues when designing national protocols to treat pediatric cancer patients.

I am particularly pleased and privileged to be an Adjunct Attending at the Children's Hospital of New York (CHONY). In addition to my CHONY affiliation, my appointment as Adjunct Professor of Psychiatry and Pediatrics at the College of Physicians and Surgeons of Columbia University acknowledges my commitment not only to clinical practice, but also to research and to teaching medical students and residents.

The Lady Davis Fellowship Trust allowed me to spend a semester in Jerusalem to complete the preparation of the manuscript of this book, to be a Visiting Professor in Psychology at the Hebrew University, and to extend my studies of pediatric end-of-life care to the Hadassah Medical Center of the Hebrew University. I thank M. Mark Sopher, Executive Secretary of the Trust, Marianna Barr, Advisor to Visiting Faculty at the Hebrew University, Rivka Tuval-Mashiach, my colleague and research associate at Hadassah Medical Center, and Michael Weintraub, Chief of Pediatric Psychology at Hadassah Medical Center, for the opportunity to continue this work in Israel. I thank Amia Lieblich, Anat Ninio, Charlie Greenbaum, and Gersohn Ben-Shacher, all of the Department of Psychology at the Hebrew University, for the care and concern they showed me and my work on this book.

While preparing this book, I was fortunate to be a member of the American Psychological Association's Task Force on End-of-Life Care of Children and Adolescents. I learned so much from the other Task Force members: Ann Kazak, Gary Walco, Elaine Meyer, Barbara Sourkes, and Ira Cohen.

Doctoral students in the Developmental, Social, and Clinical Psychology Programs at the Graduate Center of the City University of New York led me to consider innovative, provocative, and constructive ways medicine cares for dying children. While I cannot name all of them, I want to acknowledge some of them. Jennifer Dobbins and Heather Charatz carefully transcribed verbatim the audio cassettes of the narratives I elicited, and they always remained true, in every essential way, to the participants' voices. I am grateful to Lynda Polgreen, at the time a medical student at Mount Sinai School of Medicine, who began with me and Linda Granowetter narrative explorations into this field of inquiry. Being the chair of Magaret Spier's doctoral dissertation committee also helped me to recognize the value of pursuing this project on a more systematic and grander scale—her dissertation focused on dying children and their families.

I am most grateful to Joan Bossert, my editor at Oxford University Press. Right from the start, she saw the promise of my ideas about this book and supported me all along the way. Steve Holtje was all I could hope for as development editor at Oxford, as were Barbara Goodhouse, production editor, and Jennifer Rappoport, associate editor.

I regret that I have to avoid naming the hospital from which these stories came in order to preserve the anonymity of the participants (as well as the patients and their families). My deepest gratitude goes to all of the participants who welcomed me into their professional lives and spoke to me so willingly and openly about what it is like for them to care for children at the end of their lives; who showed so much concern about and trust in what I was doing; and who wanted to be a part of this book. One of the attending physicians told me how stressful it was for the staff to hear a parent of a dying child say to them, "You've got to find a miracle." Yet when a child died in their care, I found these people to be miracle workers and I felt privileged to be with them. They will recognize their stories in this book and will understand my gratitude.

I acknowledge the children who have died and their families who unknowingly were clinical cases in my study. They set the stage for me to explore how, when treatment fails, medicine cares for dying children.

My wife, Linda Granowetter, is an amazing pediatric oncologist who has had a special role in helping me prepare this book. The idea for it was a collaborative effort between us, and she assisted me each step of the way. We share a common concern for children in crises, and we derive strength from each other to pursue ways of helping them. She inspires me, teaches me, and gives me hope.

Contents

When Treatment Fails

One death moves the imagination
more powerfully than millions;
one death is a drama throbbing
with emotion; a million,
only dry-as-ashes statistics.
— LEENA BERG
quoted in Alexander Donat,
The Holocaust Kingdom

With every child's death in a hospital there are stories to be told from the variegated perspectives of those who had been the caregivers. Most often, these stories remain unspoken; very rarely are they considered as a whole. In order to better understand the issues of caring for children at the end of their lives and to achieve clearer standards of care, I want to give voice to these stories. Compared to abstract conceptual considerations of end of life care, these stories capture the nuanced complexity of issues as they evolve in the daily press of pediatric practice in all their uncertainty, ambiguity, intensity, and sense of sheer frustration. They also capture, in remarkable ways, the struggle to resolve issues about end-of-life care for children—issues that often reflect conflicting perspectives among the staff or between the staff and families. Hence, such stories help to achieve a greater sense of clarity about end-of-life care for children in hospitals.

Aside from the clinician's stories about end-of-life care for children, there are individual stories of the children who are dying and of their families, and, on a broader level of reflection, there are collective stories (folk tales) from communities, cultures, and institutions (particularly religious ones) that implicitly or explicitly promote ways of dying. But here I consider only the clinician's ways of telling the tale. Others have already given voice to children's, families', and cultures' stories of dying.[1]

Surprisingly little has been written about pediatric end-of-life care from the clinician's perspective. To date, most palliative care studies have come from the field of nursing; yet a review of 50 leading textbooks in pediatric nursing found that only 2 percent of their contents discussed end-of-life care for children.[2] The same is true for medical textbooks.[3]

Studies of end-of-life care, in general, are very limited, and systematic data are not readily available; studies involving children and their families constitute only a very small part of this limited field of inquiry. The Institute of Medicine's Committee on Palliative and End-of-Life Care for Children and Their Families considered ways of improving palliative and end-of-life care for children. In 2003, they concluded, "Throughout its work, the committee has been hampered by the lack of basic descriptive information about death in childhood," and they called for the "collection of descriptive data . . . to guide the provision, funding, and evaluation of palliative, end-of-life, and bereavement care for children and families."[4]

We need descriptive accounts, in practical day-by-day, eyes-wide-open terms, of what happens to children and families during the last weeks, days, and hours of life and how these experiences affect end-of-life decisions for everyone involved.[5] Is there a natural trajectory to how children die in hospitals? Is there any way to define a "good death" when children are involved?[6] How might children participate in end-of-life decisions concerning them? This book provides the kind of "descriptive data" called for by the Institute of Medicine.

We all would prefer to die quickly without protracted suffering, pain, and humiliation. Death during sleep is especially preferred, but this kind of death is not very common. Some patients at the end of life in hospitals are overtreated with needlessly aggressive care, whereas others are undertreated and die in unnecessary pain.[7] Conflicting advice from different nurses and different physicians confuses families about how best to prepare for and accept the death of their child. The process of "active dying" is distressing, even under the best circumstances. For example, seeing a child hungry for air is a wretched experience for everyone involved.

How a child dies is not only biologically determined but also depends on the child, the family, health care providers, the hospital, insurance providers, state and federal mandates about issues such as advance directives and ages of consent for children, and the curricula in schools that train physicians, nurses, and psychosocial staff. Taken together, these variables affect the quality of end-of-life care for everyone involved. Although no one can assure a good death, we have the means to improve the quality of care provided during the final days of a child's life.

When considering end-of-life issues, there is a need to capture the sense of immediacy and involvement of those who, day-by-day, make critical decisions regarding the end-of-life care of children, whether their deaths are from acute or chronic conditions. They have to account for how issues evolve in the press of hospital-based pediatric practice where dying may be messy, muddled, unduly complicated, bewildering, sometimes painful, possibly degrading, wildly uncertain, mystifying, circuitous, dirty, and debilitating.[8] The "roller-coaster" experience of dying from chronic, progressive, and incurable diseases has become so commonplace that medicine has coined the term *Lazarus syndrome* to describe it. A patient is expected to die, and the family engages in anticipatory grieving and prepares for the death, but then the patient goes into remission and the family may be resentful that the expected death has not occurred. The family is left with enough uncertainties to expect that it will occur but not knowing when.[9] This syndrome engenders in patients and their families loss of hope with bouts of despair, followed by some renewal of hope along with a continually increasing burden of information load.

Dying children often are highly symptomatic. End-of-life symptoms for children can be categorized according to five biological/psychosocial systems: gastrointestinal, neurological, respiratory, hematological (i.e., anemia and bleeding), and psychological (e.g., fear and anxiety). Accordingly, at the end of their lives children commonly have the following symptoms: pain, anorexia, fatigue, dyspnea (i.e., gasping for air), constipation, vomiting food and blood (hematemesis), bleeding, seizures, fear, anxiety, and terminal agitation.[10] These symptoms develop more rapidly in children compared to adults and often are less clearly localized.[11] Sometimes these symptoms are not easily controllable, and, at other times, trying to control them is inappropriate because it may complicate and needlessly prolong dying.[12] Treating children for end-of-life symptoms is complicated because choices of drugs for adults are not recommended for children either because of known complications or, more often, because of lack of findings from pediatric trials.[13] Adding to this problem is that children differ from adults in their ability to absorb, distribute, metabolize, and eliminate drugs that might manage their end-of-life symptoms.[14]

Talking to Children about Dying

Despite empirical evidence dating back to 1965 about children's understanding of the biological and irreversible nature of death, adults are reluctant to discuss end-of-life issues with children.[15] Although adults often justify this reluctance as a need to "protect" children from the fears and uncertainties of dying, it more likely reflects adults' need to defend themselves from their fears about death and dying. Children recognize this and soon sense that it is inappropriate for them to talk about end-of-life decisions. Adults then mistakenly take children's reluctance to talk as a sign of their disinterest in learning about the limits of end-of-life care. It often leaves children feeling alone in their grief for loss of functions and inability to participate in the activities of daily living. Consequently, they undertake a solitary journey in search of personal meaning and an understanding of what is happening to them. This conspiracy of silence between children and adults about end-of-life care is similar to how, 20 years ago, we were reluctant to talk to children about having cancer.[16] Today, we recognize that children who have cancer have a right to know about it and their treatment.[17]

Even though they are rarely told directly,[18] there is evidence that all children in hospitals know when they are dying and that they are able to discern the imminence of death through the extraordinary stress of the family and caregivers around them.[19] They therefore have the right to supportive and developmentally appropriate means to express their concerns about end-of-life issues. This can be done by talking alone or in combination with various kinds of play activities, including music, art, video, story writing, and creation of rituals. Those of us in pediatrics are learning how to talk to dying children in ways that preserve honesty with compassion so as to alleviate their anxieties while preserving hope through the chaos. When the medical staff does this, the children's families will begin to follow suit because children will validate such discourse.

With the encouragement of medical ethicists, difficult as it is, we are coming to recognize that "dying children should have the information they desire about their illness, including the relative merits or burdens of any proposed treatments or procedures so that they can exercise some personal choice. This is true regardless of whether they have the full maturity of an adult."[20] Guidelines have been published to determine the capacity of children to give assent with parental permission or to give legally binding consent for medical care.[21] The American Academy of Pediatrics goes even further than just endorsing the need for physicians to give children and parents the information they need to make decisions about health care, but advises those physicians who choose to withhold information to assume the burden of justifying the decision not to disclose and document it in the medical record.[22]

Parents and Siblings of Dying Children

The death of a child colors everything the parents do for the rest of their lives; the event can never be fully resolved because there is no tolerable answer to why their child has died.[23] It prematurely breaks the bonds of parent-child attachment that begins the moment a child is born, if not before.[24] The torment of this loss is captured in the following: "When a child dies, it is always out of season. When a child dies, dreams die, and we are all diminished by the loss of human potential. Although dying is a part of life, a child's death . . . is unnatural and has a devastating and enduring impact."[25]

Parents always are an integral part of their child's health care team, as is reflected in the term *family-centered medicine*, the hallmark of pediatric practice in major medical centers. However, when, in the course of a chronic and prolonged illness, parents come to recognize that hope for a cure for their child is receding, they approach a new phase in how they relate to the medical staff. Often, they begin to question, if not abandon, the premise that their child, the medical staff, and they are all inseparable in a common struggle to "fight" the illness and find a cure. While trying to protect their child from what they perceive as the increasingly more frightening realities of death and dying, most parents press the medical staff to assume ever more heroic, invasive, and uncertain kinds of treatment protocols. This press for increasingly more aggressive care means that parents (and medical staff) often begin to divert their attention from the child's feelings about death and dying. Even when physicians, however reluctant, go beyond established procedures to uncharted and highly experimental treatment protocols, it is only natural that, when their child dies, parents question whether they did all they possibly could to save their child. Whereas pediatric subspecialists often seem unwilling to accept death as a likely outcome and pursue curative intent, at all costs— even if nothing else than as an experiment from which to learn and apply to other cases—parents typically are much less able than physicians to accept the idea that treatment ought to be withheld or withdrawn because there is no realistic chance of cure.

Even when prior relations between parents and staff have been optimal, the ending of hope for cure introduces conflict and frustration into the relationship. Parents, feeling guilty for the death of their child, inevitably question whether they should have pursued other treatments or care at other medical centers. Other emotions that now arise include intense anxiety, anger, and depression, although many of these parents are grateful to the staff for their care and concern. And, too, families' relationships with each other during this time can be either mutually supportive or alienating.[26]

The agony and guilt that parents experience when their child is dying is exacerbated by the strongly held, pervasive belief that parents are not supposed to outlive their children. In our culture, the death of a child, is an anomaly. While death is so often said to be a natural process resulting from disease, when it involves children, a substantially greater momentum (compared to treating adults) is set in motion to continue aggressive treatments, even when these treatments provide little realistic hope of cure and often impose barriers to adequate palliation.[27] The success of medicine in improving survival rates for children with life-threatening illnesses exacerbates, among staff and families alike, the false sense that death can always be averted. As a recent review in the *New England Journal of Medicine* observes:

> Recognition that death is inevitable often lags behind the reality of the medical condition, leading to a treatment approach that is inappropriately aggressive. For example, a child with multiple leukemic relapses may be offered a third or fourth bone marrow transplantation to attempt to induce a short-term remission or to maintain some quality of life, but with no hope of cure. In such a setting, essential palliative care services might be rejected by the parents, who will continue to view the procedure as curative.[28]

Moreover, certain interventions may serve curative intents for some patients and strictly palliative intents for others, even for the same patient at different times. For example, pediatric oncologists speak about the benefits of palliative chemotherapy to induce a short-term remission and maintain some quality of life but with no expectation of cure. Parents, however, typically interpret it as a hope for cure. According to Cicely Saunders, the founder of the modern hospice movement, "The old acceptance of destiny has disappeared and a new sense of outrage that modern advances cannot finally halt the inevitable makes caring for the dying and for their families demanding and often difficult, but perhaps all the more rewarding as truth becomes more openly discussed."[29]

One study found that 56 percent of children with cancer were receiving cancer-directed therapy in the last month of their lives.[30] The increasing toxicities of curative treatments at end of life can compromise children's quality of life. Often, questions about their growth and development become secondary to the unwavering goal of achieving a cure. The same study reported that parents of children who had died of cancer first recognized that their child had no realistic chance for cure 106 days prior to death, while pediatric oncologists came to such a conclusion 206 days prior. They reported that "as the children's cancer advanced, parents' understanding that the child no longer had a realistic chance for cure was delayed, lagging behind the explicit documentation of this fact by the primary oncologist by more than 3 months." Parents in this study recalled having discussed with a caregiver the idea that their child did not have a realistic chance for cure, but only 49 percent of them reported that they understood from this discussion that their child was terminally ill. These findings need to be understood in the context that the median length of stay prior to a child dying in a hospital is only 7 to 9 days.[31] On the one hand, they reflect the difficulty that pediatric oncologists have in breaking bad news and clearly and honestly discussing end-of-life issues with patients and parents. On the other, such findings reflect parents' reluctance to consider the likelihood that their child is going to die.

Our cultural problem associated with publicly expressing emotions about death and dying, particularly when it involves children, has become so entrenched that the family, friends, and neighbors of parents whose children have died often are at a loss for words to express their feelings and comfort parents. This phenomenon has come to be known as *disenfranchised grief* wherein parents (and siblings) are left feeling marginalized and alienated from their communities in their grief and mourning.[32] Institutions involved in child and family welfare have been negligent in helping parents (and siblings) cope with the process of their child dying and their grief and mourning after death. Only institutionalized forms of religious rituals and funeral rites explicitly and systematically recognize the restorative roles of grief and mourning. Religious rituals of mourning capture the family's profound need to seek spiritual succor when dealing with death and dying, regardless of the family's prior extent of religious observance.[33]

Medical Staff

Medicine is conservative and physicians generally are reluctant to consider anything but clearly tested methods of care because, if they are wrong, the consequences are too great. However, end-of-life care presents physicians with inescapable opportunities to move beyond established methods of medical practice. When it involves children, such opportunities rise exponentially, but caring for dying children is one of the most stressful situations for medical staff. For many complex reasons, the death of a child is seldom addressed in medicine beyond the idea of the so-called good deaths and bad deaths. Good deaths are thought to be quick, uncomplicated, expected, progressive, without pain and suffering; all staff in all subspecialties are on the same page regarding end-of life decisions. Bad deaths are the opposite of all that. Bad deaths, along with intractable pain and chronic problems with symptom management, involve the loss of the patient's (and the patient's family's) sense of autonomy, loss of control of essential bodily functions, decreasing ability to enjoy simply being alive, and undue agitation. Among the medical staff any death is seen as a failure of treatment because treatment always is viewed as a cure from illness.[34] Contributing to this sense of failure is the knowledge that the promise of a cure through genetic engineering and yet-discovered biological means is all around, like distant rescue ships that are too far off today to be of any assistance but are due to arrive tomorrow.

The death of a patient, especially when that patient is a child, can be a powerful impetus to seek new and more effective treatment protocols. Hence, the seemingly controversial title of this book: *When Treatment Fails*. This title captures the gut-wrenching aspects of having to finally relinquish expectations for cure of a child with whom you have emotionally bonded and then you have to continue to care for this child and others who will die.[35] It often is as tough a lesson for the medical staff as it is for the parents of the child. As we will see in chapter 6, physicians who are unable to save a child experience a profound sense of failure. They repeatedly (almost endlessly) question, "What if I had done something else? Could I have saved the child?" However, *When Treatment Fails* focuses on the failure of treatment and not the failure of the staff.

Ninety percent of us will die from an intractable illness.[36] Consequently, how we die and the quality of our dying will most likely be in the hands of medical experts who will prescribe therapies based on their training and the institutional policies where they practice. Until the early part of the twentieth century, most serious diseases, including cancer, took a fairly rapid course to death. Over time, however, medicine has become increasingly more complex. Despite substantially improved prognoses, greater complexity has led to more uncertain consequences for dying patients and their families. The introduction of increasingly more effective treatments, medications, medical imaging technologies, and surgical procedures has produced remarkable improvements in prognoses and longer survival times. But with the chances of cure and survival in individual cases becoming more unpredictable, new uncertainties and risks have appeared. These uncertainties constitute the psychological impact of having to cope with increasingly protracted and complicated ways of dying. The growing sophistication of advanced medical practices (which are increasingly becoming known to patients and families on the Internet) means that people are living longer with knowledge that they may be dying while they are simultaneously struggling to deny it. As a result, dying has become a more profound and protracted process for more and more people.

Pediatric Hospice Care

The specialty of palliative medicine grew out of the principles and practices established by the hospice movement.[37] Although most hospice care is provided in the home, 75 percent of children who die from medical causes do so in hospitals,[38] and only 0.4 percent of dying children receive hospice care.[39] Among adults, less than 30 percent of dying patients receive hospice care, and the median length of care is less than 1 month (often, only days or hours before they die).[40] In the Netherlands, by contrast, approximately 80 percent of children dying of medical causes do so at home or out-of-hospital hospice care[41] and, in Britain, 40 percent.[42] Current regulations in this country pose significant barriers to pediatric hospice care. To be eligible for hospice care, it is required that a child (like an adult), have 6 months or less to live. Even among adults, relatively few diseases fit neatly into such a prognostic model and, given the greater prognostic uncertainties in pediatric care and children's greater recuperative abilities, it is even more difficult for pediatricians to ascertain as much.[43] In addition, to enter hospice care, the patient must agree to forgo any care that has curative intent and to receive strictly palliative care. In pediatrics, however, the boundaries between palliative and curative often are blurred in the eyes of patients, families, and staff (palliative chemotherapy, for example). This fragmented model of hospice benefits was developed for adult patients and not explicitly for children and adolescents.[44]

Further barriers to out-of-hospital care for children at the end of their lives are the fears and culturally grounded reluctance of U.S. parents to allow their child to die at home.[45] In a country such as ours with diverse cultural beliefs and values about death and dying, it is difficult to establish uniform standards regarding the dying process and end-of-life decision making. Consequently, parents are inadvertently offered a greater sense of security managing their children's potentially frightening end-of-life complications (e.g., seizures or hemorrhages) in the hospital rather than at home. Also increasingly, greater technological advances in medicine are offering options that further medicalize death and dying—options that preclude home-based care at the end of life. Furthermore, because so few children are admitted to hospice care in this country, hospice providers lack adequate expertise in pediatric care.[46]

Most of the medical staff in tertiary care hospitals do not recognize the extent of children's suffering at the end of life because they are trained to focus on cure as a goal of aggressive treatment and they have inadequate training and clinical experience in caring for dying children. For example, today in the United States, 75 percent of children and adolescents with cancer, the leading cause of illness-related deaths in children, are cured. But cancer remains a relatively rare disease in children (1 per 600)[47] and accounts for only 4 percent of deaths each year.[48] This rate of cure is vastly different from that in developing countries where most children with cancer will die either because their disease is too far advanced by the time it is diagnosed or because curative therapies are not available owing to limited resources.[49] The goal of treatment shifts from cure to palliation only when staff and parents together recognize that the struggle against cancer is lost. However, the remarkable and continuing new discoveries and medical breakthroughs make it exceedingly more difficult for staff and parents alike to come to this recognition.

Discussing End-of-Life Options

Discussing end-of-life options with parents when their child's hopes for recovery are rapidly diminishing is a formidable task. A survey of pediatric oncologists by the American Society of Clinical Oncology (ASCO) reported that they generally were anxious about discussing the likelihood of death with children and their parents. For example, "47 per cent of pediatric oncologists do not initiate a discussion of advance directives; instead they leave this to the family to initiate."[50] Pediatric oncologists reported that their greatest barrier to more supportive and comforting end-of-life care were parents' unrealistic expectations of cure and their denial of their children's symptoms as terminal. This, in effect, confuses curative and palliative intent as parents push for ever more aggressive treatment protocols and contributes to physicians' anxiety about discussing end-of-life care options. Yet, 55 percent of parents whose children died in ICUs, after forgoing life-sustaining treatment, felt that they had little or no control of situations during the child's final days. Nonetheless, 76 percent agreed with staff regarding the decision to discontinue life support.[51] ASCO concluded that caregivers face substantial challenges in integrating curative intent, symptom control, psychosocial support, and palliative care in the routine care of seriously ill children. According to some researchers, there is a "mismatch between the standard aggressive tertiary pediatric care practices and the philosophy of hospice or palliative care"[52] Others cite such logistical obstacles as a shortage of medical staff trained to provide palliative care, inadequate funding, and insurance benefit packages that sharply limit palliative care.[53]

At a recent meeting of the Supportive Care Committee of the Children's Oncology Group (COG), it was reported that parents claimed that they were not adequately informed that the purpose of allowing their children to participate in Phase I cancer treatment protocols was for experimental research rather than for finding a cure for their child's cancer.[54] Reluctance to so advise parents (and patients) of the transition from curative to palliative care may reflect providers' general disinclination to deal with end-of-life issues and palliative care options in pediatrics. To help overcome this reticence, COG is preparing a paragraph that will be included in all Phase I protocols, reminding providers to discuss end-of-life issues when enrolling patients. This paragraph (in draft) in part states, "At this time, as Phase I therapy is being offered, the possibility of a cure of the child's underlying disease is quite small. While not giving up all hope, the patient/family must be informed that the balance of primary approach needs now to be moved to the goal of providing for comfort."[55]

Palliative Care

Unlike hospice care, palliative care seeks to maintain a patient's quality of life alongside the active treatment of the underlying disease, regardless of the prognosis. The specialty of palliative medicine dates from the mid-1980s,[56] and its emergent growth today is a response to the aging of the "baby-boomer" generation, which also has fostered the development of geriatrics as a significant medical subspecialty.[57] Issues of palliative care in geriatric medicine have led to innovative ways of handling death and dying and of making end-of-life decisions. They have raised heretofore unthought-of bioethical questions about the uses and abuses of dramatically advancing medical protocols, technologies, and genetic engineering. Among geriatricians, decisions about end of life are being considered as moral and bioethical imperatives of how medicine cares for those for whom a cure is no longer possible.[58] Current debates about physician-assisted suicide and euthanasia are dramatic illustrations of end-of-life bioethnical concerns.[59] As an aging baby-boomer myself, I welcome this interest in how we die, how we might be comforted when facing death, and how we might be empowered to make our own decisions about ways of dying, when we are terminally ill.

However, in pediatrics, unlike geriatrics, dying is still considered a failure of medicine. When a child dies the staff typically question, "What happened? What did we miss? What did we do wrong?" Hence palliative care options are not as easy to approach, discuss, or resolve. End-of-life decisions regarding children are different from those involving adults (particularly the elderly) and, therefore, require their own sets of standards apart from geriatric medicine. Some of the issues that distinguish geriatric from pediatric end-of-life care involve the course of disease in children, decisions about withdrawing or withholding care, means of introducing advance directives, and recognizing guardianship over the best interests of children. Caring for children (and their families) at the end of their lives can never be approached as a kind of dumbing down of standards derived from geriatric palliative care. For example, a recent study of interventions with ICU physicians to improve their communication with patients and enhance "deliberative decision making about care plans" reported that among elderly patients the interventions led to decisions to limit treatment and provide greater comfort care but they had the opposite effect among pediatric patients.[60] Therefore, despite significant advances in studies of adult palliative medicine,[61] similar studies are warranted for pediatric palliative care.

As in any emerging inquiry, there are different definitions of palliative care. These differences revolve around questions about when, in the course of care—from a potentially life-threatening diagnosis to the time when end-of-life decisions are considered—palliative care should be considered. In this regard, there are broad and more narrow definitions of palliative care. The Institute of Medicine's Committee on Palliative and End-of-Life Care for Children and Their Families, for example, adopts a broad view. It defines palliative care as "care that seeks to prevent, relieve, reduce, or soothe the symptoms produced by serious medical conditions or their treatment and to maintain patients' quality of life."[62] From this kind of definition it follows that palliative care need not be limited to people who are thought to be (or have a high probability of) dying. Nevertheless, symptom management and concern for the patient's quality of life are parts of competent medical practice at any time. Hence, such a broad definition of palliative care obscures the particular and pressing needs of patients and their families in end-of-life care. The World Health Organization's narrower view of palliative care is preferable. It defines palliative care as "the active total care of patients whose disease is not responsive to curative treatment . . . [when] control of pain, of other symptoms, and of psychological, social, and spiritual problems are paramount."[63] The American Academy of Pediatrics promotes an integrated model of palliative and curative treatment such that physicians and families do not have to exhaust all curative options to reverse the disease process before considering palliative interventions to relieve symptoms, regardless of their impact on the underlying disease. They further recognize that, at times, "it may be difficult to define individual therapies as either curative or palliative. For example, mechanical ventilation often is viewed as a life-prolonging or curative therapy. . . . However, such support . . . may provide symptomatic relief from dyspnea and significantly improve a child's quality of life."[64] Cystic fibrosis presents another example where aggressive treatment without curative intent has prolonged and improved the quality of children's life expectancies from several years to decades.

Although effective pain management, symptom relief, and maintenance of quality of life are integral components of medicine at any stage of treatment, from diagnosis to death, end-of-life care presents special challenges (often overwhelming and paramount) to effect a balance between needs for comfort and quality of life with hopes of extending life. Contributing to the challenge is the difficulty of assessing and managing symptoms and suffering in children and the paucity of developmentally appropriate methods available to reliably measure the suffering and quality of the life of children with life-threatening illness.[65] Even for adults, "complete remission of pain, however fortunate when it is achieved, is not the preeminent clinical objective in palliative care, since increased medication doses have side-effects that include decreased lucidity. The preferred treatment is to alter the patient's experience of pain so that less medication is necessary."[66] Obviously, this is not as easy for children (and their parents to accept) as it is for adults experiencing pain.

Specialties and subspecialty areas in medicine evolve when we recognize that other fields of medicine have not adequately addressed the needs of special classes of patients. The evolving discourse about palliative care may be a way of telling those physicians who find nothing left to do—when cure no longer is an option for them—that there remain ways for them to be involved as physicians in the care of their patients and families. Having said that, we probably should establish a pediatric subspecialty because end-of-life care presents unique scenarios that transcend the initiating diagnosis.[67] At its best, palliative care is always multidisciplinary, including physicians, nurses, social workers, psychologists, psychiatrists, child-life specialists, and multidenominational chaplains.[68]

End-of-Life Care

When the attending physician finds that treatment no longer benefits the patient and should be forgone, it usually is documented in the medical chart and sometimes with reference to DNR (do not resuscitate) status, when consent for such status has been obtained from parents.[69] When and how this conclusion is arrived at and communicated to patients and families is a continuing, even controversial, concern in pediatrics. Parents cannot compel a physician to provide any treatment that the physician judges as unlikely to benefit the patient, nor can parents withhold treatment from a child if the physician thinks it will substantially benefit the child. The latter case requires invoking the intervention of child protective services to contravene parental authority.[70]

Particularly difficult questions in pediatric end-of-life care occur when patients (typically adolescents) choose end-of-life treatment options that go against their parents' or siblings' wishes.[71] In such cases, physicians, along with the rest of the medical staff, have to negotiate between conflicting interests in order to consider the best interests of the patient. Although 20 years ago, this hardly ever was the case, the increasing range of options for end-of-life care today increases the likelihood of conflicting interests between patients and their families.

End-of-life decisions about caring for children in hospitals never are simply a matter of right or wrong. They stretch the limits of medical practice (something we prefer to think of as systematic and utterly rational), and, although medicine is an applied science, there is a dearth of reliable empirical evidence to guide us when considering these decisions.[72] As scientific uncertainties regarding outcomes escalate, the principles of evidence-based medicine begin to dwindle and physicians find that they can rely on only a limited range of statistical probabilities. The scientific community, often with a disdaining nod to the contingencies of practice, describe this as moving from nomothetic to ideographic science. This breach between the science of medicine and clinical practice is increasingly and inevitably expanding as we move toward end-of-life decisions; it pushes medicine to its limits to reveal its best and worst aspects.

There can be no theory of dying, if by a theory we mean a set of principled hypotheses that apply across individuals and situations. Because there are few empirically validated answers to questions that arise at end-of-life medical care, particularly when they involve children, end-of-life decisions rest on bioethical concerns that, in the most profound sense, capture the cultural and moral lessons by which we live. Accordingly, there can never be a correct or incorrect way of dying. Those who promulgate such a coercive orthodoxy about ways of dying are at best misled or worse, imperious. All standards of practice seem to boil down to exploring ways to respect and honor what patients, within the purview of family-based practice, find is best for them. In this sense, every patient for whom death is becoming increasingly more probable has the right to know and understand the status of his or her illness, consider treatment options, and choose with whom, if anyone, he or she wants to share this information. While advance medical directives, power of attorney documents, and DNRs address the legal aspect of dying, they say little about its biological, psychosocial, and cultural aspects.

Narrative Theory, Medicine, and Methods

> How people die remains in the
> memories of those who live on.
> — CICELY SAUNDERS

Recent narrative inquiries in medicine, the social sciences (especially psychology and anthropology), and philosophy are derived from advances in postmodernism, culturally contexted and distributed cognition, phenomenology, feminism, discursive and dialogical processes, and inductive and ethnographic research methods. Such approaches rest on the premise that it is best to understand people (and how they behave) on their own terms instead of posing a priori hypotheses and analytic presuppositions, as is common in more traditional positivistic methods of studying human behavior.[1] In medicine, narrative approaches focus on the holistic treatment of the person instead of the disease alone—a biopsychosocial approach.

A narrative is a story about people, events, settings, and times told from the narrator's point of view. All narratives hinge on what Aristotle, in the *Poetics*, described as the principle of peripeteia. Jerome Bruner, a leading advocate of narrative methods, describes peripeteia as "a sudden reversal in circumstances [that] swiftly turns a routine sequence of events into a story."[2] It is a transgression in what we consider to be the normal course of events. This sense of peripeteia, as a narrative force, is well expressed in the following tale:

The road to Jerusalem was dark and wet. I was ten at the time, sitting in the passenger seat. A partner of my father, a family friend, was driving me back home from somewhere. He had an imposing bulbous nose, laced with purple veins. I avoided staring at it, choosing instead to gaze through the rain drops at the emptiness ahead. We were quiet. There was not much to say. Suddenly, bales of hay from the overloaded truck ahead of us started to tumble onto the road. Our wheels screeched, as one bale squeezed under the car and another landed on the windshield. The car shook to an abrupt stop. The driver turned to me, looked me in the eye, and said: "You see, Solly, either things go according to plan, or there is a story."[3]

Kenneth Burke describes a narrative in terms of a pentad (what he calls story grammar) involving (1) an agent performing (2) some activity to achieve (3) a goal in (4) a setting by using certain (5) means.[4] The stories in this book, told by physicians, nurses, social workers, and child-life specialists about end-of-life care for children, reflect Burke's story grammar. They are about medical staff (agent) providing care (activity) to cure the patient (goal) in the hospital (setting) according to protocols based on science and medical expertise (means). For Burke, the perpeteia is the incongruity among these story elements occasioned by an unforeseen change of circumstances.

The present stories always involve some breach or transgression between goal and means. They are always about something that has gone awry—the curative goal was not achieved by the available means. It is an incongruity (peripeteia) because the means chosen were expected to satisfy a goal and they did not: a conflict between what was expected and what happened. In other words, the death of a patient presents an incongruity between means/end relationships, which, inevitably produces a dramatic and compelling narrative involving agents, activities, and settings. Bruner conveys this sense of narrative by describing it as "a recounting of human plans gone off the track, expectations gone awry. It is a way to domesticate human error and surprise . . . Stories reassert a kind of conventional wisdom about what can be expected, even (or especially) what can be expected to go wrong and what might be done to restore or cope with the situation."[5]

Stories about caring for children who die in hospitals capture the messy particulars, beyond the biological imperatives. They give voice to the quotidian pain and distress that children invariably endure, the shifts and struggles among providers to pursue a cure, the dashed hopes for a cure, and, most significantly, how it is understood and what it means for the staff. Narratives about end-of-life care assume their full fecundity only upon reflection after the death of the patient, in the struggle "to restore or cope with the situation." Constructing a narrative about oneself as agent during the evolving and seemingly interminable process of caring for a dying patient does not fully capture the struggle to understand and make sense of the conflict between the means and the goal. Only when knowing death as a consequence is the agent prepared to capture the full emotional and rational weight of having cared for the child. Accordingly, we have found qualitatively and irreducibly different kinds of narratives of end-of-life care when we elicit them prospectively—prior to death, when the staff is still actively engaged in decisions about end-of-life care—compared to retrospectively—after the child has died. The prospective narratives focus primarily on the day-to-day course of medical decision making—what to do, when to do it—and the need to justify or defend the decisions. It is more a "job-related" kind of story that is too practice oriented and embedded in medical jargon to be of much reflective value in capturing the breadth of concern about having cared for a child who died.

"Narrative is both phenomenon and method."[6] It is less a way of simply expressing past experiences than constructing present interpretations and giving meaning to our experiences. In this sense, narratives constitute how we organize, cognitively structure, and make sense of our lives rather than simply being expressive of prior narrative-independent realities.[7] Narratives are constructed in the context of interacting with a listener, whether physically present or imaginary. They represent and adhere to social, cultural, ideological, and historical presuppositions that enable us to professionally and personally relate to one another reciprocally. Narratives also evolve and develop—they change with time as new experiences influence the understanding and deeper interpretation of prior experiences in anticipation of future experiences.[8] They are not passive memory storage devices, and their purpose is not to present historical accounts or factual reportage. Considering narratives in this way (i.e., their ontological status) does not negate the existence of a material reality apart from narrative interpretations of it, but it can never be directly understood, in any culturally meaningful way, apart from the lens of narrative discourse.[9]

In medicine, story telling is a time-honored means of thinking about illness and disease, formulating interventions, and recognizing staff and patient relations.[10] The medical case history is a narrative that structures ways that medical knowledge and practice are advanced. Its canonical form and structure have not varied much since its inception in the 1890s.[11]

Because end-of-life care of children in hospitals is so traumatic for everyone involved, the struggle to make sense of the situation and find meaning lends the narrative a dynamic force that dramatically captures the social, cultural, emotional, and cognitive issues involved. Because narratives assume the particular perspective of each narrator, by eliciting narratives from several members of the medical team involved in caring for a given child, we are able to capture a range of differing perspectives and study what they have and do not have in common. The lack of commonality, if it is consistent across disciplines and clinical cases, will reflect the disciplinary stance that different caregivers, having different professional roles, bring to the events and how their training and experience inform them about death and dying.

Compared to other kinds of more quantitative tools used by social scientists to study knowledge and ways of knowing (such as surveys, questionnaires, tests, and rating scales), narratives are particularly effective in the study of issues about which we are uncomfortable or anxious, and find difficult to articulate. Because narratives give participants the freedom to explore their own ways of approaching issues without undue concern for saying the "correct" thing, they honor the integrity of each participant's particular ways of speaking and finding meaning in their experiences. In this regard, several studies have shown that, as a tool for guided reflection, constructing a narrative is a highly adaptive way for us to deal with loss and trauma.[12]

Eliciting narratives is very different from conducting interviews. By choosing questions beforehand (often standardized across participants), framing them in particular ways, and deciding when to direct a change of topic by posing the next question, interviews invariably reflect the interviewer's rather than the interviewee's areas of interest, topics of relevancy, and ways of speaking. With interviews, the interviewer's questions inevitably shape the responses. By contrast, narratives shift the focus of inquiry from the interrogator to the narrator. This is because they are elicited according to a clinical method by which interrogators are trained to follow, as much as possible, participants' own lines of thinking and ways of speaking without imposing their own judgments and reactions.[13] In clinical psychology, this is known as entering the psychological space of the participant. Participants are probed in nondirective ways to elaborate on issues and events that they themselves deem important and relevant. Such kinds of probes include, "Tell me more about that." "What was that like?" and "What did you mean when you said that . . . ?" A final probe might be, "What else should we talk about?" Probes never are designed to elicit "yes" or "no" kinds of responses, nor are they ever leading or suggestive. Leading and suggestive kinds of probes presuppose an answer and contain inferences about feelings, events, or conditions that had not been previously established by the participants. Because questions have not been prepared beforehand, the challenge for interrogators is to interpersonally negotiate within the psychological space of each participant, knowing when and how to respond without challenging or prematurely changing the participant's topics of discourse or deflecting new ones. This is not a totally passive process on the part of interrogators. There remains an interactive and dyadic relationship that is propelled by the myriad ways by which we unconsciously use body language (kinesthetics) and vocal intonations within the dialogic framework of eliciting narratives. Therefore, investigators have to lean how to maintain a sense of unconditional positive regard for participants and the contexts in which they are eliciting narratives. Without unconditional positive regard, our biases, beliefs, and values are covertly conveyed via these paralingual modes and flavor the narratives in subtle yet profound ways. Despite a sense of unconditional positive regard, investigators always influence, to some extent (preferably less than more), the kind of narratives being elicited. The investigator is not simply a conduit from which the narrative flows, and his or her relationship with the narrator is always somewhat collaborative.

In simpler terms, eliciting narratives encompasses the skills of empathy and good listening and, by so doing, validates the experiences as understood by the narrators. This has sometimes been called "witnessing listening, and in medicine, it reflects on the staff's competency to empathize with their patient's suffering."[14]

This book is less about the experiences of children who are dying and their parents than about the practices of the medical staff who have to make difficult, painful, conflicting, frustrating, and sometimes contradictory decisions about end-of-life care. To capture the immediacy and emotional texture of the range of issues that inevitably arise in medical centers when caring for children at the end of their lives, these issues are illustrated on a case-by-case, day-by-day basis in the form of narratives using the staff's own words and ways of speaking. By focusing on stories from the medical staff, to the exclusion of those from children and their families, this book offers a particularly biased perspective of death and dying in pediatrics. This perspective is not meant to diminish in any way the place of children and parents but to offer medical staff the autonomy to us tell their own stories.

Eliciting the Narratives

Narratives were elicited from the staff at a major tertiary care pediatric teaching hospital affiliated with a preeminent medical school in a large city. All pediatric specialties including oncology, hematology, cardiology, pulmonary care, neurology, neonatal intensive care (NICU), pediatric intensive care, and infectious diseases were represented. Approximately 135 children die in this hospital each year (including 60 in the NICU). Most deaths are from cancer, accidents, respiratory diseases, and congenital malformations. I was notified, usually by the chief residents in pediatrics, within hours of a child's death (excluding emergency room acute traumas) along with the names of all of the clinicians who had been involved in the child's care at the end of life. The clinicians included senior attending physicians from one or more subspecialties in pediatrics, fellows, medical residents, interns, medical students, nurse practitioners, floor nurses, social workers, psychologists, and child-life specialists. Each of them individually met with me, and typically the meeting began with the simple question, "What was it like for you to care for [name of child]?" I met with 110 clinicians concerning the end-of-life care of 20 children.[15]

Although the narratives were elicited on a case-by-case basis, they are largely presented according to different themes that arise in end-of-life care for children. The themes usually transcend specific cases, although each case provides an opportunity to illustrate the nuanced complexity of collaborative or contradictory issues in the press of practice. As narratives, the themes and issues they raise are no longer limited to standardized sets of variable-specific abstract principles and uninstantiated guidelines that are so often found in standard texts on end-of-life care in pediatrics. Instead, they are confounded by the particularities of any given disease, its progression, the patient and family, the medical staff, and the institutional resources, at any given time (i.e., praxis vs. theory). Because the narrators usually referred to patients by name, the patients have been given fictitious names. Table 2.1 lists the case number of each child, his or her name, age at time of death, diagnosis, subspecialties involved in their end-of-life care, and the proximal cause of death.

Road Map

Here is a brief road map of the rest of this book. Chapters 3 through 7 are the narrative chapters.[16] They convey not only common and compelling themes but also the incredible diversity of experiences in end-of-life care. In the press of practice, even common themes are acted out in uncommon ways, and it is important to provide descriptive evidence of how and why that is so and why it often is such an incredibly messy and uncertain business.

By and large, the idea behind the narratives is to speak to the reader without the intrusion of my interpretations. Readers may consider their own interpretations and arrive at their own conclusions. The interpretive stance of the present work is evident in the choice of narrative segments included to portray and promote what was considered critical topics in end-of-life care.

TABLE 2.1

Clinical Cases by Number, Name (Fictitious), Age at Death, Diagnosis,
Subspecialties Involved in End-of-Life Care, and Proximal Cause of Death

No.	Name	Age (yrs./mos.)	Diagnosis	Subspecialties Involved	Proximal Cause of Death
1	Karen	14/2	Liver transplant, liver failure—cirrhosis hepatocellular carcinoma	Liver transplant, ICU	Liver failure, renal failure (due to medication to prevent liver rejection and sepsis-blood infection)
2	Devon	5/4	Neuroblastoma (NB)	ICU, Oncology, Pain team, Radiation oncology	Relapsed NB & complications of bone marrow transplant (BMT) incl. adenovirus infection & graft versus host disease (GVHD)
3	Elsa	11/1	Neuroblastoma	Pain team, Oncology	Relapsed NB
4	Danny	3/3	Wiskott-Aldrich syndrome	BMT, ICU, Pain team, Radiation oncology	Leukoencephalopathy (possibly due to immunosuppressive medication) & multisystem failure
5	Ricardo	5/6	Acute lymphoblastic leukemia (ALL)	BMT	Sepsis, liver failure & GVHD
6	Abdul	7/3	Automobile accident	ICU, Neurology	Brain dead
7	Carol	0/11	Undifferentiated sarcoma	Oncology, ICU, Pain team	Tumor (in neck and chest) causing respiratory failure
8	William	1/4	Hemophagocytic lymphohistiocytosis	Oncology	BMT engraftment failure & sepsis
9	John	12/10	Ewing sarcoma	Oncology, Surgery, Radiation oncology	Respiratory failure (due to pulmonary metastases)
10	Sarah	4/0	Brain tumor	Oncology, Surgery, Radiation oncology, Neurosurgery	Brain tumor—causing respiratory failure
11	Susan	1/1	Mucolipoidosis Type II (metabolic disorder)	BMT, Genetics, Cardiology	Cardiac failure (due to underlying disease & BMT conditioning chemotherapy)

(continued)

TABLE 2.1 (*continued*)

No.	Name	Age (yrs./mos.)	Diagnosis	Subspecialties Involved	Proximal Cause of Death
12	Alice	5/0	Neuroblastoma, Stage IV	Oncology, BMT Radiation oncology, Surgery, PICU, Infectious diseases, Pulmonary	Respiratory failure (due to multifactorial chronic lung damage & infection)
13	Rebecca	16/2	Wilms' tumor	Oncology, BMT, Radiation oncology, Surgery	Respiratory failure (due to pulmonary metastases)
14	Roberto	11/7	AIDS (vertical transmission)	Infectious diseases	Progressive multifocal leukoencephalopathy
15	George	3/2	Rhabdomyosarcoma	Pain team, Surgery, Oncology, Urology, Radiation oncology	Respiratory failure (due to pulmonary metastases)
16	José	16/11	Desmoplastic round cell tumor	Oncology, Surgery, Pain team	Respiratory & liver failure (due to metastases)
17	Christianna	15/1	Osteosaracoma	Oncology, Surgery, Orthopedics, Pain team	Respiratory failure (due to pulmonary metastases)
18	Baby A	3 days	Respiratory distress syndrome (RDS) of preterm (28 wks.) & intraventricular hemorrhage	Neonatal intensive care unit (NICU)	Respiratory insufficiency (due to RDS)
19	Simone	0/3	Critical aortic insufficiency causing left ventricular heart failure	Cardiology, Cardiac surgery, ICU	Cardiac failure & sepsis
20	Babies B & C	3 days	Preterm twins (24 wks.) with Grade IV intraventricular hemorrhages	NICU, Radiology	Respiratory insufficiency

The purpose is not to resolve problems in pediatric palliative care by advocating a particular set of practice guidelines or, worse yet, promoting particular, canonical ways of how children ought to die in hospitals. Rather, the deeper intent is to raise critical and relevant issues in the dynamic contexts of practice-based perspectives that allow readers to understand and appreciate the problems from a bottom-up instead of the more typical top-down approach to pediatric end-of-life care.

Among the 20 narrative cases (outlined in Table 2.1) are children who died from a range of conditions stemming from different diagnoses. As with most children dying in hospitals, the majority of the children in these narratives had various kinds of cancer and often, with relapses, had bone marrow transplants. Others were neonates who had congenital anomalies—one child had a liver transplant, another a kidney transplant, one child had been in an automobile accident, and another had aortic insufficiency causing heart failure. Other diagnoses included Mucolipoidosis Type II (a metabolic disorder) and acquired immune deficiency syndrome (AIDS). The diversity of end-of-life care experiences for the medical staff, the children, and their families was occasioned, in part, by the presenting diagnoses and biologic consequences of different kinds of treatment protocols. However, the cultural milieu of different cohorts of staff, working in mutually reciprocal relationships with different families that have different needs and ways of coping, at different times, also had considerable impact on the diversity of end-of-life care experiences. Therefore, the narratives have been parsed to arrive at five essential themes about pediatric end-of-life care as presented in chapters 3 to 7.

Chapter 3 documents, case by case, 20 stories about what it is like for children dying of medical causes and what is happening to them and their families and medical teams caring for them along this circuitous trajectory.

The narratives in chapter 4 concern issues about withholding or withdrawing care at end of life—when is enough enough? When caring for a child who is not responding to treatment intended to cure, there always is a point where death shifts from an "if" to a "when" proposition. The significance of this shift is not only in the emotional baggage that comes with this change in expectations but in how we alter practices between treating for curative intent and treating for comfort. Despite what we hear about palliative care and curative care going hand in hand, as we will see, they simply do not. Decisions about when to continue to proceed with invasive procedures hoping for a cure and when to step aside and simply provide palliative care to comfort a child are the most difficult and constitute the core issue in end-of-life care. For many reasons, it is a very different kind of consideration when applicable to children compared to adults.

The narratives in chapters 5, 6, and 7 convey how complicated and uncertain are children's ways of dying in hospitals and how difficult, emotionally draining, and heart wrenching it is for the staff caring for them, as well as for the children and their families. Chapter 5 considers issues about pain and suffering at end of life. They are particularly poignant because most of us today believe that, with sufficient pain medications, no one need die suffering and in pain. How the staff reacts to caring for dying children in regard to the children and families as well as among themselves is the narrative focus of chapter 6. The chapter considers (1) how the staff communicates with patients and families; (2) how the staff relates to one another in both complementary and conflicting roles; (3) how the staff is able to cope with the stress and challenges of pediatric end-of-life care and find ways of moving on; and (4) the educational and training needs of the staff doing this kind of work. Chapter 7 considers how the staff experiences their patients' and families' ways of reacting to and participating in end-of-life care. Finally, chapter 8 offers some conclusions.

Twenty Stories About | 3
How Children Die

I expected death to glimmer with
meaning, but it doesn't. It's just there.
— HAROLD BRODKEY
The Wild Darkness: The Story of my Death

I begin by providing stories of what it is like for children to die in hospitals and what it is like for their families and the medical staff. These stories were not chosen to exaggerate or play upon the drama and poignancy of pediatric end-of-life care. They simply are the cases sampled during the months when I was eliciting narratives. Some cases had to be forgone because of logistics: the death of some children occurred too close in time to that of others. Also, in terms of sampling, the chapter includes less than the proportionate rate of deaths occurring in the neonatal intensive care unit. But by and large, the 20 stories presented here constitute a fair and representative sample of the pediatric end-of-life issues encountered in any tertiary care hospital in the country. They are the full sample; none has been omitted.

A recent study estimates that, in the United States, among the 50,000 who die each year from medical causes,[1] "15,000 infants, children, adolescents, and young adults die from conditions that suggest that they and their families might benefit from pediatric supportive care services. On any given day, 5,000 of these patients are living within the last 6 months of their lives."[2]

The medical causes of children's death include cancer, AIDS, metabolic disorders, end-stage organ failures, cystic fibrosis, severe congenital anomalies, and complications from extreme prematurity. Ways of dying follow the biological course of these different diseases and the arsenal of available treatments. As the process of dying progresses, it becomes more individualized. Although a child might have begun treatment with a common diagnosis and treatment protocol, his or her death will be highly particularized and will increasingly stretch the boundaries of medicine from science to the point when scientific findings and rational discourse no longer dictate medical decisions. In other words, death is rarely explained by abstract conceptual rules substantiated by sets of empirical proofs; it always is specific to the particular situation, and as we shall see, the situations are unduly complicated and widely uncertain. Dying almost invariably involves a spiraling number of medical subspecialists, raises new and daunting issues about patient and family involvement, and encompasses an ever expanding range of uncertainties about whether and how to proceed. For reasons involving biological, cultural, psychosocial, familial, and spiritual considerations, a child's death follows a more circuitous trajectory than that of an adult.

Sherwin Nuland begins a discerning discussion about how adults die in *How We Die* by claiming, "Everyone wants to know the details of dying, though few are willing to say so," and, "To most people, death remains a hidden secret, as eroticized as it is feared. . . . Moths and flames, mankind and death—there is little difference."[3] We take it as a mark of our civilization that dying is never permitted to be banal or prosaic. Instead, we expect, indeed demand, that medicine heroically mount a struggle to fight against dying at whatever costs to the patient and family. According to Nuland, this is because dying is not simply our collective fear; it is our "looming terror" in life. Case by case, he incisively illustrates just how messy, dirty, ugly, degrading, deteriorating, complicated, fluid, and uncertain it is to die from a variety of diseases that ultimately result in stoppage of circulation, inadequate transport of oxygen to tissue, or failure of brain functions and other organs. As a physician, Nuland finds that the idea of the "good death" or "death with dignity" is, and always has been, a Western myth, and never more so than in today's medical climate of advanced technologies and pharmacologies. Ultimately and inevitably, he states, "The quest to achieve true dignity fails when our bodies fail."[4] Our single-minded focus on cure often leads us to inadvertently disregard the need for greater palliation at the end of life.

A century ago, most people died of infectious diseases (e.g., pneumonia, tuberculosis, diarrhea, and enteritis), which entailed a fairly rapid and certain trajectory to death.[5] Diagnoses were made late in the course of disease, and, more often than not, no effective treatments were available. Since then, medical advances have dramatically changed and complicated the trajectories from diagnosis to either cure or death. Today 70 to 80 percent of people die from chronic or degenerative diseases that have a slow onset and an extended period of decline. In addition, a growing number of deaths are based on medical decisions to withhold or withdraw treatment.

The death of children from medical causes is now viewed not as something that just happens but as something that happens despite all efforts to prevent it from happening. One of the social workers in our sample described it this way:

> We are brought up, especially in America, to believe that this is not supposed to happen. Outside of America, children die all the time and the parents don't suffer this way because it is kind of a given that, if they have five kids, maybe two are going to be lost to diarrhea, to vomiting—to stupid things that we don't even think about because of no running water, no electricity—an act of God, if it is a hurricane or earthquake, or whatever the heck it may be. That is not supposed to happen here. Here, we have the money, we have the technology, we put a man on the moon, we got so that a child is not supposed to precede a parent in death or a grandparent; that is just not the way we are conditioned. It simply is not what is supposed to happen. We are not prepared to accept the death of a child. . . . Children are our future and, when children die, our future and the future of those families are forever compromised.

Following Nuland, this chapter provides descriptive information in order to demythologize the way children die. Only by first understanding the complicated ways by which children die—and not in just any kind of hospitals but in the very best ones in the United States—can we begin to appreciate the issues that need to be addressed as we seek ways to improve current standards of care and recognize current constraints of care for children at the end of their lives.

When Is Death?

As if the complicated and messy uncertainties of dying were not disturbing enough, we also need to consider the controversy in medicine surrounding the very definition of death. Today, because more and more people require organ transplants, it has become important for physicians to verify how and when someone is dead. Is a child dead when his or her heart stops beating? In the typical course of dying, first the heart stops, then the lungs, and finally the brain. If we consider death further along these lines, we find that medical decisions about when life ends are as elusive as decisions about when life begins. If we conclude that a child is dead when the heart stops, does that mean that it cannot be restarted? How long ought we try to resuscitate before concluding that it cannot be restarted and has ceased contracting (i.e., asystolic): 2 minutes, 5 minutes, 15 minutes? There are no standards; it depends instead on the medical contexts of each and every case. Although there is a legal definition of brain death, not every practitioner or parent accepts that standard. Hours after a child's heart has stopped, sparks of electrical activity remain in the brain. That doesn't mean that there is consciousness in any human sense involving thought, affect, and sensory perception, yet there still are some brain functions. Laws about how to define death have evolved largely outside of patient (and family) concerns about dying. Questions about what death is today are tied into the practical considerations of when it is morally and ethically acceptable to remove organs for transplantation—"Okay, can we turn off the respirator now?"[6]

Organization of Medical Care

In order to appreciate the complicated process of how children die in hospitals and what it is like for their families, it is necessary to have a sense of how major medical centers (i.e., teaching hospitals or tertiary care facilities) function as hierarchically organized institutions mandated to provide medical education, research, and patient care and be financially solvent. Children and parents who enter the system face the daunting task of mastering the differing levels of expertise and lines of communication among medical staff.

Medical Divisions

The medical care offered children in major medical centers is organized among divisions according to different clinical specialties. The divisions, in turn, function within two departments: surgery and medicine. The department of surgery includes divisions of surgical subspecialties such as general surgery, ENT (ear, nose, and throat) surgery, ophthalmology (surgery of the eye), and neurosurgery. The department of medicine includes all of the pediatric medical subspecialties: oncology and hematology (the care of children with cancer and blood disorders, respectively), gastroenterology, pulmonary, cardiology, emergency medicine, pediatric intensive care (PICU), and neonatal intensive care (NICU). In a children's hospital, the staff use the terms PICU and ICU (intensive care unit) interchangeably because for them the intensive care unit is necessarily pediatric.

Divisions such as oncology provide continuing care for children (often for many years) in both the inpatient units of the hospital and the outpatient hospital offices (referred to as clinics). Two exceptions are: (1) emergency medicine, which provides emergency care only and then, when warranted, transfers children to one of the other divisions, and (2) pediatric intensive care, which cares for children referred from the other divisions of medicine when children's medical conditions exceed levels of care available in those other divisions. Other departments are concerned primarily with assisting in diagnosing disease. The radiology department produces and interprets ("reads") images such as X rays, CT scans, and MRIs. The department of pathology and laboratory medicine perform and interpret laboratory tests on blood, urine, and tissue biopsies. Sometimes, at admission, only a single division is involved in providing care while, at other times, depending on the presenting symptoms, several divisions are involved, usually on a consulting basis. However, when a child's disease does not respond to curative treatment, other divisions become more centrally involved because biological deterioration often affects other functions and organ systems. For example, a child recovering from a bone marrow transplant may need to be transferred to the intensive care unit because of respiratory failure. However, it may not be clear if the respiratory problem is due to infection or to lung damage. Thus, attendings from the pulmonary and infectious disease divisions will become involved as consultants to the intensivists. If the child then requires a lung biopsy to determine the cause of the problem, a surgeon will be consulted as well. The following organ systems are involved in the dying process: cardiovascular, respiratory, musculoskeletal, and renal. Depending on how these systems are affected, specialists in these areas of medicine will need to be consulted for symptom management.

General pediatricians in the community may refer children with complicated disorders to a medical center in order to obtain specific diagnostic tests and/or therapies. However, parents may choose, on their own, to bring their child to a center because of the reputations of its medical divisions and subspecialists. Other children may be brought to a center by ambulance after an accident or acute onset of illness.

Physicians

Within the divisions, physicians have varying levels of training and experience. At the lowest level are *medical students* who are in their third or fourth year of medical school and are learning clinical medicine under supervision.

Medical students have limited responsibilities and are carefully supervised, yet they may be important team members and develop strong relationships with the families. *Interns* are physicians who are in a postgraduate training program in their first year out of medical school. The intern is usually the first person called to the bedside when problems occur. Interns are supervised by *residents* who have completed their internships and are obtaining 2 years of additional training to be qualified for board certification as pediatricians. They, in turn, are supervised by *chief residents* who have been selected to do a fourth post-graduate year. *Fellows* are physicians who have completed general pediatric training and are training in a subspecialty for 3 years in order to become board certified (for example, board certification in pediatric hematology/oncology). The most senior members in the divisions are *attendings*, who are board certified in their pediatric subspecialty areas beyond pediatrics. Attendings are children's primary care providers and are the ones ultimately responsible for medical decisions regarding diagnosis and treatment. The same hierarchy of physicians functions in the surgical division, except that surgical residents and fellows spend considerably more time in surgical training (i.e., 5 to 8 years).

Interns and residents spend nights on-call in the hospital, and, when problems arise at night, the intern calls the supervising resident and they make joint decisions as to whether to call the fellow on-call, who then may decide, depending on the severity of the situation, to come to the hospital. It is the fellows' decision whether to involve the attending on-call. In the ICU and the NICU, fellows remain in the units during the night. This pattern of night service raises issues of rotation of medical personnel. In the past, hospitals would require their interns and residents to work during the night for days on end without sufficient rest; today most state laws limit them to 25 hours of continuous service. Hence, interns and residents serve every third to fourth night.

Most attendings have at least four responsibilities: outpatient care, inpatient care, medical education, and research, either basic (i.e., laboratory) or applied (i.e., clinical). Attendings also might have significant and demanding administrative responsibilities. Although every patient has a primary attending physician, he or she is not always on-service. Different attendings are on-service on different days, and those on-service are in charge of all the children in a given division. When on-service, they conduct patient rounds with nurses, residents, interns, and fellows at each child's bedside and enter findings, for each child each day, in the medical charts. Attendings on-service will consult with a child's primary attending when significant situations arise so that the child's primary attending can make the ultimate decisions concerning care.

I am the first to admit that this organizational hierarchy of medical care must be confusing for children and families because I've been married to an attending pediatric oncologist for 15 years and she still chides me for forgetting the difference between when she is "on-service" and "on-call." In the former case, she'll get home 3 hours later than expected, while in the latter, she will have to be in the hospital on the weekend to do patient rounds, make treatment decisions, and enter notes in the children's medical charts.

Nurses

In many respects, nurses are the most consistent health care providers for children. The majority of parents who had a child die in the hospital rated nurses as the ones most involved at their child's bedside at the time of death.[7] There are three kinds of nurses in the divisions. *Registered nurses* provide bedside care ranging from helping to bathe a child to running multiple machines to infuse complex medications. Registered nurse/patient ratios vary according to the severity of children's medical conditions. On an ICU or an NICU, the ratio is 1 to 1 or 2 to 1. In the other divisions, ratios may be as small as 2 to 1, for example, for bone marrow transplant patients, or as large as 5 to 1 in the general pediatric division. Registered nurses (at least those involved in these narratives) work 12-hour shifts, 3 days per week. Then there are *clinical nurse specialists* who directly assist the attendings (e.g., participating in patient rounds with them) and educate the nursing staff about the different clinical specialities in pediatrics, ways to perform procedures, and the different treatment modalities. The third kind of nurses are *nurse-practitioners*. They are qualified to examine, diagnose, and treat under the direction of an attending. Aside from direct patient care, nurses have considerable administrative responsibilities in the divisions.

Psychosocial Staff

Social workers assist parents through the quagmire of insurance claims, assist them in securing community resources that will help parents care for their children, and provide emotional support and counseling. A very special service in pediatrics is provided by *child-life specialists*. Through talk and play activities, they help children understand why they are in the hospital, the nature of their illness, treatment, and medical procedures. They often are at the front lines in helping children cope with their fears and uncertainties about being hospitalized because different modes of playing, under appropriate adult guidance, is a relatively safe outlet for children to express and resolve their fears. *Pediatric psychologists* and *psychiatrists* become involved when children and families come to a medical center with preexisting psychiatric problems that become exacerbated with the stresses of hospitalization. They also become involved when children act in ways that undermine their treatment (e.g., medication or procedural noncompliance), become unduly angry or withdrawn, show signs of clinical depression or anxiety (sometimes leading to suicidal ideation), or behave in ways that generally exceed the levels of psychosocial support social workers and child-life specialists can offer.

Over and above the healthcare providers, often and for different reasons, children and families might become emotionally connected to other people in the hospital setting. These people might be part of the cleaning, dietary, or security staff, or they might be medical technicians or elevator operators. Children's and families' connection with different people in hospitals becomes very individualized, especially when care becomes prolonged and children and parents spend increasingly more time in the hospital. Pediatric medicine always has been an intensely interpersonal endeavor, and advances in medical technologies have not lessened this intensity in any way.

Although children's recoveries from life-threatening diseases usually follow a fairly orthodox prescriptive standard, every case of caring for children at the end of their lives is unique—cures are nomothetic, deaths, idiopathic.

Narratives

Each narrative segment, in this and succeeding chapters, begins with two numbers with a colon between them. The first number refers to the patient's case from which the story was derived and as outlined in Table 2.1. The second number refers to the participant's discipline as listed in Table 3.1. Readers who want to identify the patient and the participant's profession can refer to these tables. Because at times there was more than one participant from the same discipline in a case, the same participant number might refer to more than one participant. For example, in almost all cases more than one attending or resident was involved (from different subspecialties).

TABLE 3.1
Participants According to Discipline

No.	Discipline*
1	Attending physician
2	Fellow
3	Resident
4	Intern
5	Medical student
6	House physician
7	Nurse practitioner
8	Registered nurse
9	Child-life specialist
10	Social worker
11	Psychologist

*In most narrative cases, two or more participants are identified as being from the same discipline.

Story 1

The first story is about a 14-year-old girl who died unexpectedly following a liver transplant. Her mother was the donor.

———

1:3. It's 6:00 and I notice that she had a wide pulse pressure because she had that over the night and we had started Dopamine. She was still having it, so I went and got the fellow. He came and said, "We have to give more fluid." Then they started this whole thing to give more fluid and then the nurse was like, "She needs another access, she needs more IV access," so the fellow put in another IV and it was so hard to put in. Then we started giving fluids. Then her blood pressure really went up. Then I realized she's starting to arrest. Her blood pressures didn't stay up. She's gotten a lot of fluids and then everything was starting to happen and the crash cart was being pulled into place. The attending and the fellow were putting in a catheter and so they were starting to do that and I knew this was bad. Then everyone was starting to come in. That's when they started putting the catheter in and she started to bleed and her pressure was going down and her heart rate was going down, everything was getting doubled. All her pressures were getting doubled, her vent settings were going up. By this time, the other resident who's on call came over and they were like, "We need blood. We need blood." So I was calling the blood bank and then I got the other resident to call the blood bank and I started paging the liver team, and the surgeon who had been involved in her transplant. Then I started the whole process of keeping them up to date about what's going on and trying to get blood. So basically, that's what I was doing and I'd go in and then someone would say, "We need calcium," and I'd go—since the cart is outside and the curtains are closed—I'd go there to get it and kept going back and forth. From this point on, for an hour and a half, she was not doing better and her coags [coagulation profile—a battery of tests measuring blood clotting] came back and they were so high and she's oozing blood from her mouth and then, during the code, she started oozing blood from her nose and it started going into the tube. It just looked horrible.

Toward the end, it was getting to the point where, "Are we going to stop or not?" One of the head nurses came over and she was like, "When are you going to call it? You can't keep doing this." What she did then, which was very disturbing, was she pulled open the curtain and the mother and her other family that were there that evening saw what was going on and you heard the mom scream. They were doing chest compressions and one of the nurses was like, "They need to see this" and then another nurse was like, "No," and she pulled the curtain back. And then the other one pulled it open again. I'm standing there and I know I can pull it closed but I'm not. I can't get involved with this. And then finally it stayed closed. They gave her Fentanyl so that she had enough sedation and then finally they just stopped. I was going back and forth calling the liver team and whatever and then I just stopped. By that time, the family had gone somewhere else—I don't know who took them somewhere else but they weren't there.

1:1. There was a lot of commotion in the room and people were coming in and out because it was a continuous resuscitation for over an hour and we needed equipment and drugs and things like that. The family literally was watching as if they were in a theater and this was happening on the stage. I told somebody to close the curtain. Usually this is a controversial issue and it is a philosophical issue, if you wish, because some people would argue that it's their child's last moments; it's the last moments that this child is alive and who are you to deprive the family from being with her? The counterargument is a practical one. In these cases, they cannot be at the bedside because they are taking somebody's place who's performing something hopefully helpful and life-saving. From a strictly emotional standpoint, my feeling is that to hear and see all this, as the last image of your child, blood splattering literally from every orifice of her body and 10 people sticking needles and doing compressions is not necessarily what you want to remember about your child. Clearly there may be a lot of people, either the family itself or other individuals who may disagree with my approach, but this is the way I look at it. "Your presence is going to clearly obstruct what I'm trying to do. If you really care about her life, let me do what I need to do. Remember her when she was smiling, not when there was almost nothing human left."

Story 2

This story is about a 5-year-old boy who had a malignant abdominal tumor (neuroblastoma) and who, after being hospitalized for 2½ months, died from complications of a bone marrow transplant. In the last weeks, he was in chronic, intractable pain.

2:2. The resident called me at home because the patient had high blood pressure and was having a seizure; he needed to get certain things at certain times and we totally missed the boat there. He was meant to get a CAT scan at 6:00 A.M., and he didn't get it until 9:00. I had to take him down there myself, with the mother and, when we came back to the ICU, they told me that the bed was not ready and to take him back from where he came from in the hallway, with the mother by his side. So then we went back to his room on the floor [i.e., the pediatric oncology floor instead of the ICU] and his room was being set up for somebody else. So not only did I have to deal with the medical issues going on, I had to deal with the mother screaming, "My kid is not going to die in the hallway. I know he's going to die but not in the hallway!" It was the worst day of my life, if I can say that. It was hard enough knowing that I had a kid that was going to die; but it didn't have to be that dramatic and that stressful for me and for the mom; the poor lady who was taking care of this boy was running around like a chicken without a head. It was a horrendous experience. . . . When I came in that morning at about 9:00, I took one look at him and I knew he was going to die; I knew. He was still seizing subclinically, his pupils were dilated, and I knew that if he hadn't gotten his platelets up, he probably had bled [into his brain] and, if he had bled, then that was going to be the beginning of the end—you get a sense. I've known him since he came into the hospital a year and a half ago; he was my primary patient. He was just completely out of it; not responding. You get a sense after all. You hope that it won't happen but. . . . He got to the ICU finally around 11:00, but by then he was still having seizures so, whatever was going on, was progressing and after a while the mother stopped talking and was very, very silent. She was just by herself and keeping away from everybody. When he finally died, the dad was there and most of the people who knew Devon in the hospital had come to spend more time with him, like the nurses on the floor, the doctors in our group who were pretty close with him, some of the residents, the NPs, the social worker, who was very close. The social worker spent the whole day with the mom; she had got there at 10:30 and spent the rest of the day with her. And you could see that the mother was being more of her normal self, stressed but not angry or livid or whatever. When he died, he actually looked better dead then he did when he was alive that last day and everybody was commenting on it. Like, "My God, he looks so peaceful. He looks so different."

2:1. We were planning to have a family meeting to discuss advanced directives and DNR and, possibly, even stopping the care that we were giving so that they could take him home with the understanding that he would die but he never got there. They wanted to take him home because they thought he was suffering too much and they wanted to let him die. Part of that was driven by Devon and what he was saying and part of it was by what I clearly recognize now as their faith, where they truly believe in an after-life and he was to go on to greener pastures, so to speak. I thought what they were asking was not unreasonable, and, in the end, he was made DNR about 2 or 3 hours before he actually died. The nice part about that was that he was not intubated; he had very minimal stuff attached to him in the way of tubes and things in him so, within about 5 minutes of his having died, they were able to take everything off of his face and you were able to see him looking the way we all remembered him to have looked but haven't seen him look for 6 or 8 weeks. We were all relieved by that. I was really pleased that at least that much had been put in place that he wasn't intubated because it really makes those moments so much more difficult.

2:2. When I walked into the room, the mom wanted to know the CAT scan result. The mom's a nurse, so I brought her the printout and I showed it to her. She saw it and I said, "He's not going to survive this. Even if he does, he's going to be a vegetable." So, you can see her come to that realization. Then the attending in charge of the transplant went in and spoke to her and said, "We need to talk to you. We don't think he's going to make it from this,"and the whole DNR discussion ensued and she said that she didn't want him to be intubated or anything heroic and that she knew that this was the end—it was her reading the CAT scan that broke the news. She knew all day—you could see from the way she was talking and stuff— but she needed that one thing to put it in perspective for her. He was sick but, up until that last day when he had that seizure, he wasn't at death's door. He's been in the hospital for 80 something days; he came in to get his transplant and he never left. He got sick, he went to the ICU, he got better, he came back down, he got sick, he was chronically sick, and then he got a little bit more sick, and then he got a little bit better. Every time we had a family meeting with the mom we told her that, if it got to the point when we thought we could no longer do anything for him, we would let her know and, if she felt that she didn't want us to try anymore, we would respect her wishes.

2:7. Devon was a wise little kid, not a typical 5-year-old. Every day he would say, "My belly's hurting, can you fix it? Can we go to the belly store and get a new belly?" Every day he would just tell me what was the matter with him and ask me could I help him. Every single day, it was the same. Part of me would think, "Why do they keep asking me? I'm not prescrib- ing this stuff." I often thought that I'm only the order-writer and that's all I am. But I know that I'm a part of the team and, though I would think that, I would never say that to them, but yes, that was often how I felt. I knew that the attendings didn't have the answers either—no one did, not even the program director—so I would just try to calm them down as much as I could and give them as much information as I could, but it was frustrating day after day. I was one of the more consistent people who were there with them, whereas the attendings changed every week and there were different people covering on weekends whom they didn't know that well. I think they asked everybody who walked into that room, but the floor nurses and I got probed a lot more because we were there all the time. The pain was not getting better, the scans were not getting better; he was just sitting there wasting away, physically and emotionally. He was just constantly miserable, his family was miserable, and that was about the point when they started hinting that they wanted to stop and asking, "Why are we doing this?" especially the grandma; she's a pretty religious lady, and would say, "God didn't intend this for him. Why are we doing this? I don't want any more tests." She'd get very upset when we added new medicines or wanted to take him for another test so, when he died, it was probably helpful. I think it's harder when the family is hanging on so hard, and I think they knew it about the time we probably knew it. The family wanted that release for him, so it was hard. I don't think Devon knew it until a couple of weeks before. He just started saying, "I can't do this anymore. I can't do it." It was hard to see him give up like that. He wasn't articulating his pain any more, he was just saying, "I can't do this anymore." I didn't know what I could say at that point. I probably said stupid things to him like, "Why don't you try and sleep? Here's your bear. We're going to help you take care of the pain. Your Grandma's right here," just nonsense things. I didn't really know what to say to him. I wouldn't feel comfortable saying something like, "It's okay, it'll be over soon," even with the family probably on board to that way of thinking. I didn't know if the family would want to see their health care providers giving up. I didn't know that they would, so I would never say that. Maybe more supportive care people like social workers would, but I certainly wouldn't.

2:9. He was a lot of fun, very intelligent and very articulate. He was able to express anything he was feeling and be very honest about things and was never really lost for words. He's very up front about everything. He would say, "I'm getting very tired and I can't take this pain any more." There's not very many children who would be able to say those things. When he was in a lot of pain about 2 or 3 weeks ago it was, "My belly hurts, my belly hurts. Why does it have to hurt this much?" As it was getting toward the end, it was more, "I really don't want this anymore." He wasn't that active anymore. One of the more frustrating things for me was that, a lot of times, some of the physicians wanted me to provide distractions for Devon—like are distractions going to work at this point? We knew him well enough to know that distractions just weren't working for him; it was true pain, and I know the difference between when you can distract somebody in pain and when you just need to be with him and there's a very big difference there. But it was always surrounding what they were doing, like, "How much morphine is he getting? How much should he get? Maybe there's ways we can distract him so he feels better." . . . In some sense, Devon resolved himself to the fact that "I don't want to do this anymore" and I'm not so sure what death meant to him at that point. With the older ones it's a little easier, but, at his age, it's not as concrete and he wasn't afraid, let's put it that way. He was definitely not afraid. He was more afraid of pain than he was of dying, so when he said, "I don't want to do this anymore," it was a little easier than what happens to somebody who, no matter what's going on, says, "I don't want to die." So, you can ask me how I knew Devon wasn't afraid to die and I don't know, I just felt it; I really don't know it for sure. For some kids I do, but I didn't feel that kind of anxiety from him. The biggest thing he was anxious about was his pain, and the truth of the matter was that we couldn't stop it no matter what we did.

Story 3

This is a story about an 11-year-old girl who battled neuroblastoma for 6 years and finally succumbed with multiple bone metastases.

3:1. Taking care of her was about the hardest thing I've ever done, particularly in the several weeks at the end of her life. I had worked intensely with this family for 2 years and, for 8 months, we had known that she was going to die. We said it to the family in so many different ways, gentle and not so gentle. I had always promised them when the writing was on the wall, I'd let them know; that I would fight as long and as hard as I could but when it was clear that there was nothing more to do, we would take care of Elsa. What was so hard about this case was that they maintained hope for a miracle, and they fought me for what I felt was beyond the line of care and doing no harm and playing God for too long. It had been ugly from a hospital standpoint as well. I'd gotten a lot of pressure from the hospital to have her die at home, but the family wasn't comfortable with that either. So it started back in about December, when she started actively dying. I had her on an oral palliative chemotherapy regimen. We weren't doing anything and were really just watching her deteriorate, which is a very hard thing to ask the family to do, especially when their child has been through the most intensive chemotherapy that I can give with the goal to cure, then do absolutely nothing vis-à-vis keeping the tumor in check. It was incredibly hard for the family. They were of the mind-set that, when you need platelets, you give platelets and, when you need blood, you give blood. I tried to explain to them how it had been and the situation we were in now. In the past, we were supporting her because her low platelets and low counts were something temporary that I had caused by the therapy I was giving, but, now, her platelets and red cells were low because the tumor had invaded her bone marrow and her bone marrow was no longer capable of making it themselves and wouldn't ever recover that function, but they wanted things like daily platelets. Even up until the night before she died, they were fighting me that I wasn't transfusing her enough. I said to the mom, "In the event that Elsa's heart stops or that she stops breathing, do you want me to pound on her chest, put a tube down her, put her on a machine or can I let her go peacefully?" She finally—and she only could verbalize it once, because that's the kind of woman she was—said, "Let her go peacefully." I know that was what she wanted because she had said it in so many ways, but she was unwilling to commit to anything in writing. But I knew those were her wishes because I'd been working with her for months and months.

3:1. Elsa had always been very body conscious, and she had been living with these tumors popping out of her head for a while. That bothered her a lot and she'd wear a hat and she managed to deal with that. But then, what happened was an end-stage neuroblastoma where what she got were tumors behind the eyes, retrobulbar disease, and, initially, it caused proptosis [protruding eye] and we had treated her with radiation so she didn't have one bulging eye. But then, at the end stage, you get what's called "raccoon eyes." You get black eyes bilaterally and you can't do anything to take it away, no amount of platelets would take that away, and she was also having intractable pain. She must have had a tumor in her spinal cord, and she became essentially a paraplegic from the waist down. But this also took away the pain because her pain had been in her leg. She used to complain to me that she had terrible pain where she was rigid and couldn't get control. She was on everything; I've never seen a child on so many adjuvants. She was on steroids, she was on a tricyclic, she was on methadone, she was on morphine, she was on Neurontin, she was on Vioxx, and then they put her on Calcitonin. We used everything to try to get her pain under control, but it wasn't until whatever happened in her spinal column that caused her to lose the feeling below her waist that we could ever keep it controlled, to some extent. At least she didn't have these escalated bouts where she was rigid and weeping totally out of control.

3:1. I said to the mom, "This is the end. Talk to her, I'm sure she can hear you," and she started to weep. The mom knew and, while she was uncomfortable with it—she'd flip between anger and denial—there was some level of acceptance. But that day, when her aunt arrived and when Elsa was moribund and had agonal breathing, she shook her and said, "Wake up, wake up, wake up," trying to pull her back. We had told the family a number of times that, if somebody just told Elsa that it was okay to go, that she would go because we'd seen it before. She was doing all the things that I've seen people do just before they die, hallucinating, having visions, speaking to friends in native tongue, seeing children in the distance. She had told the child-life specialist that she had seen children, and when she said she had seen the children again, the specialist said, "Do you want to go with them?" and she said, "No," and gripped her hand. I think that was on her mother's behalf because I've never seen a bond this strong between her and her mom. I had begged her mom to give her permission to go, and I had begged her mom's sisters to tell Elsa, "Don't worry about your mother. We'll take care of your mother." That last day, they never asked about the transfusion, they never asked me for anything more. They just sat and held her hand and had prayer ceremonies around the bed and the chaplain was there most of the day. A lot of people had worried that there would be a scene because the DNR that I had gotten [gestures in quotes] wouldn't hold. I knew that's what they wanted, they just were never going to give up until it was clear. If there were any spark of life in her, they were going to keep her going. It was so difficult to watch.

3:10. This was a kid who clearly met all the criteria for home hospice care. She was the classic textbook case for that, but the mom did not want to go home until I could get her more hours for home care. Every hospice package which I researched only offered 20 hours a week of home care services. The mom was terrified to take this child home so I said to her, "If I can get you more hours, will you go home?" I thought that would be great and would be meeting the needs of the patient, the mom, and the hospital because we are an acute care facility so we needed to get her out. I found a way with a private foundation that was set up by a family who had lost a child and had put up a lot of money for any kind of private financial needs that patients have. I was able to get her 75 hours of home health care a week. But that took a lot of coordinating, a lot of time, and a lot of paperwork so, when after only two weeks she was readmitted, I was personally frustrated. I was a little self-centered, at that point, because I thought, "Oh my gosh, look how much work I did and it all went for nothing." But then I was able to look at the whole picture. First of all, she did get home for a few weeks, which was what the child wanted, so I felt good about that. When she came back, since there was nothing for me to do because I was done with all my concrete services, I spent a lot of time just sitting in the room and just providing emotional support and a lot of hand-holding and encouragement, and that was very difficult. It was very hard for me to watch her die here—I was actually in the room when she died, which has never happened to me before. That was pretty intense; it was hard. Her breathing was very labored for the last few hours before her death and I saw her go [demonstrates a couple of gasping breaths and then a deep sigh] and then some beep went off. I went to the nurse practitioner and asked, "Did she die?" and she said, "Yes." Her family just threw themselves on her.

I would have preferred that she had died at home because I knew Elsa wanted to be home, and it would have been nice if all the stuff I did worked but it did work for a little while. I did get her home for two weeks, but it just became too much for the mother. She got very scared because Elsa was dying and she couldn't handle it at home. She wanted to treat her fevers, she wanted her to keep getting transfusions, and it was too much to bring her back to the clinic all the time. What particularly brought her in, at the end, was that she had a fever and we called the hospice people at night to see if they could go in and assess the situation and maybe advise the mom this is kind of where we can maybe let go. She really didn't want to let go; she was not ready. She did everything short of resuscitation. She was doting on Elsa. Every time Elsa moved a half an inch, like turn her head a little bit, her mom would just jump up and start rubbing her face, "Are you okay? Are you okay?" She couldn't give Elsa any space; she was hovering over her and rubbing her everywhere. I know the mom needed to do this, but I felt that Elsa was very tense and there was no talking mom into just sitting back—she couldn't. She wouldn't allow Elsa to have more morphine. She kept blaming it on cultural issues, saying, "In my culture, we wouldn't do that." She thought it was going to kill her; to suppress the pain would suppress breathing or something. We were very concerned and we were thinking, "Should we bring this to the ethics board? Is this barbaric?" even though it wasn't because she was not doing it maliciously. She just didn't want her to die. It was very difficult, but we kind of let it go because we knew she was going to die any second. It was such a sharp contrast to the way this mother had been. She was an unbelievably committed woman to this daughter but was so immersed in it that she just could not see objectively that she was hurting her and prolonging her suffering.

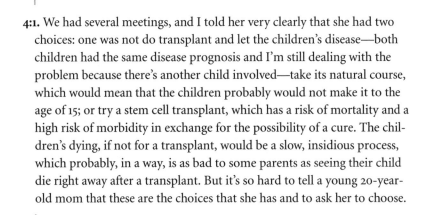

Story 4

Story 4 is about one of two siblings, 2 and 3 years old, both of whom had Wiskott-Aldrich Syndrome, a genetic disease for which there is no curative treatment, except bone marrow transplant (BMT). Without transplant, both would not be expected to make it beyond age 15—even with continuing supportive care. The mother consented to BMT for her older child, who then died from complications of transplant, and was left to decide whether to give consent for her only surviving child to have a BMT.

4:1. We had several meetings, and I told her very clearly that she had two choices: one was not do transplant and let the children's disease—both children had the same disease prognosis and I'm still dealing with the problem because there's another child involved—take its natural course, which would mean that the children probably would not make it to the age of 15; or try a stem cell transplant, which has a risk of mortality and a high risk of morbidity in exchange for the possibility of a cure. The children's dying, if not for a transplant, would be a slow, insidious process, which probably, in a way, is as bad to some parents as seeing their child die right away after a transplant. But it's so hard to tell a young 20-year-old mom that these are the choices that she has and to ask her to choose.

4:7. After a while, we started putting pressure on the mother to make a decision. I always told her that if she decided not to transplant it was all right; it was her choice. It was not the choice that we recommended, but it was a choice that she could make but, if she wanted them transplanted, the earlier the better. If you transplant a child after the age of 5, the complications are much higher. A lot of people believe that the age of 3 is a threshold, so that's why we were pressuring, and she would waver back and forth. We pressured her, and pressured her, and pressured her, and she made a decision, which was to go to transplant.

4:10. Toward the end, it was a tough situation for all the health care professionals as well as for the mom, who was always there. The most difficult part was knowing that the care we were giving was not going anywhere; it was just prolonging his suffering and prolonging mom's suffering. It was difficult that every day you came in, little problems came up and we took on these problems knowing very well that it wasn't getting us anywhere. I spoke to the mom a few times trying to establish what the issues were. She never gave me very straightforward answers, but I think she felt she had made a wrong choice for her son. She would pursue every possibility, probably to deal with the guilt that she felt. She had told me once before that she didn't think he was going to get better but she still wanted to do everything and I think it's all because of the guilt she felt.

Story 5

This is about a 5-year-old boy who had a bone marrow transplant and was in remission from leukemia. He died of complications of treatment.

5:1. I started taking care of Ricardo in April when, at that point, I was just serving as a consultant to help figure out how best we could transplant him, which turned out to be to give him cells from his mother who was an almost perfect match. I spoke rather extensively with his mom about the transplant. We had a number of very nitty-gritty conversations about it. She heard about all of the potential bad side effects and potential bad outcomes of transplant. . . . This mom understood better than most moms I've encountered. I was impressed right from the start with her degree of realism and pragmatism. In the two lengthy consultations I had with her to discuss the ins and outs of transplant—consultations that lasted well over an hour and the second one where I explained the whole consent for the transplant and went through it pretty much line by line with a translator—she asked very pointed and insightful questions. She wanted to know what the chances were of survival, chances of survival without relapsing, and for me to break that down, not in a nitpicky way, just that she really wanted to understand. His chances were decent but not great and she went into the transplant knowing that and every bad thing I presented to her about morbidity and posttransplant complications, sterility; all the things that this child was going to have to look forward to, if he survived.

5:1. Ricardo got sick a few times and he could never have a break. Every time something seemed to be getting better, he'd get another wham. When he had graft vs. host disease and that seemed to be getting better, then wham, it affected his gut and his liver. That seemed to be getting better and wham, stuff got worse again. It was one thing after another. From the point at which he was sick enough to even entertain going to the intensive care unit to when he was finally being moved there, there were several times when the family talked to us very seriously and said, "We want to do everything, but if you ever feel that, you know, we don't want him to suffer unnecessarily. We don't think that's what's happening now. We want to fight for his life, but if you ever feel like it's at a point where there is no hope, please let us know. Please don't keep us in the dark." Since they put that up front, every conversation we had along the way I would say, "You've asked for this. You've asked us to tell you when we're at a point when there's no hope and I don't think we're there yet. The things that worry me most about your son are X and Y. These other things I can see getting better." At every point up until quite close to the end, the medical team thought that certain things were potentially correctable. At the very end, we wanted to give the situation a few more days to declare itself in a very final way, but the family thought that we were there already and we really had to admit that they were pretty much right. We did see the situation turning itself around by sort of number parameters, so we couldn't really say we were there yet, but, by everybody's Gestalt, we were heading there. We would easily be there the next day. So, in a sense, you could say that the family was ready to throw in the towel before we were but not because we didn't see the writing on the wall. It was just because we'd sort of picked this arbitrary number parameter to let's wait till day X before we stop. What I mean is that at the last week of his life, Ricardo had gotten much better and then he suddenly took a nosedive again. It looked like he had some kind of serious infection, and we couldn't figure out what was causing it. He was covered with antibiotics, antivirals, antifungals, everything under the sun to fight infection. But all of his organs started to fail, his kidneys, his liver, his lungs so we were supporting all his body functions. We said, "If this doesn't turn itself around in the next few days, we will know that there's no hope of return." What ended up happening and, we expected that to happen, was that everything just got progressively worse—his lungs got a little bit better or maybe were stable; they weren't going down the tubes real fast. But his liver got worse, and his kidneys were hard to evaluate because he was being dialyzed. So his numbers got better, but it was not because his kidneys were working; it was because we were successfully dialyzing him. So he could've gotten worse across the board, but, as it was, he didn't get worse across the board. One of the two scariest things was that his liver dysfunction was getting worse and he wasn't able to make his blood clotting factors and he was starting to bleed out. So, if you just look at his numbers, certain things looked a little better the day he died than they had the day before, but the patient didn't look better. So, it was totally realistic to respect the parents' wishes and withdraw support when we did.

5:1. I offered the family an autopsy[8] of the child to figure out what had really gone sour at the end, and they ultimately took us up on it. That's one of the uncomfortable things that you're faced with sometimes because you're there comforting the family through their child's death and everybody's there hugging them and saying they're sorry and they're packing up the room and then you bring up this unpleasant thing. Not only is it unpleasant to discuss it, but if they agree to it, you have to go through this paper-signing process, which is tacky, under the circumstances, to be asked to be signing papers. I don't think it came off awkwardly, but it was an awkward moment for me, especially because I don't speak Spanish, so somebody else had to translate. It can be very awkward, pat someone on the shoulder and say, "By the way, now that your son is dead we'd like to get an autopsy." In this case, the mother wanted it very badly and the father first said, "No," and then thought about it and said, "Yes, I really want to know."

Story 6

This story is about a 7-year-old boy who died of brain injuries sustained in a car accident.

———

6:1. I met him about 3 days after the car accident. He was comatose with no neurologic function, and he remained in the same condition until the end. During the course of the week that I took care of him, I had the chance to discuss his condition with his mother on several occasions. The last time I talked to her was just a few hours before he was physically removed from all ventilatory support when I told her that his studies had shown evidence of being brain-dead. Part of the mother's reactions was very understanding of the situation and very matter-of-fact. At the same time, she was hoping for something to happen. She never expressed it very specifically to me, but she was asking me questions: "How can you be sure of about this?" "Is this definite?" and "Have you ever seen anybody recovering from these kinds of things?" always with a very appropriate matter-of-fact tone of voice. She told the nursing staff, "I will not withdraw support; only God can take care of him." The most striking aspect about her was that she had, from the beginning to the end, exerted the same affect. It was very flat—not indifferent—she was clearly very much involved, she practically never left the bedside, but, no matter what I was saying, her reaction was exactly the same. She had a polite, tiny little smile; it was almost an ironic kind of smile, like, "Okay, I know what you're going to tell me, but I know something you don't" kind of situation. She did not react in any different way when I told her that he was brain-dead, officially. Up to that point, we were talking about the high probability that he was going to end up brain-dead. I had been very explicit from the very beginning with her judging from his presentation and his course. Up to that point, the chances that he would recover even the slightest neurologic function went from minimal to impossible. I said, "Unless there is a miracle—about which I don't know and I cannot control—based on my experience, there is no way that he could recover." I tried to put it, from the beginning, that we were only talking about timing outcomes. In the first meeting that we had, I said, "One of the possible outcomes is that his vital functions, especially the heart, remain intact and, unless they express the desire to withdraw support, he could stay in that state essentially, indefinitely. In that case, we would have to think about doing a tracheotomy and a gastrostomy." That was the bottom line of the conversation. When clearly the days were passing by and he was not recovering any function at all, I introduced the concept that, for all practical purposes, if he's not already brain-dead, chances are that he will undoubtedly be brain-dead. Then, in the final meeting, there was the conclusive evidence. . . . It was a straightforward very severe brain injury, and you just provide support and you keep your fingers crossed. Neurology was the service that was, by definition, involved, but, even in that case, they just came daily to say, "Yes, he continues to be completely devastated," and, as far as the prognosis, every day that passed, he was getting worse and worse.

6:1. Instead of saying "brain-dead," I prefer to speak of the death of the brain. I explained that the brain is the organ that controls the functions of everything else, and, when the brain dies, it's a matter of from seconds to minutes to hours before everything else dies. I also made the point, very specifically, that the heart—that, of course, is the obvious thing that everybody can see on the monitor, beating—is an organ, technically speaking, that can survive even by itself. You can take it out of the body, put it on the table, and stimulate it, and you can make it contract in the absence of a living brain so that should not be perceived as a sign of life. They seemed to understand that. They did not ask anything that was either inappropriate or that would indicate that they were completely off the subject. They seemed to understand, but they seemed also to have some hope that something might actually change. This is always the situation, and we cannot take this hope away. We can tell them that, on the basis of my experience, on the basis of literature, or on the basis of whatever evidence we have, but we can't say for sure that nothing may ever happen.

Story 7

This story is about Carol, a "miracle" baby born to parents who were told that they were infertile and were about to begin in vitro fertilization. She died from a sarcoma after a last-ditch surgery.

7:1. She was 15 weeks old when she came to me. She came to me about 6 weeks after I had returned from maternity leave so she was 5 weeks younger than my new baby. She came billed as a neuroblastoma and had a rapidly expanding mass in the left supracurvicular fossa the night she came in. I knew that babies under a year of age with neuroblastoma did well and everybody, along the line, had said they thought it was neuroblastoma, so I was excited that I was referred this baby that would do well. I mobilized everything, and I had the baby in the operating room that night. It was a very difficult anesthesia because it was basically around her trachea and, even from the CT scan that we got that afternoon, it was clear that this was not your typical neuroblastoma, if it turned out to be a neuroblastoma. But I had her in the OR that night and we did an awake procedure; I did awake bone marrows. We wanted to try to get an answer by Friday so we could start therapy right away because her airway was potentially compromised. But by Friday, we knew we weren't going to get an answer and that put me in a very difficult spot. I started meeting the family and learning that this was basically a miracle baby born to two parents who were told that they would most certainly be an infertile couple. They had been about to start in vitro fertilization when, miracle of all miracles, they found out they were pregnant. I spent a lot of time with them. The service happened to be quiet those 2 days, so I probably gave them 5 or 6 hours each of 2 days and we bonded very quickly. But then the diagnosis became a real issue and actually took almost a week to establish that basically we weren't able to establish a diagnosis other than it was a malignant small round cell tumor that looked much like a sarcoma [because the tumor was so undifferentiated]. Beyond that, we weren't going to get much more information, and, in many ways, what was most frustrating to the family was that we could never pigeon-hole a diagnosis. Undifferentiated sarcoma just means the tumor looks like a sarcoma, but beyond that no one knows what tissue it came from. As time went on, the baby initially seemed to do a little better, although I had been very up front with them that the less we knew about this tumor, the less we were going to be able to make any prognostic statements about it. But I would never close the window to hope because we all go for the miracle. But the less we knew, the less I could tell them specifically and the only thing we could do then was to treat it empirically and see how she did and then go from there, but then the tumor was in a bad place as well. She did well enough initially that they enjoyed some time with her. She tolerated the chemo remarkably well but it became clear, over time, that the sarcoma wasn't melting away—it would respond initially, but it seemed to grow in between chemo cycles. So, functionally she was doing better; clinically she didn't seem to have much trouble with the chemotherapy, even though it was tremendously aggressive chemotherapy, but it wasn't melting the sarcoma away. The parents wanted frequent CT scans, and I knew we weren't going to see tremendous shrinkage because I could still feel it. So it wasn't worth subjecting the child to additional diagnostic studies. What was also clear was that they knew from the outset—I'd always been completely honest about this—that if it were sarcoma, in the absence of a curative surgery there was really no hope of cure; they knew that.

The surgeon here was adamant that the tumor was unresectable and would not agree to do an operation. They asked me what to do and I said, "There is a person in the city who is a very aggressive surgeon and I happen to know him to be a decent man as well. He'll give you an honest opinion and, if anyone would do it, he would do it. I trust the surgeons here with all my heart, and it was the chief of surgery here, who's an expert surgeon, who said the tumor was unresectable." The family said, "I respect him. I understand him but, if there's any shred of hope here, in order to live with ourselves, we need to know we did everything." I spoke to the surgeon at this other hospital, and he was very honest with me. He felt that the family was so proactive, so interested, so engaging—they live in our neighborhood kind of thing—and the baby was so engaging and just so young that everybody wanted to do whatever they could for them. The way he figured, it was that either this baby has surgery or the baby dies; the only chance was with the surgery. That's what he said to me and that's what he said to the family. He was very excited after the surgery because it took him much less time to get it out but he knew he left some behind. We all just wanted some good news. Two days later I got a call from the surgeon that the pathology report came back on the pleural fluid and it had malignant cells in it. That basically meant that there was no way of cleaning anything out and he'd known he'd left tumor behind too. As far as I was concerned, that was a deal breaker. I spoke to the oncologist at the other hospital and said, "That's a deal breaker," and he said, "Oh, I don't know. Let's wait for the rest of the pathology report to come back." I don't know what he thought it was going to show. I knew that the pathology report was going to have no surprises. I was hopeful that maybe they would see some differentiation which would help us put a better name on the tumor, but I knew that the margins were going to be positive; the surgeon had told me so, and I knew that the fluid was positive. So the only thing I was looking for was maybe a clue as to what it was that might help us change the chemotherapy. The other oncologist was hoping that there would be something even more positive then and that he would be able to come up with a very elaborate radiation treatment plan that was potentially curative. I didn't know what his hopes were, but the pathology reports were not out yet. The next day happened to be my daughter's birthday, and I was on my way to give cupcakes out at the public school when I got a call from the oncologist at the other hospital saying, "Well, we had the talk." I said, "What do you mean, 'You had the talk?'" and he said, "Well, I went over for a completely unrelated issue and, on my way over there, I checked the computer and the pathology report was back. So, when I got there and they said to me, 'Do you have the pathology?'" I felt like it was my moral duty to tell them the truth, that I had it, and so I told them that it's undifferentiated sarcoma, less than 50 percent necrosive, highly malignant, positive margins here, positive margins there, and that she would surely die." The baby was still intubated in the ICU and that was the Friday before a long weekend and there was nothing we could do about it. He had had this whole conversation with them without ever discussing it with me, after I'd had a 6-month relationship with them. So between cupcakes at the school and family cake at home, I went to the other hospital to see them. We met for over an hour and tried to put things in perspective and calm them down. They had been getting angrier and angrier at the other oncologist. He said that he had taken them into a room and sat them down, but they say he broke the news to them in the hallway and they suggested they go to a room. I don't know what went on, but, in the end, I was very honest with them. I said, "In some ways it makes my job much easier because the bad news was coming and it's much easier for me not to have been the messenger." They understood that and the mom even said to me, "Yeah, I don't think you could have gotten the words out."

Then, we began talking about other options and I said, "I would give her palliative therapy that's reasonably well tolerated" and they said, "When should we start?" and I said, "She's in no shape. She was intubated for 10 days, she had just gotten off, extubated 3 days prior," and they said, "Can we take a trip?" I told them to go and they went to Florida for 10 days to be with the grandparents and, on the seventh day, she got admitted to a hospital there. I got a call from the doctor that she'd been anemic to a hemoglobin of seven and they transfused her. When she came back, I got a CT scan and a chest X ray and it was clear that her left side was completely filled with fluid. In 10 days, she filled up her chest with fluid to the point where she was already in moderate distress, so we started the chemotherapy and I got her through the first cycle. For symptomatic purposes, I admitted her for a therapeutic tap that took off some of the fluid once and I did it again a week later. At that point, I started saying "No" to them when they said to me, "Shouldn't we just tap her again for comfort?" I explained to them that I got the cycle of chemotherapy into her, and either it's going to work or it's not, but I cannot justify giving this baby more aggressive chemotherapy and I cannot justify doing any more invasive procedures. Either the chemo will work or it won't and we're just going to have to wait and see. It was clear that she was popping out new little tumors everywhere along every surgical excision; anywhere she'd been instrumented and, growing along the track, was a new tumor. It was very hard to watch and it happened so rapidly. I'd never seen something grow that fast. And they always had the question—for example, they'd show me baby pictures and say, "See, it was there all the time, right?" We just didn't know, and I said, "They looked at a sonogram in the twentieth week of pregnancy and didn't see it." Yes, it presented at 15 weeks postpartum and it was quite large, and they were very mad at their previous pediatrician because they felt he'd missed it. They'd gone to him for breath-holding spells and reflux. In retrospect, it probably was the tumor sitting on vital organs, but certainly not what the general pediatrician sees and thinks of first. By the time it was poking out of the left supraclavicular fossa, he initially thought it might be a broken clavicle with callus, but then they got to an orthopedist who said, "Oh, no. It seems to me that, by the time it had declared itself, it had declared itself." So, yes, the pediatrician was late on picking the ptosis and the brachial plexopathy. Given these symptoms, the kid should not have had a diagnosis of brachial plexus palsy, but I don't think it would have changed anything. They had always said to me, "Was it there all the time?" and I said, "Well now we know the natural history of this thing." Left untreated, it is extremely aggressive. They kept saying to me everyday, "So how much time do you think she has left?" and I didn't have an answer to that question. I made a home visit when I heard that she'd had dusky spells—she'd turn a little blue and get agitated and have trouble catching her breath—that was a week after the chemo had been completed. She was already on home oxygen, she was already on nebulizers, she was already on methadone for pain, and we were doing palliative care. That was the true test of whether she's going to get better after the chemo or is the chemo not going to keep this in control? When I went to see them that night, she actually looked pinker and was rolling over. She wasn't well, but I knew that she wasn't going to go over the weekend; I also knew she was going to die sooner rather than later. They asked me, "Should we call hospice?" and I said, "There's no down side to calling hospice. People notoriously call them too late. There's no down side. If she recovers from this, fine, you'll just say, 'Thanks, we'll get you later.'" They set it up and had a hospice worker in by Tuesday and she died on Wednesday morning, the day I moved into my new home. So the other very sad day for her was another significant event in my life. I knew when she had dusky spells that she was going to die the day I moved into my new house because I believe in my own strange, weird, spiritual way that Carol came to me, in part, so that I would keep my own life in perspective. I have three healthy kids, and I have a lot of things going on that I have to manage, major nuisances but no major tragedies.

Story 8

This story is about a 1½-year-old child who died from a second bone marrow transplant after a relatively long and complicated illness.

8:1. He had hemophagocynig lymphohistiocytosis, which is both a congenital and an acquired type of illness. When it is seen in small babies, we presume that it is congenital. It has an unknown etiology and is generally fatal without transplant [i.e., bone marrow transplant]. So transplant was recommended, but the only option for this infant was cord blood transplant, which is, overall, a higher risk in terms of outcome and length of time it takes to recover from it. He received this transplant in December—the first of two transplants. He had a near-death experience because he got critically ill, was in the intensive care unit with respiratory failure, and everybody managed to pull him through—it was actually pretty miraculous. Unfortunately, the transplant did not work, in the sense that there was not permanent engraphment, and so we were left with basically rejection of the transplant and persistence of his disease. It is known that transplant may be accompanied by rejection of the graft so that re-transplanting, in such circumstances, is well recognized. We used that as justification to describe to the mother that this wasn't the first time that somebody had been in this situation and we recommended doing another transplant. But it was also clear that it was high risk for the first transplant and it was going to be doubly high risk now. I remember going over that consent form with the mother in extreme detail, to make absolutely sure that she understood that this wasn't just a repeat permission from the first time, that every risk that pertained to the first transplant was going to be multiplied more in the second transplant. So taking care of William was challenging and involved dealing with a mom of limited intellectual resource—she was essentially illiterate and didn't speak English. Whereas we probably should have been doing the second transplant in 3 months, it turned out to be more like 5 or 6 months. Part of this was that the mother was hesitant to go through with it, but not severely. She saw him come close to death before and she probably estimated, correctly, as it turned out, that he might be going through the same exact thing again. Transplant is so demanding that, whether you are talking about adult patients or families of children, the idea of going through a second transplant really puts you off right the minute you hear about it because of all of the implications of things that could go wrong. The transplant would have happened about a month earlier except that he had an infection. One of the problems that he ran into, early on in the transplant, was severe pneumonia with parainfluenza. This is not a big deal in healthy people but is often life threatening for transplant patients, so we knew that we had a serious problem. We were now a couple of weeks into the second transplant and blood counts were still low, some problems with diarrhea, bloodstream infections, and other medical complications—many of the types of things that we, from our point of view, accept as anticipated but that are always a lot for the families to accept. But this was a new problem and there was a recommendation to use Rybovirin, which was an available medication but the intravenous form of it, which was what we wanted to use, was still by compassionate use basis so we had to present to mom to agree to such therapy in the midst of all the other problems. We had to get the drug from the company and, when he got it, it seemed to help but then he proceeded to worsen. There were bacterial infections and some kidney problems too, and, ultimately, he was transferred to the intensive care unit, which was very frightening for mom because it was where she had been with him before. We met with the mom on a Friday, 5 days ago: myself, the transplant hematologist, who was on-service, and the social worker, who was fluent in Spanish. We discussed that we had a lot of complications now, and we were very concerned about whether William could survive but we were doing all we could. We wanted to make sure that that was exactly her wish too—the usual sort of discussion. She was calm, not frantic, and the immediate suggestion had been to begin yet another supportive therapy which was a venovenous hemofiltration, essentially a dialysis kind of therapy. By now, the father was there much more often, and, it became apparent, from further discussions, that dialysis had a bad connotation for this family because the mom's first husband had kidney failure and had been on dialysis and died. Hence, they simplistically interpreted that any such machine was basically a death sentence. Well, he was close to death so we were concerned, but we thought there was still a chance that it could help so we encouraged them to consider it and they accepted it, although, I would say, with some reluctance. But it was absolutely medically indicated. So we instituted dialysis, but he didn't get better and was probably more unstable as the day went on so we were in the ICU to basically offer the option of withdrawal of active care, if that is what the mom wanted. They wanted to see a priest, and it was frustrating because the best we could offer was the fill-in, a non-Catholic person from the hospital chaplain's office. So we couldn't even meet their most immediate need to have a priest there. Apparently, the Catholic priest who usually does it was out sick, and they didn't have any relation with the neighborhood churches to have temporary people fill in or anything. So you could sense the discouragement; they were asking for something that seemed pretty simple and we couldn't even do that; they just were looking for some spiritual help with their difficult situation. I think they needed some confirmation that all these things being done were still the right thing to do as opposed to deciding that it was too much suffering for their child. I think the mother, at least, was able to consider that, somewhere along the way, there was going to be too many things and too much suffering for the child. She couldn't really define it and we didn't really define it either. I think her asking to talk to a priest was her way of finding another person to talk to. That was our discussion that Friday, and, on Saturday, it sounded as if he was holding his own. Also on Saturday, he had gotten onto a new kind of ventilator, the oscillator type of ventilator, and we had discussed that with the mother who initially thought that it was yet another device, but we explained to her that it was meant to do the same job with less damage to the lungs because of less pressure. It seemed like it was having some benefit for him, but then, the next day, Sunday, he got into heart failure and had signs of myocardial damage that was looking much more irreversible. That evening he died.

The social worker was with them and, if called, I would have come in but since on Saturday it sounded like he was probably stable and would make it until Monday, I didn't say, "Call me" and, I guess, it was assumed that there was nothing more to do. I found out about it Monday morning. In retrospect, looking at the medical issues, such as the blood pressure and the need for valentory support, it is possible to create a scale as the likeliness of surviving all of this and the percentages would have been pretty low, based on hypotension, need for valentory support, and renal insufficiency.

By the time you add them up, you get a score that is pretty low for survival. It used to be that the ICUs wouldn't let transplant patients in because they all died. So it used to be that that was a major issue because the outcome was so poor. Now, we know that some patients can survive, especially if their problems are dealt with successfully early on and we were hopeful that, between the Ryboviron and not having developed respiratory failure immediately, maybe this would be a process that could be turned around. And he had gotten better in the winter from what looked about as serious, so we still had some hope that it was appropriate to go ahead. But you always have to question all of this because of what goes on in the ICU in terms of the intensity of the treatments and, if it is absolutely predictable that the child can't possibly survive, how much of it really makes sense. These are always difficult situations.

8:2. She [the mother] had a limited educational background and so her thinking was like, "He has fluid in his lungs so why are we giving him more fluid?" and "Is it because we are giving him fluid through the IV that his lungs are wet?" It was hard communicating with her, and you had to keep trying not to get upset with her because she didn't understand. She couldn't really understand a lot of what we were saying, even though we tried to speak to her in Spanish. Even the last day, she said, "If his heart stops, don't make it start beating again but, as long as it is beating, do everything to make him better." That is why we kept going, and we kept going, and we kept going. Toward the end, the doctors in the ICU told her that as much as we were still doing everything, he was not going to get better. He had a heart attack, his heart was going to fail, today, tomorrow, maybe the next day, and we have done everything we could do at this point. She accepted that and that was when she went to his room, and was just talking with him, and staying with him, and sitting at his bedside for 36 or 48 hours and he finally expired.

8:8. Saturday, I was telling the mom that we didn't think he was going to make it through the night. Friday night, his stats were 66, his heart rate was in the hundreds, his blood pressure was down on the floor, we were maxing on just about all the meds, the ventilator was maxed, there was not much room to go and, all of a sudden, he just got back up through the night. By that point, they were able to wean him off some of the medication so that if he got into trouble later on, we would be able to go up again. But when I came back on Saturday, just to say, "Hi, I am here if you need me," his stats were up 30 points, his blood pressure was great. The sad part about this child was that, when you looked at him, he looked like there was nothing wrong with him—usually, children at this stage, look horrendous—they are bleeding from all over the place and they are so swollen that it's easier to say, "This is enough, please, enough." But it was hard to see this child without thinking, "My God, he looks great" if you didn't look at all the equipment that he was on. That was the hardest part, and that was the reason that the mom had such a hard time. When you see a child bleeding out of the eyes, bleeding out of the nose, and you're packing the nose because it is pouring out, you are packing the mouth because the blood is pouring, it is coming out of the ears, their eyelids from the inside, and they are so swollen that the eyelid has reverted this way. The whites of the eyes are like balls of water just hanging; they are completely deformed. When you look at a child like that, you know that this was not the child they had brought in. They have no hair, their skin is peeling off, the tape on their face just rips their skin off, they are bleeding from everywhere. Their hands are like 10 times their size, it's horrendous. They look like a piece of meat that went through a blender or something. That is what they look like. This child, on the other hand, was not swollen, he was not bleeding that you could see, his face was clean, the tape on his face was clean. He looked like he was just waiting, like he was sleeping, and that made it so hard for the mom, because he really did not look that sick.

8:8. The doctor, one of the fellows, kept listening for a heart rate and blah, blah, blah and I said to the parents, "He is gone. I am really sorry but he is gone," and it took like another 10 minutes and I said to the doctor, "He is gone. I am taking him off the monitor because he is gone. I don't care how long you are going to look for this pulse, you are not going to get one and he is gone." He said, "No." He wanted to wait for somebody else, and I said, "What are you waiting for? He is gone and I am turning off the monitor right now." Before I turned off the monitor, I again said to the parents, "I am terribly, terribly sorry, but his heart is no longer working. I am going to turn off the monitor. I am going to take off all the stuff he has on him, and I will give him to you." So that is what I did. I turned off the monitor because, as long as they looked at the monitor and they saw anything—like the little brother, a 10-year-old, was asking the doctor, "What does zero mean?" That's when I knew we had to stop. So I started turning off all the pumps, the monitor, and the valve, and I disconnected the lines.

I was not going to give the fellow a chance to continue. No, we were not prolonging this any longer. The fellow knew me, he trusted me, and he knew that it was futile to continue to attempt to look for a pulse because there was nothing there. I guess he just wanted to make sure. The other nurse, on the other side, listened and she didn't hear a thing and now you were going to get a Doppler and do this? I said, "No. It is over." The fellows don't understand that as much as we do. We see it more. They are afraid, like, "Oh my God, what if I pronounced him and he comes back?" I don't know if that is their fear. There was nothing there; everything was flat all the way across. You would get a blip but it was because we were moving the cables. It wasn't him, he was gone, and you could see it in his face that he was gone. I could see it in the child's face without the monitors. The whole time, when patients are intubated, there is this tension—I don't know how to describe it—it is this mask of pain. It's not pain, in pain; it's like tension, it's like a mask, as if you would put on a mask like those peeling masks that you put on to clean your skin. The skin is very supple, very gentle, very soft. Sometimes you can see that, between here and here, they are frowning. Everything just moves up. You can see it in their face because, although they are not there, sometimes you can see like a smile. It is really weird; you could see a smile. Sometimes, they can smell, like a fruity thing. Others said that, but I have never smelled it; but I have seen them smile when they have died. And the whole room can just sense this peacefulness that just came on. I sensed it especially. It was there, when I walked in. I was very like, "Oh my God," and then, as I got to the head of the bed and I saw him and I touched him, my shoulders were like killing me, my back was killing me—I guess I had all the tension from the past 3 days—all of that was gone. And you could see it in everyone, even the mom. She was sobbing and all of that, but when I put my arm around her shoulders—when I had done it on Friday, her shoulders were like cement, she was that tense—her shoulders came down. She knew that the suffering was over. She could begin to grieve, and grieving is different from suffering.

8:8. Once a child dies, you take away everything that you can—all the IVs, all of that, the breathing tube—and you immediately give him to the mom because he is still warm, so you give him to her immediately. She held him and screamed, sobbed, carried on. It was horrendous; it was awful. I was here until midnight that night. This is the first thing you do when a baby is born—you give it to the mother because it is her baby, and then the other thing that they do is a bath. That is a ritual that is very maternal and paternal and what parents do all the time. After the bath, we dress them, usually we put pajamas on them or whatever and then we rewrap; we put them in a baby blanket. I asked the mom, "Do you want to give him a bath?" and she wanted to. That is the last thing you can do for your child. It is a bed bath, so you put lotion on them, you wash their hair, comb their hair, make it pretty, kind of. Usually as they are doing that, they are crying. It is really very emotional because everyone is sobbing at this point; the mother is sobbing, the nurse is sobbing, the father, everyone. But it gives you a time to just do something that is not a suffering thing. Once you finish with your bath and you dress him and you put a diaper on or whatever, you give him a clean blanket and you have them hold him. They hold him usually until they are very cold and the warmth under the body goes out. Often, other family members come and you essentially hold the first wake right there; it is very intimate. After that, we clean out the room. We take everything out, the pumps, all that stuff and move the bed out of the way. We take anything that would remind them of a hospital; we try to, anyway. We put chairs in the room and just wait for the rest of the family and let them be alone. You just kind of be there for them and stay outside. If they want you in there, and sometimes they do, they ask you questions; they want to know certain things. Not all families are ready to leave the hospital so you give them a time frame. Six hours seems, to me, good; by 6 hours they are kind of ready to leave. I always say, "You could be here as long as you want." They usually say, "Well, how long do other parents stay?" and I say, "Well, they usually stay between 4 and 6 hours." There was a little boy there, his 10-year-old brother. That was the saddest thing because the parents were screaming and wailing and this poor kid was left all alone sitting in a chair.

Story 9

John was a 12-year-old boy who presented with a standard low-risk kind of cancer from which everyone expected a relatively quick and easy cure. However, he relapsed and developed an incurable lung metastasis. While he was being treated, his father also was being treated for cancer of a different kind. His mother was a cardiac transplant nurse.

9:1. During the early part of his treatment, I was very optimistic and I expected him to do well, so when he relapsed, I was not only devastated but really shocked. Usually, it's just the parents who are shocked and we kind of know what to expect. We often know when a patient is high-risk, even if the family is in denial, but this time I thought he was the standard low-risk kind of patient who would do well with standard therapy. When somebody's relapsed, it's always very disturbing but there are kids, for example, who have metastatic disease to begin with or present with extraordinarily large tumors that can't be removed and I kind of find a way to brace myself for the fact that they may relapse at some point because the chances of that happening are moderately high because of the way they started out with their illness or because of the kind of illness they have. When a patient has an illness that in the beginning looks like it's curable, you look the parents in the eye and say that you're aiming for cure. You don't promise it, you know that even people who have a high probability of cure sometimes are not cured, but when it's a patient who has the statistical probabilities in his favor and the treatment goes well and the family does everything they possibly can and there's no hitches along the way, then, when they relapse, it's more of a shock. It's also more of a shock when it's a patient that you particularly, for whatever reason, just resonate with; that you just feel close to and John was just one of those kind of kids for me.

9:1. When John was first diagnosed, his attitude was that he had a lump, it was biopsied, and then it was completely removed. So his attitude was that the cancer was out of his body and he was getting some medication to just sort of prevent any further problems. He felt that he was going to be fine. At least that's what he expressed. I'm not sure that that's exactly how he really saw it because one of the things that made taking care of him even more poignant was that his father was being treated for cancer at the same time. He was diagnosed a little bit before him, and so John had already seen the ups and downs of his father's course and, at one point, thought his father was going to die, although he did not. He's had other older family members die of cancer, so even though he kept up this positive outlook, there was a part of him that knew things were not necessarily going to work out so well. Then, when he relapsed, he was at first very angry, which I was glad to see. He wasn't trying to be the good, perfect boy. He cursed a little, there was a bit of "Why me?" all of the normal kinds of expressions,

"I don't want any more of this blank chemo. It doesn't do any good." However, within a short period of time, he started to calm down and gathered up his resources and talked about how he was going to fight it and be well. Even as he was getting much sicker and we knew that he must be aware of how sick he was—he was losing weight, he was short of breath, he had pain, he was getting less medicine instead of more—he didn't directly address the fact that he was going to die. In one of the last meetings I had with him, I met with him without his mother and father in the room. This was unusual because usually he was perfectly content to have his mom there, so I thought he was going to bring up some difficult issues. He was talking about having pneumonia, and I said something to him to the effect of, "Do you ever worry that it could be something more than pneumonia?" and "Do you ever worry that your illness can get worse?" and he said, "No" and changed the subject so I didn't push him. I had thought that that was what he wanted to talk about but actually, when I got near that area, he changed the subject. I went there once and then retreated and then did it again, and both times he backed off so I didn't push it. We never really directly talked about him dying.

———

9:9. Once we realized that the tumor was in his lungs and that it was still there after radiation, things quickly went downhill. At first, his mom didn't want to tell him, but we were able to get her to tell him that the tumor was still in his lungs and gave him the opportunity to understand what was happening. The mom would tell him certain things, but there were other things that she wouldn't tell him. But this was important for him to know because it wasn't a good sign that the tumor was still there. There's a way to kind of segue into what will happen, what could happen eventually, and what we could do about it to help him feel better. So it was easier for me once she had told him that the tumor was in his lungs because then we could talk about what kinds of things he wanted to do. Like, "Okay, you're going to get more radiation and we're going to try to get rid of this tumor. While we're doing that, what kinds of things do you need? What do you want to talk about?" One of the things was that he wanted to go to Puerto Rico to visit family. I remember one of the last conversations I had with him before he went to Puerto Rico. I said to him because I knew that the tumor was still there and it didn't look good, "Well, John, you're going to go to Puerto Rico and I know you're going to have a good time. You're going to get this inhalant that you're going to take with you, but what's going to happen if the inhalant doesn't work?" and he said, "All

I want to do is go to Puerto Rico. I want to go knowing that I don't have to take any medicine that's going to make my hair fall out because I don't want to have to go through that again and whatever happens, happens." I thought at that moment that he knew that his days were numbered and that he didn't have a lot of time. He realized that he was just going to have to make the best of it. He realized that things weren't going to get better; he was smart enough to realize that. They were giving him other medications, but they weren't as aggressive as before so he was smart enough to realize that what they were trying to do was make it go away but maybe it can't go away.

9:10. He said, "I'm not dying" when his mother said, "You know, John, it's okay to let go." He was like, "No, I'm not dying, mommy. God, I'm not dying. I'm not dying." The mother was saying that it was so hard for her because she's like, "I knew what you told me to say was right to say to him, but it was hard to say that to him when he kept telling me 'No.'" At that point, she was deciding if she should call 911 because he was saying, "Mommy [his mother is a nurse] give me CPR. You can make me better." And she's like, "I can give you CPR, but if I give you CPR, I have to call 911 and then, if you call 911, they're going to put a tube down your throat." He's like, "No, mommy, I don't want a tube" so she goes, "Well then, I can't do that. If I do this, I can't do that" and he was like, "Okay" but he was kind of back and forth also. He must have been delirious at some points. She realized, at that point, that she had to walk out of the room, so she walked out and called the oncologist and said, "The time's coming." She also said that her sister-in-law told her that—I guess Sponge Bob is like his favorite cartoon—that, at the end, he opened his eyes and started laughing and said, "Hi, Sponge Bob" and he just took his last breath and that was it. So she said, "At least I know he was happy when he died. He had a happy something. Wherever he was going, he was happy going there."

Story 10

This is about a girl who presented at 2 years old with a brain tumor and died 2 years later.

10:1. She had a good response to the first 21 weeks of chemotherapy, but then she got started on the second phase of chemotherapy and, with that, she had tumor regrowth. This was in the frontal lobe of the brain, and she had presented with seizures. We discussed trying a different chemotherapy because we still had, in front of us, the possibility of completing the chemotherapy with a good response to the remaining tumor and then being able to do a single hiatus of chemotherapy treatment or stem cell transplant. That was the overall plan. But then, from that point on, she progressively lost her response to the chemotherapy. So then we got into secondary treatments—and this was frustrating because we seemed so close—we seemed to be at a point where there had been pretty much almost complete disappearance of tumor. It seemed that surgery would continue to be helpful so she had many brain surgeries, but instead the tumor progressively got more refractory. We had discussed with the family in the first place that the chances that she could be cured were probably not more than one in three, and objectively they understood that, but still they remained very hopeful, especially in the beginning part. Then, as we got into additional chemotherapies, we explained that, even though we were not quite at the point of suggesting radiotherapy, we were going to want to consult on that. Radiotherapy felt that if we could possibly continue with chemotherapy, that would still be preferable, at least till we got maybe to her third birthday because such radiation would have involved the whole brain. A lot of the dynamic here was these back-and-forth decisions about conflicting goals of treatment—trying to eradicate the tumor but also trying to do it in such a way that we didn't create a 30-point IQ deficit at the same time. These are sophisticated, complicated decisions, and the parents were conflicted even between themselves. The father had job issues as well and his life was not easy. There was also a small baby in the house. So you had to guide the parents along in making decisions. There was also a consensus that radiotherapy should be deferred, if possible, until a child is at least 3 years old. So that was directing the decision. However, in order that the family at least have the chance to hear about radiotherapy, we sent them there so that if that had sounded like something that they specifically wanted, they had the chance to hear it. I think, at that point, they still felt that they didn't want to go away from the chemotherapy plan in the direction of radiotherapy, but then she was worsening neurologically too and that got us into more surgery, which was complicated by postoperative problems, including fluid imbalance and so forth. We got into a few weeks where it was impossible to make any other decisions about any other kind of treatment because we were stuck in this postoperative period, and I think that really made the parents, especially the mother, realize how really sick she was. She had probably half a dozen surgeries with the goal of removing the tumor because it had crossed to the other side of the brain and was causing shifts in the brain and was obstructing and causing fluid accumulation. It was hard for the family because when surgery is recommended, it implies that it is going to be a big positive step forward but the further along she got, the chance that surgery could contribute to cure was definitely getting less and less. Radiotherapy ultimately was started in September with the hope that she'd at least get some stabilization. We explained to the parents that we still expected that she would succumb to her disease, but the mother was still hoping for some miracle; the father was absolutely realistic. Then, a week or so into the radiotherapy—because she was, among other things, requiring sedation for the radiotherapy treatment—her breathing became an issue. She was requiring pain medication for tumor-related head pain, and so her breathing was beginning to be a little irregular and a question arose as to whether there could be some emergency. Two weeks before she died, I went to the family—the radiotherapy had been going on for a few days—and said, "We really need to discuss some things. Let's suppose she has some kind of emergency with her breathing, especially if she is down in radiotherapy, because I am concerned that this is beginning to be a problem." Families all have different feelings about what they would want done, so you need to know what this family would say if she really had a period where she ceased breathing. Would they interpret or feel that God was telling them or, somehow, that it was a message that this was the point where it was not reasonable to bring in machines or other levels of support above and beyond what was already being done because it was not going to work in the end? I told them that, if they felt that way, they needed to let us know. The mother had a puzzled expression, so the father said, "He is telling us we have to decide if she should go on a ventilator or not." They didn't make a decision immediately, but, within the next few days, they decided. They said, "We can see that she is sicker, and we can see that she is certainly comfortable with the pain medicines and we can imagine how she might not be comfortable if other things were being done, so we don't want that." Four days later, they decided they wanted to discontinue the radiotherapy because they had concluded that it really wasn't helping her and we indicated that we were okay with that decision. The point of radiotherapy at this stage was to give her a prolonged symptom-free period so that she would be able to go home. It was palliative basically, and we told them that, in spite of doing this, she was not going to survive but she might very well be able to go home. We thought that they might like to have that choice, rather than being imprisoned in the hospital, if it became that way for them. But I don't think the parents really sensed that the condition was terminal and that the treatment was palliative. They spoke of radiation as if there was still hope for a cure, and I could understand how it had, for them, the appearance of a definitive treatment that might still be enough to kill the tumor. The mother still felt that, and she was also even asking for chemotherapy with the radiotherapy. She was asking whether there was another chemotherapy she could get. She had all those questions and I am not sure that she couldn't understand, but I think it was her way of fending off the notion that was too uncomfortable for her. I think that she just didn't want to hear that this child, sleeping peacefully in bed, was going to die soon. She couldn't accept that, and she couldn't accept that radiotherapy or some other combination of treatment that we could come up with would not be helpful. We were surrounded by critics who said, "This family really doesn't understand what's going on." But the diagnosis of a life-threatening illness in a child is at the top of the list for stress for parents; I don't think there's anything that exceeds it. So it's kind of gratuitous for people to expect us to bring these families down to a level to accept a situation that they were never prepared for and cognitively may not be able to deal with.

10:1. I had gone over, a couple of times, with the parents about what I thought her death was going to be like. I told them that her disease was going to slowly make her less and less responsive and slowly make her breathing slower and slower until the point where she would just not be able to oxygenate normally and, therefore, the rest of her organs were going to die. I told them that I did not think that she was just going to automatically stop breathing. On Friday morning the parents had left the hospital to get some lunch or to go home to take a shower and refresh themselves, and the nurse came and said, "She stopped breathing." She stopped breathing and she completely desaturated, but her heart was functioning fine, her blood pressure was okay; the only thing she did was stop breathing. So even though she was DNR—and we did not intubate her— we used a bag valved mask to kind of breathe for her body until her parents got back to the hospital so that then, when her heart stopped, they would be at the bedside holding her. And that is what we did. We basically bagged her [i.e., placed an oxygen mask over the face which is attached to a bag that the physician presses to fill the lungs with oxygen] and kept her alive until they got there. We called them up and told them that she had stopped breathing, and so they came within 15 or 20 minutes. When they arrived we stopped bagging her, and she slowly desaturated over the course of a few minutes and she died.

Story 11

This is a story about a 1-year-old child whose death was sudden, totally unexpected, baffling, and devastating for the staff.

11:1. She had mucolipoidosis, which is a metabolic disorder that is life threatening. Most children live only until 3 or 4 years of age. The one treatment that we've started to try, as with other storage diseases, is stem cell transplant. The idea is you replace with donor or normal white blood cells which carry the enzyme they're deficient in. The last time I saw her was Sunday night—cute with her rattles and playing, like, "Googoo, googoo" kind of thing—normal. I examined her from head to toe, and she was totally fine. She had issues in terms of what we needed to watch for the transplanting. We were trimming her fluids and being very careful about what we were doing in terms of medical management. Monday, I was out but came back on-call Monday evening and got reports from the oncology attending and resident who had seen her all day. They told me what were the issues I needed to look out for, but there was no sign that anything imminent was going to happen. I usually call the resident around midnight to see how everybody's doing. I was sleeping, and I got up around 12:15 and checked my beeper. Apparently, my beeper had gone off at 12:13 and I didn't hear it so I called the floor and said, "This is the oncology fellow, did somebody page me?" and she said, "Yeah, Susan just died." I said, "What do you mean she just died? Where is my resident?" So she put the resident on the phone, and I said, "What's going on?" and she started telling me, but then she put the PICU fellow on the phone. He ran the code[9] and he told me that he didn't know what the issue was but that he came right away and they tried and tried but they couldn't—she died. I was like, "You've got to be kidding me." I was in shock; I literally was in shock. I said, "Let me speak to the resident," and she gave me her side of the story of what happened medically. And I'm like, "You've got to be kidding. You can't be serious. You can't be serious," and I'm trying to think, "What should I do next?" This was so unexpected. It wasn't like, "Okay, let's decide on how to take care of a problem with a patient"—there was nothing to do. They had called the code, certified her dead, and I'm like, "So how come?" She said that it happened so fast they didn't have a chance to call me before they started running the code. Her voice was trembling, like she was out of it. As I was on the phone talking to her, I was getting dressed and said, "I'm coming. I'm coming. I'm coming, just hold on tight. I'm coming, okay? And, how's the mom?" She said, "The mom is as good as can be expected." I then told her that I would call her back when I'm in the car, and I just put on my jeans and my sweatshirt and I just jumped into the car and I paged the attending on-call and the primary attending for the child. Then, in the car, I called the resident back because I was very concerned about her. She wasn't hysterical, she wasn't crying, she was very calm but you could hear, in her voice, that she was completely frazzled by what was going on. She's very competent and very confident; she never sounds like she doesn't know what to do, but, this time, it was so different from how she usually sounds: "I don't know. I don't know." I'm like, "Okay, just hang on. Is everybody else okay?" She said, "I don't know." She couldn't focus on anybody else. I called her three times on my way in the car just to see how she was doing. The third time I called, the attending on-call was there already, and I told her what I knew and that I'm on my way in and she asked if I was okay and I'm like, "Yeah, but I want to speak to the resident," and so we talked a little bit and, by that time, I was just about there. I came into the hospital and rushed to the floor and I guess I was in such shock. I kept thinking, "What happened? What did we miss? What did I do wrong? What did the attending do? Should I have stayed late?" I was confused and really had no idea. I went over what happened. She had a fever Sunday night and I made a judgment call and gave her antibiotics, but I gave her a one-time dose and said, "Let's see how it is the next day," because it was a very skimpy fever and it went away. Now, I was double-checking everything I did. When I got to the floor, I saw the nurses, and they were so upset because they hardly ever get codes on the floor. Usually, when our kids die, we expect it; we know that they're on their way out. I gave the nurses hugs and said, "You guys just hold tight. You did a great job." Then, I went to the resident and asked her how she was doing. She kept saying, "I don't know. I don't know." She was just sitting there and staring into space. It was so hard for her, and I felt so bad because she had just come on-service and she didn't know this girl from Adam; she had never seen her before.

She saw the kid when she came on the floor and did a checkup, and then the mom came out and grabbed her in the hallway and said, "Something's wrong with my kid," and that was it. The resident had been going from room to room to see how the kids were doing. That's when the mom called and she was close to the room, so she was the first to get into the room. The mom said, "Her belly is distended. Something is wrong," and she just reached out all of a sudden, like she had a pain or something and then just collapsed. As the resident was examining her, the kid's stats were dropping—it happened so fast. She just grabbed the bag and started bagging and told the mom to get the nurse. The nurse came and they called the code. It was very quick. There wasn't a chance to sit down and think it out. The next thing was, "What do we do with the body?" The mom was alone, and they had to call the dad. I let the attending deal with all the talking to the family, getting the paperwork signed, and all that stuff. The issue about the autopsy and what to do with the body came up, and it was very confusing because nobody seemed to know what to do, how to go about the whole procedure. It was very hazy in everybody's mind, and it may have been that they were all in shock and not thinking straight. Normally, when somebody dies, we take good care of the family, their medical issues, and the body and morgue—all that stuff is taken care of by the social worker who's on duty or the nurse in charge. I've never had to deal with it before. We signed the form and tried to figure out what to do next. The nurse in charge tried calling the nurse manager, and it was like a circus. It wasn't negative; we just needed to find out what was going on and what to do so that we could do it right and make sure that we had everything all set up. We didn't know if the body should go to the morgue or should go to the medical examiner. Nobody was clear about that. We called the administrator on duty who had no clue, and she said to call the social worker at home. Somebody paged the person on-call that evening who said, "Well, I'm not supposed to be there at night." It was a circus. It was very frustrating in terms of needing somebody to help us through this, and we didn't have anybody and everybody you'd call was upset because we're waking them at 1:00 in the morning. I don't think it was so much that they didn't know what to do with the body but that they needed somebody outside of what was happening to say "Do this, do that and that," somebody to direct the flow of things. The nurse in charge was frazzled, and somebody else stepped in to help her. I don't think she knew all the policy in the hospital or whatever, and I had no idea who to call. Every time I've had a kid die, I've had my social worker right there beside me. I've never had somebody die at 1:00 in the morning. Even though the mom wasn't hysterical, she was in shock and she needed somebody by her side. When we called, they told us that nobody was supposed to be on-call for social work, but because of the abruptness of how it happened, we needed somebody to help us out. We called the geneticist who had been following her and she said, "You got to be kidding. You got to be kidding." She couldn't believe it. She was like in shock. Same for the primary attending. He was in shock. He was on the phone like, "What? What? What are you talking about? Are you serious?" . . . The mom was going to wait for her husband to come because she said he wasn't sure he wanted an autopsy. We told her that, because it was so sudden, we won't know what happened or have an explanation for it and that we'd like to know so that we can all learn from it. So she gave her consent, but she had to get her husband to agree also. The overwhelming feeling of that night was confusion. I kept questioning what happened; where do the pieces fit? We went into the computer and checked all her labs, all her numbers, all the fluids that she was getting. I called the pharmacist to check what chemo we gave her, "What was in the bag? "Let's calculate it again." We were going over and over what could possibly be the reason for this happening, and we came up with nothing and that was very, very frustrating. The nurses were confused, and the resident was like, "I should have gone in before this happened" but, on a 29-bed floor, you can't be everywhere at once, and Susan wasn't even on the list of who were the sickest kids, not at all. It's been two and a half days, and I'm still wondering in my head. First, I thought that maybe she was septic and so maybe I should've given her a bigger antibiotic, almost double the antibiotics that day that she had the fever. I asked the attending, "How did she look on Monday?" because I wasn't here on Monday and she said, "She looked fine," and that if she thought she was septic, she would have upped the antibiotics. You keep questioning and thinking and thinking, "Was her white count okay?" Her white count was fine; it was normal. "What about her heart?" We read the cardiology notes back over, and they were not excited about the heart. She had the myopathy (weak heart muscle) and we had to be careful, but would it give her a sudden death, without any notice? No. She was on digoxin, so the myopathy was well controlled, her levels were fine, and we took her levels a hundred times that night. You just kept on looking for something—did she bleed into her belly? She wasn't bleeding before this happened, and why would she bleed into her belly? We never gave her anything that would cause her to bleed, and she was not on steroids. I still wonder why, every day. I talked about it again this morning with the attending trying to figure out what happened. It's very weird.

By the time the father arrived, I couldn't go back in the room; I couldn't deal with it. So the attending, unfortunately, had to be the one who dealt with the father and mother. It was hard because the mom was saying how she couldn't say good-bye because it happened so suddenly, and the attending came out and she fell apart. She started crying and said, "What am I supposed to do?" She just lost it, so we went to a room in the back; we gave her a tissue and sat with her. The nurses were all talking about it among themselves—how they couldn't believe what happened and, "Oh my God, this is terrible." They were all like paralyzed for the rest of the night. You always think, "Did we miss something?" The tendency is to blame ourselves. Maybe we should have put her on a monitor. As they get older and get sicker, they end up having respiratory problems and as-pirate and choke and have sudden death like this. Did she have any of those signs coming in? No. Should we have assumed that she has this diag-nosis and cover every single thing that could happen? Is it a realistic thing to do? Probably not, but you keep going over this—should we, could we, did we, why didn't we, kind of thing. I don't think you ever get over the fact that the kid has died; you've lost a patient. You get over that part, but what could you have to done to have prevented it? If somebody else dies, you're going to bring back part of this and say, "Okay, why didn't I learn from this to prevent that from happening?

Story 12

Alice died when she was 5 years old of respiratory failure after a long and pro-tracted illness with numerous complications.

12:1. I first met Alice shortly after she had her primary tumor removed. The surgeon was a pediatric urologist and thought he was getting into a kidney tumor and, instead, got into a large neuroblastoma. He removed her kid-ney, which probably would not have been done had he realized it was a neuroblastoma. So, from the get-go, there were disappointments for this family, and a learning curve in terms of dealing with this kind of an event. They were surprised and overwhelmed in the beginning, like most of the families, and they came to understand the gravity of her situation as she embarked on chemotherapy here; her surgery was elsewhere. They had just come back from a trip to Europe, and, while they were there, Alice had strep throat and then she had a blister and these were all taken care of and they had no idea that she had any kind of serious illness. Then, all of a sudden, they went from having strep throat to having a kind of cancer that was against the odds of being cured. The next thing you knew her kidney was removed and she had some minor complications after surgery. Then she came here and tolerated the initial chemotherapy very well but then developed an Aspergillus infection which was thought to be something that she caught from the environment in the hospital. All sorts of hospital people came to explain that to the family, and she went on an experimental drug in addition to the usual antifungal things. Then she took longer than most to recover from the chemotherapy and required a lot of supportive care. So, from the time that she got the Aspergillus infection, she was on an experimental drug, which had to be given in the hospital, so she was here every single day either in the clinic or as an inpatient for just about a year. She was known to everybody and was one of the patients that everybody was involved with. I was her primary oncologist. She was unable to complete the entire course of chemotherapy. It turned out, later we found out, that she had hemophagocytosis, which means that she had some cells that were eating up her white cells and her platelets. She went on to have a transplant [bone marrow transplant], but in the course of things, a couple of more things happened. For one, she had CMV [cytomegalovirus], which made her a bad candidate for transplant and, second, she never produced enough white cells of the right type to be collected for an auto-transplant, which would have been a much safer procedure for her. One thing after another happened along the way. I feel very proud that I was able to get her down between some of the things and get everybody to agree that she could have 4 days off of this experimental antifungal therapy so that she could go to Disney World; she had a great trip and really enjoyed it tremendously. So she went to transplant, and going into transplant, she was a very high-risk patient because of all of her lung damage that had been done before. Although the transplant team is very careful about what they say, the overall presentation was a little bit more optimistic than what you can expect the outcome to be. So I didn't think the family was as prepared as they could have been because, for me, the expectation was that she would be very lucky to come out of it alive. But there were no choices; they were in a corner between a rock and a hard place. There were no good choices for this child because, if they didn't do what they did, the disease would have recurred and she would have died from the disease. As is, she died 110 days posttransplant.

This was a girl who had 9 lives, or 10, or 12. She made it through all these terrible things: a bad fungal infection when she was immunosuppressed; CMV when she was immunosuppressed; they even had trouble getting her off the ventilator when she went to the OR for a procedure; and she was intubated from the anesthesia, and she came right off of it two days later and some people were saying, "Gee, we don't get kids who have been transplanted off the ventilator so soon." She did well and she had some very good days after that. But then she had pneumonia, and her lungs deteriorated rather acutely over about a 4-day period. She went from being completely alert to requiring a ventilator that required her to be sedated to the point where she couldn't respond, and her breathing was paralyzed so that the ventilator could not do its work. She was on that ventilator for 3 weeks. My experience with ventilators is that, once you're on them for more than a week or 10 days, you sustain additional damage to the lungs and the lungs are unlikely to recover. So I started preparing myself for this outcome when I saw that she was not improving to the point where she could be weaned off the ventilator. About 10 days before she died, it was clear to me what was going to happen.

12:1. The ICU attending, who had been the one who had been following her over the course of the whole week, was the one who decided that the time had come and he moved her from the jet ventilator to the conventional ventilator. They then picked her up and put her in mom's arms and, while mom was holding her, they turned off the monitor and left the room so the family could be alone together. Alice had been in their arms for maybe 10 or 15 minutes, not much longer than that and the family was all assembled. Alice was nestled in mom's arms, getting bluer, but they were holding her and dad went in, half to the side but half holding her too. And she died very comfortably in the parents' arms and everybody else was in the room, crying and stuff but not wailing, just quietly crying and everybody was hugging each other. The child was still hooked up to all the leads and everything and they were monitoring them. I had to leave the room, at one point, because one of the monitors was buzzing and we needed somebody to come in and turn off the alarm because that was really annoying. We knew it was slowing down and didn't need to hear some kind of a buzzing noise. So, when I went out, I saw the ICU attending and all of the nurses huddled around Alice's monitor and they could see it slow down. When she flat-lined, they quietly walked in and the ICU attending listened to her and he shrugged his shoulders and they understood.

Story 13

This story is about a 16-year-old girl who had a prolonged illness and who died despite pursuing many treatment options.

13:7. Whatever we gave her never worked. Her disease just continued to progress and progress and progress. But through it all, she always remained a very bright spot in my day and in everybody else's day. She never questioned, "Why isn't it working? What's going to happen to me?" She just always was, "What's the next plan?" She was very driven, but toward the end, I could see that she was starting to fray; she knew what was going on. She was a very bright girl, so it's not as if she didn't realize what was happening, but she chose to put her energy into other things, like school. Denial worked very well for her, and I don't think that she ever really grappled with the "Am I going to die?" question. She certainly never discussed it with me or her mother. Mom and I had talked about having her talk with our psychologist, but Rebecca was really against it so we didn't see any benefit in shoving it down her throat—if she was ready to talk about it, we felt that she would.

13:7. On Thursday, Thanksgiving day, Rebecca was in a lot of pain. Her feet were very swollen; she was just very uncomfortable. She spent most of her day in her room but was able to come down for dinner and be with her family and enjoy that time. Friday morning, when she woke up, she was working hard to breathe and was very out of it. Her mom described it as a dreamlike state where she was talking to people who weren't there. It was very frightening for her parents, and I definitely had the sense that her parents knew she was dying. The mom said to me that she missed Rebecca so much already that it was as though she was already gone. The mom and I were pretty close, and we cried a lot together.

13:8. The time came, probably in the last month of her life, when she began to realize that hope for a cure was getting pretty dim and there was a good chance that she was not going to make it. Her attending physician worked very hard to get approval from the FDA for an experimental treatment that he had very high hopes for. We gave it to her, and she had terrible side effects and couldn't continue receiving it. It caused such a major bleed that she ended up on a chest tube. The mother said, "Well, in essence, that is what you wanted the medicine to do; it did exactly what it was supposed to do—it broke up the tumor. It is just too bad that it caused this other side effect because the risk of the side effect was too great to continue the treatment, even though the treatment was actually working." After that, I noticed Rebecca seemed much more anxious. She was sicker at that point too, and after that drug, we didn't have much to give her. She would focus on her symptoms more, and she would tell me more about little things that normally she probably wouldn't have told me about. Also, she seemed quieter when she was here in the clinic. She seemed more easily tearful when normally she wasn't very tearful at all.

Story 14

This is a story about a 16-year-old boy who was born with AIDS (vertical transmission) and was in foster care. Toward the end of his life, when any attempt at resuscitation was considered futile and particularly onerous, he became entangled in a legal quagmire regarding who could consent to a DNR order for him.

14.1. Roberto had been previously in our care [at a nursing home facility] and was discharged about a year and a half ago to a foster mom. Then he came back to us about a month before his last hospitalization when he died because his HIV had progressed. He came for basically skilled nursing and rehab care in the face of his neurologic progression. His presentation led to the diagnosis of Progressive Multifocal Leukoencephalopathy [PML]. With that, unfortunately, he began to suffer a fairly rapid progressive course. He became hemiparetic [paralysis of one side of the body] and was having difficulty speaking. Then he developed respiratory problems and then fever and illness in the face of excessive diarrhea, for which he had to be hospitalized. We had started him on a new anti-retroviral regimen, and he didn't tolerate it in terms of the side effects of diarrhea and became significantly dehydrated. Then he came back to us after about a week in the hospital, but he became febrile and had to be readmitted to the hospital. During this last hospitalization, it became evident that it wasn't likely that he would ever be able to return to our nursing care facility because he wasn't, at any point during this hospitalization, medically stable enough in terms of the care he needed for us to meet him here. One of the issues was that he ended up requiring respiratory support— and that wasn't something that we could do here. But Roberto was caught in a legal limbo. With this rapid deterioration of his course, it became fairly clear to all of us who were involved in his care, including his foster mom, his foster care agency, and the city's Agency for Children's Services [ACS] that we couldn't treat his HIV. He couldn't tolerate, in terms of the diarrhea, a last-ditch effort at constructing a regimen that might have been potent enough to treat his resistant virus. So we couldn't treat his HIV, which was advanced. He began a rapidly progressive neuro-devastating course. So, here was a child with a terminal diagnosis who had significant neurologic progressive compromise and, in the last weeks of his life, was essentially unconscious or nonresponsive. We felt that resuscitation would have been futile and a burden on him. All of us agreed that this was a child who should have a DNR order, but there wasn't a legal way to obtain that consent. His mother had HIV and, according to the foster care agency, was not in contact with them. They didn't know where or how the mother was, so they did a search and were able to find her death certificate. She had died the past year in the city. While doing the search, the case workers identified the name of the father, but they didn't know his whereabouts or whether he was alive. So the agency had to go through a process of trying to figure that out because, to be able to sign a DNR consent, the child has to be solely in their custody. If there's any question that there may be a parent alive and reachable, then ACS cannot consent. So they tried to find out if his father, identified in the foster care agency case records, was findable. They looked in the city for a death certificate but didn't find one. Then they got in contact with Roberto's mother's family, who indicated that maybe he had died but in Florida. So they did an expedited request for the death certificate of the father in several of the main counties in Florida, but they didn't find a death certificate for the father there either. Ultimately, the pediatric infectious disease attending met with the agency, and they agreed to take everything that they had to court to present to a judge and to say, "Mom is dead. We think dad is dead, but we can't prove that with a death certificate, but here's what we've done to try to find him," and then request that Roberto be placed in the sole custody of ACS. With that, ACS was able to sign a DNR consent. It came just in the nick of time because, after having signed the DNR late in the day, 10 hours later Roberto died. It was amazing. The nurse who was there with me said that she thought Roberto somehow heard or knew it was time give up. It was as if he was waiting for it to be signed so that he could finally die because, if his DNR hadn't come through that day, we would have had to resuscitate him and that would have been awful for everybody, but especially for Roberto. So, on one hand, it sounded like it came in the nick of time, but it really didn't because the decisions that needed to be made for Roberto involved more than what to do at the moment of a cardiopulmonary arrest. There were decisions to be made all along the way in the face of a terminal illness that we can't treat and with a severe neurologically rapidly progressive devastating course about what is appropriate for him and what is medically futile. How aggressive do we want to be about fevers? How aggressive do we want to be about nutritional support? How aggressive do we want to be about investigatory or diagnostic procedures? You normally would have discussions about those decisions, outside the specter of medico-legal considerations, in conversations with the family, and Roberto had family, his foster family and many people who cared about him, but he didn't have someone who could legally be responsible for guiding those clinical decisions with us. This was complicated because this was a child who should be DNR and would be DNR, if he wasn't in this legal limbo, and it made it uncomfortable for everyone.

14:1. When I came on-service, we were led to believe that he would qualify for a "medical futility" because he didn't have a guardian to sign a do not resuscitate [DNR] order. That didn't sound right to me, and on the chart they had written, "Don't intubate this patient. Don't do any heroic measures, quote, unquote, slow code"—that doesn't exist. But the foster care agency and his guardian and his legal advocate weren't willing to sign the DNR, and there was no note on the chart about what the ethics committee said. It didn't make any sense to me, so we ended up having a meeting with the hospital lawyers who said, "There's no such thing as medical futility in pediatrics." So, if he had died and people had done what was said in the chart, I'm not sure that the hospital would have backed us, because we didn't follow medical policy. Everyone kept looking at me like, "You're such an ogre. This kid needs to die. Why can't we just let him die?" I'm like, "Yeah, he needs to die. I think that he should die because he's suffering now, but, guess what, I'm not putting my license on the line. You have to follow policy." We eventually ended up getting it resolved and getting the DNR, which was a good thing because he died 4 hours after the DNR was put on the chart. Isn't that weird? I don't know. I'm a true believer in karma and the way things are supposed to be, and I don't know if he was aware of the situation or what was going on but it just seemed so unusual that that would have happened. But waiting to get that DNR was horrible for us.

14:7. His mother refused to name his diagnosis or talk directly with him about his illness, but she had this awful habit of speaking about his illness in front of him. So it was kind of this Catch-22 where he wasn't allowed to talk about it but everybody could talk about it in front of him. So that set the tone for Roberto's ability to talk about his diagnosis. Even later on, when he was not with his mom and we did talk about his diagnosis, he didn't feel comfortable asking questions. He would sit in my office and there was a pamphlet or something I had that said, "How, how does it feel to have HIV?" He looked at it and he said, "Well, I wonder how it would feel to have HIV" and I said, "Well, you have HIV. What do you think?" and he kind of got surprised and looked at me and said, "Oh yeah, right" and then changed the subject. This was when he was 10. It wasn't too far before he deteriorated so he never really felt that he had permission to talk about his diagnosis. He knew his mother was sick, and I think he knew he and his mom had the same thing. But I'm not sure because we never got into the details of where he got his HIV because he never asked. He started having neurologic symptoms, and that was really a horrible thing for him. He had a couple of seizures when he was in Costa Rica, and he was terrified and very happy to be back here. He wanted to know what was happening with his body, and I explained to him that he had an infection in his central nervous system because his soldier cells were not very strong right now and that we were looking very hard for new medications to make his body stronger; that we were doing everything we could to find new medications and, as soon as we found them, we would offer them to him. He was satisfied with that, but obviously, as he deteriorated more and more, I think he knew that we didn't have anything to treat him. He was neurologically deteriorating so fast that we weren't sure what to tell him then and at what point. Then we lost some opportunity because, within the course of about a week, he lost the ability to speak, and, once that happened, we couldn't get a response from him and had no idea what was going on in his head; it was horrible for him. We found out, at one point shortly before he died but while he was still verbal, that his mother had passed away. We had been looking for her, and, when it came to light that she had died, we had this big discussion about how to tell him and when to tell him. But then he lost the ability to speak and we were like, "How do we tell him now because he can't even verbalize his own upset and fears and concerns?" It was very sad. We had mixed feelings about telling him about his mother. Part of me really wanted to tell him because I felt he was holding on, hoping that she would arrive and appear. He had a real religious framework—he was Catholic—and I thought that maybe knowing that she had died would be something he could use; something helpful like maybe an image of her being in heaven and waiting for him or something like that. But we never really resolved that because he just deteriorated so quickly.

14:4. The saddest thing was the night that he died he spiked a really high fever and his stats started dropping rapidly, and that was worrisome so I tried calling his foster family. But they never made it in time, which was sad. In the end it was just me, his nurse, and a nurse's aide. Even though he was completely unconscious, when you think about it—you bring yourself away from it and look at the situation—it's so sad that an 11-year-old kid died with no one there who had known him for more than a couple of weeks.

14:3. There were times when his eyes were partially opened, and there were other doctors who came and felt that he could respond—like, when they would call his name, he would open his eyes just a little bit wider. I never experienced that, but then, just on that off chance that he was still conscious, I would, when I did things, talk to him and explain things. But my feeling was that, for most of it, he was unaware of his surroundings. We had his favorite little teddy bear that the nurses would put in his arm, and we'd have music playing for him so it was the general feeling that we would try to make him comfortable. And if he was at all alert, to any degree, we should do these things to keep him comfortable. I told the interns to do the same, in terms of whenever you are going to do anything, talk to him and explain to him what you are doing.

14:4. I don't remember whose idea it was, but we made sure that physical therapy was coming to see him even if they could just massage him. He was unconscious, and we don't know how much he was aware but I'm much more into the idea of pretending that they are aware; that's just the better way to go about it. When he was dying, I had them put on a tape recorder and play some music. I don't know if he could hear anything, but, just in case he could, I'd rather he hear that than all the beeping and everything.

Story 15

This is a story about George, a 3-year-old boy, who was diagnosed at 9 months with a rare, high-risk cancer and then, in the midst of his treatment, his 4-year-old sister also was diagnosed with a virulent form of brain tumor. His parents were going to lose both of their children, their only children. When George died, his sister was dying in the next bed.

15:1. I started taking care of him a few months after he was diagnosed. The first year was pretty much okay because he did quite well with his chemotherapy and he had a good quality of life. But then the problems started the beginning of this year. A few months after he had finished chemotherapy, he relapsed, because the probability to be cured was really low. It was a big stress for the parents because it meant a lot of hospitalization and chemotherapy again. The mother at the same time was having some health problems, and she was illegal in the country so she didn't have insurance. It was a lot for her to take care of, and she also had another child. We started chemotherapy again, and it seemed like things were going okay. He was always very playful and was tolerating it well. But

I really had very little hopes from the beginning. I thought he was not going to last much and was not going to do well. But thanks to another attending, who is much more aggressive than I am and wanted to try every single chemotherapy that we had, no matter what, he lasted another good year. So she was right to be so aggressive, and, overall, he had a very good quality of life. If we had stuck to the kind of usual routine where we keep in the back of our mind that there is not really much to do for him, his chances of survival would have been very little. We were happy that his cancer was not progressing, and we can probably give him at least a couple of years and, who knows, maybe something else was going to come out, in terms of treatment. Then the worst came, and at that time, the sister was diagnosed with cancer. That was really a disaster. From that point on, I didn't even know what to tell the family; I just didn't have any words. The mother kept saying, "Why is this happening?" It is such an unfortunate thing that you really have no words. The mother was obviously devastated, although she was a very strong person and had a very strong faith. She was able to go on, but you could tell that she was just too tired and too disappointed with a sense of guilt and a sense of like, "Why is this happening to me?" I am not sure how much support she had because the father was not around much. He was the kind of person who just doesn't want to come to the hospital. He gets too upset to see the kids like that. The sister got a tumor that basically was not curable at all, so at that point, it was basically the death of the only two children they had. That was the time I realized that I was in a bit of denial. On one side, I knew I had to be close to this family and just be with them, even if I had nothing to say; just to sit there and just keep company or whatever. On the other side, I had to push myself to do it because I was like, "Oh, maybe I will do it tomorrow. Maybe I will go tomorrow." It was because it was very uncomfortable to be there and not being able to say anything. I couldn't say, "This is going to get better. This is the worst part and then it is going to get better." I couldn't say that. I couldn't say how long they were going to last, how they were going to die, who was going to go first. There was nothing for me to say, and I couldn't even say why this happened because I was afraid that she was going to feel even more guilty than she already was. We knew George was going to die, but he was doing very well and then, all of a sudden, he had a respiratory decompensation that was totally unexpected. Suddenly, it was even hard to say how long he was going to last, maybe only a couple of days. We needed to get a DNR, but we couldn't do it then because they were not ready at all, even if they knew he was not going to last, this was too quick. Then, when he lasted a little bit longer, we had that time to ask for a DNR and the mom had time to realize that he was going to die and adjust herself to that. It was the worst thing, for sure, that I've seen, although I have only been here for a couple of years. I cannot think of anything else worse than that; it was just a sense of failure. Everything you did was a sense of failure.

15:6. The mom agreed to a DNR after we had an unsuccessful plural effusion—a malignant plural effusion from a large metastatic. This was the precipitating event. After one of the radiologists took that fluid off, it clinically re-accumulated within a half an hour. He was fine for about a half an hour, and then he just went back to exactly the same as he was beforehand. At that point, it was discussed with mom that there was nothing left for us to do and what did she want us to do in the event he was not breathing or that his heart stopped beating. From the beginning, dad's opinion—he said it flat out—was that the machine was not going to make him better and it was not going to cure him, so he didn't feel that there was any point to it. On that day, mom finally was able to articulate that. I think she wasn't willing to give up just yet but that each and every one of these events, the plural effusion, the DNR, and the medication, was another step toward her letting go, and so she came to agree with dad that the machine was not going to make him better and that she didn't want to see him on the machine.

15:1. An event like this is exceedingly rare, so I suspect that these kids had some kind of genetic defect, probably something called P-53. In the midst of all this grieving, it didn't seem like the right time to press this issue, but to not raise it with the mother may be unethical in the long run and unfair to her. So, at some point, it needs to be raised but not because we need a model for how to deal with siblings dying simultaneously—I don't think I will see it again in my lifetime. The assumption was that they didn't necessarily have separate problems but that they inherited something that, for some reason, showed itself in the children but not in the person who gave it to them. Although there was no proof of this and it could have been just random anyway, the hypothesis would be that there was a known gene, called P-53 and, when you have it, you have a higher risk of getting certain cancers. Usually, it is passed from generation to generation because most people can get the cancers in their 30s and 40s but younger than normal, younger than 50. So there is genetic transmission. When little children get it, they don't get to pass it on, so there is no genetic issue for them, but there might be a genetic issue if the mom were to have another child with this father or another, if she carried that gene. There would also be issues for her in terms of her own health surveillance because she was at higher risk for breast cancer and lung cancer. She was not that old a woman, and who knew if she ever had a mammogram? It needed to be sorted out if they had this P-53 or not. If they didn't, then, maybe, a lab that could work on it so the serum could be stored so that, if new things are developed and there are new genes properties discovered, we can find out about it. It just seemed too much of a coincidence.

The mother had some sense of this because, from the beginning, she thought it was her fault. She said, "How come my husband has two other children, two other grown-up girls from another woman and they are fine and both of my kids are sick? She was not an educated person so she didn't tell us, "Is this a gene?" but she asked me, "Is it something in me that I am giving? Is it something in me that I am transmitting to them?" So she didn't talk about genes, but she had a transmissibility sense of disease. She didn't feel guilty for having done something wrong to the kids, but for, somehow, being unlucky, "I had something that I transmitted to my kids and there was no way to know."

15:6. Over the past 6 months, since his sister was diagnosed with a brain tumor, he has been in the hospital more visiting her and was getting treatment as an outpatient. Then, over the past couple of months, he had just gotten sicker and sicker. He was 3 and he had his cancer diagnosed when he was 9 months old, so he has been basically a miracle baby for 2½ years because the kind of cancer that he had is just an awful, awful cancer to have. It is really rare, harder to treat, and invariably fatal. But the thing with George was that, until the very end, he was just a funny little kid. He would always be running around the floor. He was also so loving, especially with his sister. The last time I saw him 2 weeks ago, his sister was in a wheelchair and he was with his mom and his mom's pushing the wheelchair and then you see the wheelchair go by and there's George with his hands up on the handle helping to push the wheelchair. He was just such a cute little loving kid. Some of the nurse practitioners would take him down to the gift shop to get candy on days when he was stuck here with his mom and sister. He didn't really talk about his disease or about being in the hospital much. He was a developmentally delayed 3-year-old and didn't speak to us very much. He would speak to his mom, but, for us, it was just like he would play and smile and interact but not really speak so much. The hospital was sort of like, unfortunately, a second home to him. He didn't like it when he was in the hospital as a patient. He was usually pretty cranky when he was the one in the bed, but when he was just the one visiting his sister with his mom and running around, he was fine and happy, doing whatever. Like when his sister came in the first time around and was in the ICU, I remember him standing on tiptoes hitting the open-door button to the ICU and thinking that that was the coolest thing because he could just barely touch it—this much of his fingers reached—and he would just hit it and watch the doors open, and he would stare and look with a big grin on his face. Then they would close, and he would do it again. He just stood there for a half-hour doing that with the doors. He was just a little kid living his life, and then he had these horrible times, when he was in the hospital, where he was a cranky kid who just wanted to get the heck out of bed and run around again.

15:6. Three weeks before her daughter was diagnosed, you could tell that she was more and more afraid that something was wrong with her also. She kept bringing her to the emergency room with vomiting, and she started going to the pediatrician when she had a little fever. They said it was just gastroenteritis, and then it went away and she was better. But 3 days before George was discharged from the hospital, his mom had us look at Justine's hand because it was shaking. We were all in denial and said, "She might just be a little nervous or scared or whatever." Then, when she came back 2 days later, they did the CT scan of her head and found this huge tumor. We all were in complete disbelief. Then they got the pathology back, and it was neuroblastoma which, of all the brain tumors to get, is absolutely the least survivable. And so now she has these two kids, her only kids. The clerks in the ICU were all very much like, "Well, George can't stay the night here. We don't allow siblings to sleep over." At which point I was like, "This poor mother has this horrible thing that has just happened to her other child and we are going to let him sleep here. If he needs to come into the call room with me that's fine." The nurses were fine with that.

15:1. This was the part of this that was so unbelievably tragic. His sister, Justine, was in the room the whole time he was dying. Sometimes she wanted the curtain drawn, but most of the time she wanted it open so she could just see George from the corner of her eye. You have to understand that this was the most verbal, charming 3½-, 4-year-old you'd know. Now she was this massively cushingoid, obese child, due to all the steroids we gave her. She was nothing like that before her illness; she was gorgeous. She had a severe physical impairment from the brain tumor. She could hardly move her left side, and her right side had a tremor. Her eyes didn't move normally, and she didn't swallow entirely well. She got headaches, and sometimes her conversations were a little off. But at the same time, she could still be very sharp; she had not lost all of her cognitive functions. The way I dealt with it was mostly to deal with Justine with Justine, and George with George, and not ask Justine about George, unless she gave some entrée. Except once I did and she just changed the subject. Another time she said he was very sick, but basically she didn't want to talk about George with me and that was okay because she had a lot of other people she worked with. When George was clearly dying, we planned that someone from our child-life program would be on call to come in and be with Justine and talk her through it, and that was what we did. Most of the time the curtain was drawn but, toward the very end, Justine asked to have the curtain open; she just wanted to keep asking about George. It was one of the more difficult mornings with someone dying that I've ever experienced, and yet one of the most dignified. The mother was an extraordinarily strong and gracious woman. I walked in in the morning for my regular check and found most of the family gathered around, and there was a priest just praying and praying over the bed. I stood for a minute or two behind the mother. She was holding George in her arms, as if she was completely oblivious of everything else. I was looking at the machine, the bi-path, and all I wanted to do was turn it off so this didn't keep going. But the way people were positioned around the room, I would literally have had to move through people and fight my way through people to turn it off and ask mom's permission. I felt that was inappropriate. So, I spent time with Justine, just socially; there was no way I could examine her—I just couldn't bring myself to do that. Through the morning I came in and out and then, late in the morning, the house staff officer told me that George had died. Toward the end, he had gently told the mom that we needed to take this (bi-path) off because it was bothering him; it was the right thing to do. I went into the room, and mom just cried over him and held him but gently cried. Sometimes, when people die, there is a wailing and screaming and it's scary, if it happens, but this was not like that at all. This was just pure, calm grief. I didn't know if she did it because Justine was in the next bed or because that was who she was. I think it was both because she had always comported herself in a very dignified way. Then, the thing that was the most unbelievable thing that I have ever seen is that Justine, in a little voice, said that she wanted to see George, so the mom took George in her arms, like an infant, and brought him to Justine's bed, and Justine just moved to touch his head and mom said, "Kiss him" and Justine just kissed his forehead. I didn't catch it all, but then Justine kind of pushed him away, as if to say, "Enough." Which I was glad for because I was afraid she was just going to leave him there for a while, and I thought that was too much for Justine. I've seen sisters and brothers come in to say goodbye to their dying sibling, but I have never seen a 4-year-old kiss her brother good-bye when she was dying too. This was a child who was reported to have said—I didn't hear it myself—"Is mommy crying for George or for me now?" So, I would say, it was one of the most amazing death scenes I have ever seen. If someone was trying to write this for Hollywood, they would say it was impossible, too melodramatic.

Story 16

Jose was a 16-year-old who, after a long illness, knew he was dying but chose never to directly talk about it.

16:1. I followed him for 28 months, and from the very beginning, I had the sense that he wasn't going to be curable and so anything we did was just buying time. It's different than for lots of my other patients because almost all the other patients expected that I'd be able to cure them. From the very beginning, I told the family, "Look, the chances of cure are less than 30 percent." But the family wanted to hope, and I certainly was not going to remove that hope. There were times when I thought perhaps we'd gotten lucky because there were a number of months when he had no detectable disease. So we thought, "Well, we're doing okay," but, once things started to come back, it was a very slow, steady, downhill process. What I'm grateful for was that, until the last month, he had a really good quality of life. Caring for him was very challenging because he never wanted to know any of the medical details, even though he was 16 by the end. He was very clear about not wanting to hear bad news from me. He wanted to hear all the news from his mother, and his mother did not want him to know bad news, so I was stuck with not having a way to communicate. At first it was frustrating, but, by the end, I realized that it was just fine; that there was no reason to hit him over the head with it. He was coping with it in the way he wanted. He clearly knew because, toward the end, he became very depressed for a while. He wouldn't sleep and he wouldn't eat. He had been morbidly obese, at times, and I would give him a hard time because he was hypertensive, and he was eating this typical high-sodium junk food diet and, despite all the intensive chemo that he had, he would just gain more and more weight. He also was a very severe asthmatic, so it was challenging to care for him from his asthma perspective as well. So then everything made things worse. With his third sign of breaking through chemo and when things started to grow, I realized I had nothing more to offer him because he developed renal failure pretty early on and then, in the end, hepatic failure. But even before the hepatic failure, I knew that I had limited options, and, at that point, I had already gone through four different types of chemo. We were at the 2-year mark, and I sent them to the Dominican Republic because he said he wanted to go. I convinced the mom that they had to go and they had to have fun and, when he came back, I would give him some more chemo but I didn't know what. I told her that he had to go for at least 2 weeks—mom just wanted to go for 1. I said, "No, go for longer and then try to stay for more." In the end, they stayed for over a month because Jose didn't want to come back. It was very telling to me that he didn't want to come back. It was when he returned that he got depressed, and I thought he must have put two and two together because he'd never had a break from his chemo before. He must have been worried that, "Oh, why has my doctor sent me away and told me to go on vacation for as long as possible?" I worried that he understood something, but he wouldn't ask me and I gave him plenty of opportunities.

The other thing that was tricky caring for him was that his mother had a borderline personality. When he was first diagnosed, we thought that this was going to be a really untenable situation, and she threatened to throw herself out a window. The first night after his surgery, when they had opened him up and saw that his abdomen was just full of tumors, we realized that it was pointless to even try to do anything; that it was going to be impossible to treat this kid, so how was the mother going to react? But she came around relatively quickly, and she accepted it and she ended up being a great mom. At the end, she fell apart just a little bit, but my biggest concern around his dying was what it was going to do to his mom.

When I first told her that the end was very near, she was looking like she was going to be catatonic. She was expressionless and wringing her hands and wringing a cloth that she had. We spoke with the sister who said her concern was that mom was going to go "cuckoo." We went through all these very elaborate plans about how we were going to deal with her, when Jose died, because we didn't want her to have to go to the psych ER because we knew she'd want to spend as much time as possible with his body. We were worried what would happen to her once he died, even though, in a lot of ways, she was ready. We'd had long discussions and she had wanted a DNR. She brought it up before I brought it up. She knew what was eventually coming, yet, when things got very close, it looked as if she was going to decompensate. Jose then took almost two days to die, and in the end, his parents took him off the oxygen and it was still a number of hours before he died. But they had so much time to prepare that the mom and the family were quite appropriate in the end. During his treatment he had incredible amounts of complications, but he would always come through. Whenever he was fine—because I knew this was never going to be curable—my push was always to try to get him home as much as possible and, when he was home, he wanted to go out and she wanted to be very protective of him. I kept telling her, "Let him go. Let him play" and she's like, "But his platelets are low." "Well, don't worry about it. Let him have fun. Let him go out with his friends." She would always tease me and blame me, like, "Oh, you're not the one who's waiting when he comes home at 2:00 in the morning," and I'm like, "That's great. Let him have fun." I think there was a part of her that, in the end, was happy that I had pushed that, because he really did have a lot of fun. I encouraged her to let him go to cancer camp, and it was the first time he was away from her and then, by the second year, he went to camp again and had a great time. So, one of my therapeutic moves was to help mom, because I knew he was never going to be cured, so I wanted to help mom let go of him because it was pointless to try to shelter him too much and not give him the chance to have fun. That was my philosophy with him, for a lot of his care, and I'm so glad that he had a fun time until he no longer could.

16:11. I never knew he had a colostomy/urostomy bag, and one time, when I was sitting on his edge of the bed, he was saying, "My private part doesn't work and it's bothering me. I get blood clots sometimes." He was wiggling and I couldn't see anything and then he said, "Can I have a paper towel, sheet, blanket, anything?" He was pulling blood clots out of his penis. He was cleaning up and he said that he was concerned about his private part, and I said, "You mean your penis [I wanted to normalize the word "penis"] wasn't working?" and it hadn't worked in a while. They had done some surgery and he was hoping they would turn the bags off so, he said, "that my private part would start to work again." Although that was just another element of his disease, it added a whole other layer to his feelings of self-esteem, potency, and normalcy that his penis didn't work.

16:4. He died peacefully and comfortably and didn't suffer very much. We kept him medicated and that really helped. He was with his family around him—all the people who cared about him—so it was a peaceful passing. His parents knew he wasn't going to recover, and they had decided to make him DNR. He had been getting progressively worse for a few days before he passed away; every day he was a little bit sicker. When I went in to see him, he had an o2 sat [oxygen saturation] monitor and his stats were fine, but his heart rate was fluctuating all up and down. The family was focused on the numbers, so I said, "He's on the maximum amount of oxygen. He's on every breather and I can see how he's doing clinically and you can see that too, so we don't need to look at the numbers," and I turned off the o2 sat machine. They were okay with that. When I came back about 15 minutes later, the mom and dad had decided to take him off the oxygen, and that was the beginning of the end. It was a decision made by both parents and the medical staff. . . . He had been conscious up until the last day, but he didn't talk about his overall condition, just the immediate problems he was having, like feeling short of breath, that sort of stuff, but not overall, in a global sense of his disease and what that meant. He didn't talk to me about that, yet I had no doubt that he knew that he was dying. First of all, because his parents called in his extended family and he got to see every single one of his relatives. And it was becoming harder and harder for him to breathe, and he was conscious enough to know that he was having problems breathing, so he knew it was the end, but he had been through so much and had suffered so much for such a long time that I don't think it was such a terrible thing for him. Because he had been with us for a really long time and had been on patient-controlled anesthesia, he trusted us that we were going to take care of his pain. When he was okay respiratory-wise but was having problems with pain, we'd always adjust his pain meds and make him as comfortable as possible, so we established trust with him. He knew that when he had problems in the past, we had always responded appropriately and always tried to make sure that we took care of him and that he felt better. So, having had that relationship with us, he trusted us to make sure that he wasn't going to have these problems when he was dying.

Story 17

Christianna was a 15-year-old girl who arrived from Trinidad for treatment of metastatic disease. After several rounds of chemotherapy and several surgeries, her condition continued to worsen, her tumor grew, and further treatment became futile. The core issue for the staff then was how to get her back to Trinidad to die in comfort despite denials and obfuscations from her father and aunt.

17:1. Christianna was an extraordinary child in that she was charming, accepting of whatever happened to her, and endearing. She came to us with metastatic disease and her prognosis was very guarded. So it was with a sense of mixed feelings that I got involved with her, because it was impossible not to adore her and want to think positively, yet I knew, from the beginning, that she might not do as well as we liked. She came to the United States with her father from Tinidad. Her father was an incredibly impressive, well-spoken, educated man who had this deep religious faith. During the first year of her therapy, when she was doing well, we moved toward more aggressive treatment than maybe what was warranted. When, at the end of her therapy, she still had metastatic disease left, we opted to do two separate thorachotomies—to have surgeries to open her chest to remove the metastases. Even though logic told us that the number of metastases she had put her at very high risk for relapse no matter what we did, we decided to do it because it was impossible to imagine that someone as good and sweet and as responsive and lovely as she could not do well. I wondered if my decision-making capacity with this child was affected by the fact that her family, and she herself, were so lovely and so wanting and willing to try anything, that we did it. Certainly you could be less attractive, less lovely, less a sweet patient and we would still do the right thing for you, but I wondered if we went a little bit beyond the usual mark. What I'm trying to say, in a very inarticulate way, is that during the first year of her therapy, we were very optimistic and hopeful that, despite all odds, she could do well. When her planned treatment was finished and after she had the two thorachotomies, she was, at that time, free of measurable disease—meaning that, if you did X rays and CT scans, you wouldn't see any tumor, but we were very worried that she was still at very high risk for relapse, and so we decided to keep her on a maintenance program of relatively mild chemotherapy and work with her family to get her back home to Trinidad. And, indeed, that's what we did. She was able to go home, and she was feeling great and was doing well and was able to get chemo in Trinidad; it was administered under our direction here. Then, when she came back for followup, it was clear that she had recurrent disease in her lungs again and in her leg as well. Things then changed very dramatically in terms of the way we were able to work with her and her family. During the first year when she was here, her father was here most of the time, and when he wasn't, her aunt, the father's younger sister, was here. But during this time, when she was much sicker and needed much more parental support, the father needed to stay in Trinidad and so she was here only with her aunt. It was a complicated family story, but the aunt, who had no children, had a husband who had died from cancer about a year ago and Christianna's mother had died from cancer when she was about 7. So there was a great deal of emotional issues about death and cancer. We started using rather intensive chemotherapy, but she didn't respond to it at all and the tumor got worse. My fellow did all kinds of journal research and contacted people trying to find out what options there were for her, and we discussed it at length, but I already knew that there really weren't any options to cure her. It got excruciatingly painful to take care of her because if there was any child with cancer—and we want them all to survive—who just tugged at your heartstrings, she was one of the prime ones, and I knew that the medical tools we had weren't going to allow that to happen. The whole relationship got more and more difficult because, whenever I tried to discuss with the aunt anything about the child not doing well, the aunt became very defensive and told us that she knew she would survive and she had a very hard time hearing anything that was negative. So it became harder and harder for me because I couldn't work with the aunt in a way that felt comfortable to me and the aunt became angrier and angrier. No matter how much we all knew that her anger was about Christianna not doing well and not about any of us individually, it was extremely stressful and difficult. Certainly for me and for pretty much everyone who took care of her, it was incredible to see this change in the aunt, who went from being positive and loving for Christianna and loving to us to being positive and loving in front of Christianna but almost completely tuning many of us out because she didn't want to hear anything we said. She saw us as giving up, and I tried in every way to let her know that, in terms of prayer and belief and hope, I was with her, but I had to tell her what I thought was medically true. The entire thing was complicated by the fact that Christianna's father and siblings weren't here. So it wasn't just the family that was in denial, which we work with all the time, but we were with a child who was very, very ill, and no matter how close she was to her aunt and how wonderful her aunt was to her, she was separated from her family. I became increasingly distressed that one of the possibilities was that she would die here and her father and her sisters and brothers would never get to see her again and she would never get to see them and there would never be any closure and the aunt would be furious because she was stuck doing it all by herself. I think part of the aunt's anger was that she was here alone with the child, whom she adored, but on some level resented being the only one in the family with her. So it was just this terrible mess because normally when a family goes through this phase of denial, it's understandable, and even positive sometimes because it helps protect them, but in this situation, the father needed to make decisions and to be here with her. The decision was whether she would go home and be treated with comfort care at home and be able to be with her family or, if she was going to stay here, whether she would stay in the hospital or go to hospice, which was much more appropriate. I had pretty much ruled out trying to do any kind of radical treatment because I didn't think we had anything to offer her that would be useful and her condition was such that she couldn't benefit from any of the experimental trials, so I felt that the father needed to understand that we were reaching the limits of what we could offer medically, except for pain control. . . . The feeling of not being able to be straight with Christianna because she wouldn't let me and certainly because the aunt wouldn't let me was very disturbing, so the fellow and I decided that we had to get the father here. I first e-mailed him to give him a little time to think and then we called him and said, "Look, you just have to get up here and see her." The fellow, at one point, said to him something about how her sister had died when she was 16 and she had never gotten over not being able to be with her to say goodbye and that he had to get up here. So, we were pretty straightforward with him. When he got here, I chose to speak to him alone, without the aunt at first. Of course the aunt was annoyed about that, but I knew what was going to happen if she had been there. I told him that, at this point, we truly had reached a wall in terms of treatment options, that there weren't any investigational medicines that we could try and there weren't any other regular chemos that would work, and that the radiation hadn't done what we'd hoped it would do and we could see that her disease was getting worse. This time, the father was in denial. He said to me, "Well, if you don't look at her below the waist, she looks pretty good"—that's because her lower extremity was just a mass of tumor. I said to him, "I know what you mean, she's still as beautiful as ever and as lovely as she ever was but she's wearing oxygen now, she's breathing fast, and she gets out of breath when she talks. So, even above the waist, she's not so well." He just looked at me silently, and then we talked and talked and talked. He talked about how he thought that she could be healed anyway, and I said that I couldn't speak for the future but, from the purely medical point of view, that was not true. Then he wanted to know the timing, and I said, "Nobody could ever really know timing, but in the next weeks or months, at the most, she would get very, very sick and die and it could happen very rapidly." Then he told me that when he was in Canada they told him his wife only had 3 weeks to live and she lived for 2 years, and I said, "That was completely different because she was just being diagnosed then; she wasn't on oxygen, and she wasn't having trouble breathing. So, even though Christianna may fool me and live longer than I think, there's a real difference between someone being given a limited prognosis in the beginning of their illness and then living longer and someone who's been treated for a long time and the disease is getting worse." Basically, what was happening was that he kept coming forward with a soft sort of calm denial and I kept being honest. It was very painful; it was really difficult because he didn't show a lot of emotion, but I knew it was painful for him. I really felt that I had to make this clear because Christianna needed to go home or he needed to get his family up here— one or the other. I also went into a whole thing about what Do Not Resuscitate means and how she could be put on a ventilator or not. I explained to him that, in his country, there would never even be a question, but that, in this country, in this state, we have to have permission not to put people on ventilators and that ventilators are for people who have complications that we think can get better, or are at the beginning of their treatment because we don't know what'll happen, or in the middle of a crisis. I told him that to put someone on a ventilator, when the reason for going on the ventilator was that the cancer was spreading through their body would not be the right thing to do because there would be no chance that she could then get better and come off the ventilator. In every way, I've never been in a parental meeting so intensely trying to break through denial. By the end of the meeting, I didn't think he'd heard a word, and he wouldn't respond at all to the DNR issue. I said, "You really need to think about this and we'll meet again tomorrow." The next day I met with him and the aunt together, and the aunt started by saying, "You really can't talk to him [the father] alone," and I said, "I understand how you feel, but I felt, as a father who hasn't been here for a while, I needed to meet alone with him." Later, the aunt and I talked again and again about all the things that I had spoken about with the father, and we basically got stuck again. They wouldn't comment one way or another on the issue of the DNR and they didn't say anything about bringing her home. The next day I called the hospital and found out that the father hadn't come to the hospital at all and the aunt had nothing to say. I asked them to have the father call me, but he didn't. The next morning, he was supposed to go back to Trinidad, so I was devastated because I thought the whole thing would be left up in the air. So, when I got in, the first thing I did was go up to the room and say to the aunt that I wanted to call the father. She said, in a fairly nasty way, that he wasn't home; she was pretty mad at me and she wouldn't get out of bed—it was 9:00 in the morning. I said, "Could you please give me the phone number of the place where he was staying?" and she said, "The phone number's in my bag and I can't get it now" and I said "Okay, I'll be back in a little while." I couldn't deal with her being so mean, so I walked around and then went back a little later. She was still in bed, but I insisted she get up and give me the phone number. I called and he wasn't there; he was already at the airport. So I got her up and spoke with her. She started the conversation by saying, "I know Christianna's going to be cured, and her father went home and I'm in charge. You have to talk to me about everything." She was really laying it on me. I don't know if I was appropriate or not but, at that point, I just couldn't deal with her anger anymore and I said, "I can only vaguely imagine how horrible it must be for you to be with Christianna when she's this ill, but I don't understand why you're so angry at me." At that point, I too was angry, and I'm sure it came across as fairly harsh. I was angry at my own inability and lack of skills to get through the denial, even though I knew it wasn't my fault. I felt like I'd been doing this so long, I should be able to get there. I was angry that the father left without talking to me. I was angry that the aunt was so angry at us, making it difficult for us to care for her. Then, at one point at the end of one of our meetings, she just said to me, "We're taking her home." I almost fell off my chair because it was the opposite of everything she'd been saying all along. I think what she meant was, "Yeah, we're taking her home, because you're not doing anything anymore." Then everybody got into the act, finding ways to get them home—the fellow did a lot of research, and this guy did a lot of research, and one of the oncology nurses was calling nursing associations and everybody was getting a little crazy but we pulled it off. We found a commercial airliner that would take her with oxygen, and somehow the hospital came up with the money for two first-class tickets for them. There was a lot of tension among the staff about them leaving. During Thursday rounds, which was the day before she was supposed to go home, some people were saying, "She's not ready yet," and the pain team wanted her to stay a little longer so they could adjust her meds and I said, "Absolutely not. She's got to get home now or she's not going to ever get home." One of the nurses brought up, "Well, I think a nurse should go with her" and I just snapped at her and said, "We can't do everything. We can't do everything for everyone. A travel nurse will cost $7,000, and what is a nurse going to do, anyway? Listen to me, the worst thing that could happen on the flight is that she's going to die, and a nurse won't be able to change that. If she's uncomfortable, I wrote prescriptions for liquid morphine, for everything she could possibly use on the airplane. What is a nurse going to do?" I could see that part of this way of reacting was my own defensiveness because, even though I felt it was the right thing to do, I wasn't sure it was the right thing to do. The one thing that I haven't shared with you through the whole thing is this background noise that, even though I'm trying to filter it out, the hospital didn't want her to stay until she died because it blocked a bed, and her insurance company was writing letters that they would only pay for hospice, not hospital care. The whole time, I'm trying to keep that out of my mind and make all my decisions about what I thought was right for her, but because that noise was in the background, I was mistrusting myself—did I want her to go Friday because I thought she could have died in the next week or two, or was it because I had these other pressures on me? In my heart, I knew it was right for her to go home, but there was this whole thing going on in the hospital where some people wanted her to go home, but some people were worried that we were sending her home too soon and she might be in pain. There was a lot of raw emotion floating around about this, and a lot of it had to do with what were the limits of what we could do and what we should do. Some people lost sight of the fact that she needed to be with her family, even if it meant breaking down their denial. That night, I really tossed and turned and I usually don't; I'm usually a very good sleeper. I came in the morning, and I went up to the floor and the social worker told me that the aunt was really nervous and wanted to know if I could go to the airport with them and I said I would. I was incredibly glad I did because it gave me some closure. Christianna thanked me and said, "Goodbye," and gave me a kiss. She was wearing this scarf I had given her. She was going to Trinidad now where she'd never need it, but I'm sure she wore it because she wanted me to see her wearing it. The EMS people at the airport were great. They took Christianna in a stretcher, and then the airport people were great. Then I saw this incredible change in the aunt who'd been so angry and mean, even to the last minute. She was talking to the people from the airline, many of whom were from Trinidad, like they were old friends; she's talking about Trinidad, and there was a smile on her face and she was laughing a little. I realized then that she really wanted to go home, but she just never could say it. I turned to her and said, "I haven't seen you with a smile on your face like this in two months," and she looked me in the eyes and just smiled. I knew then that, no matter what had been said, no matter how much anger had gone before, from both sides, that it was right that this incredibly sick kid was going home to die. We got an e-mail from the father that she arrived well, that they got oxygen like they needed at home, that they had all her supplies, and that she had slept most of the flight and wasn't uncomfortable. So it all happened the way it should. Now we're just waiting to hear the final chapter. The one worry is that some of the pain medicine she has in this epidural might wear off, but we have contacts now in Trinidad who've been helpful with that too. I'm optimistic about that and I feel good that she'll die with her family.

17:2. She had osteosarcoma in the bone. When she came back, she had very significant disease in her leg. She had the surgery in her leg done, and she had a lung mass removed—there were two lung surgeries. When we finished her treatment, we knew that, even though she looked like she was okay, she still had disease that we could feel. We decided to continue her with the chemo. She wanted to go back home to Trinidad, so we worked with a doctor there to continue the chemo. We did a lot of faxing to the doctor there sending him medical summaries and trying to orchestrate the whole thing. We had to get everything ready for her here so that, when she went there, they knew what to do. We sent her down with some of her meds, but the chemo she got there but according to what we told him; the template and the calendar of treatment was basically what we gave him, including all the labs he should draw. He would e-mail me with the lab results and tell me what side effects she was having and stuff like that. When she came back in November, for her 3-month followup, she had florid disease. She had the mass back in her lungs, and she had a recurrence of her first osteosarcoma and a new one at her hip. She had a very bad limp.

Her aunt only wanted her to know about the things that were obviously seeable—that her leg was swollen and her hip was hurting her. That was all that she wanted us to tell her about. She felt that if we told her all that was going on, it would erode her faith and she would lose hope, and she believed that, if you lose hope, you die faster or you deteriorate faster. That's understandable, but Christianna was almost 15 and she wasn't stupid, so we were trying to protect her from a lot of stuff that she probably already knew. But it was hard to relay that to the aunt. So the way it evolved was that, when she came back, she had all the scans and we told her that the scans showed that the tumor had come back in her leg and in her hip but we didn't mention her lungs. We started on the chemotherapy and everything, but she was getting sicker and sicker and sicker. She was progressing before our very eyes. She had a couple of complications; she had a seizure, she had a clot in her leg, she lost weight, and she had really bad sores in her mouth. At one point, in the midst of all this, I asked her if she was lonely being here by herself with only her aunt. I said, "Your father's not here, your sisters and brothers are in Trinidad, and I'm concerned that you're going to be here for a while and you're not going to be able to see them. I don't want you to feel sad or depressed about it," and she said, "Oh no, I'm okay. I'm fine. Don't worry about it. I'm going to be okay." She reassured everybody and never wanted you to feel that she was inconvenienced in any way—that was just her personality. She was worried about her aunt, she was worried about her dad, and she was worried about her sister taking exams—"Oh, don't let her know that I'm so sick so that she doesn't do bad on her exam." I was watching her slipping downhill and was trying to find a treatment for her to make this cancer go away. I realized one day that, you know what? It's not going to go away, and I have to accept that because it's a different approach if you are shooting for a cure than if you're providing comfort. It took me a long time to see this; I guess I was the last person to believe that she was not going to get better. She got really sick, and the tumor did not shrink; it just kept getting bigger and bigger. The medical part of me said she was not going to get better, but the Scripture part of me said miracles happen and I'm going to let them have that as an option, if that's what they want to believe. I pray for my patients and I ask for guidance and what to do; should I keep going for a cure? At what point do I stop and know that this is what God's will is? I had gotten to the point where I knew that she was going to die. It wasn't like, "Oh my God, we failed." It was an acceptance of reality, and so I felt that my focus was supposed to be to make her feel more comfortable. The trouble was that the aunt never got to that point with us. Everybody else understood that she wasn't going to get better, and everybody else was concerned that Christianna was not going to be given the chance to understand or embrace the end of her life in a comfortable and less fearful fashion. She was really getting afraid. You could see her sometimes looking really scared, and this was not going to be a fast one-two-three death; she would be gradually getting worse. So how much does she understand at the age of 15 about what's going on? She couldn't ask any questions because her aunt was very protective and wasn't letting her and I wasn't sure if she wanted to ask questions. Every time somebody approached her, her aunt would interfere. We hardly were ever allowed to be alone with Christianna, and I didn't push it because I knew how the aunt felt and I knew that she had been driving other people away from her because of that. She would tell you that she didn't want you to be alone with Christianna and that she didn't want you to say anything about the tumor with her and she didn't want you to talk about dying with her. When you open your mouth to say something, she would cut in and talk over the discussion so that you deflected the questions you wanted to ask. It was really tough and you felt bad, but you didn't want to sneak behind the aunt's back and talk to Christianna because that wouldn't be nice either. The aunt was dealing with the idea that, in her mind, she knew that Christianna was going to die, but, in her heart, she didn't want to believe it or accept it as God's reality for her. That's understandable, up to a point.

Story 18

This story is about a 3-day-old premature infant who died in the neonatal intensive care unit. Because of religious reasons, the baby was kept alive on a ventilator long after the staff thought it appropriate to withdraw support.

18:1. This was a 28-weeker that was delivered at home—not that it was planned that way but, God, it's hard to believe that the mother didn't know that she was in labor; she had to have been in labor a lot of hours at home, although it was her first time. The ambulance brought the baby from home to the emergency room at their local hospital where the baby was resuscitated and stabilized as much as possible. I talked to the neonatologist out there who said he didn't even think the baby was going to live to be transported, but then the baby was transported again from the local hospital to here. The baby was able to be stabilized on very high oscillator settings, but we couldn't decrease the support, and it was only going to make his lungs worse. By the time I took over care of this baby, on Monday morning, it was pretty clear that the baby was going to die. Although it's not common for a 28-week baby to die, this baby was born at home and had no heart rate or pulse when the ambulance got there. The baby was resuscitated, and, by the time I saw him, he was on a high-frequency oscillator with severe bilateral emphysema and couldn't be oxygenated, no matter what we did. The only thing that made this hard was that the family was Orthodox Jewish, which meant that we could not withdraw care. So this put us in a difficult situation of having to provide optimal care to a baby when we knew it was futile. But we didn't want to just ignore the baby. I knew there wasn't anything we could do for the baby and that it would take a long time for the baby to die if we left him on the oscillator. I spoke to the rabbi and I spoke to the father, and it was, as I had expected, that there was to be no stopping of treatment. I can't remember the last time I had a baby die on a ventilator or had become asystolic [heart stops] on a ventilator; it's just inhuman, if you ask me— the baby's blue, ischemic [i.e., poorly perfused], and unresponsive. There probably was not that much suffering because the baby was comatose; he was so hypoxic [insufficient oxygen] and acidotic [excess acid in blood] that it was amazing to me how long you can live with a pH of 6.7, or at least have your heart beat. And nothing I could say to the rabbi or father could change their minds; this is pretty common. I've been through it with another baby that we're still struggling with. The baby certainly isn't dying imminently, but nobody thinks this baby's going to go home from the unit; it's just a matter of religion. The mother only came in once to see the baby, and the father didn't spend a lot of time with the baby; he just asked, every time he saw the baby, whether things were better or not, in spite of the fact that I'd tell him, "No, they're not going to get better. The baby's going to die." I'd tell him that and the rabbi would come by or call me and say, "You know the father didn't really understand what you meant." I'm thinking to myself, "The baby is going to die. What doesn't he understand?" But I didn't say, "What doesn't he understand about that?" Instead, I said, "If we don't take the baby off the ventilator, which I know you won't agree to do, it will take a long time for this baby to die. But the baby's oxygen is inadequate, the baby's severely acidotic, and there's nothing I can do to make it better." I found it very unusual that the mother only came in once to look at this baby, and the other thing that was unusual was that, when I called the father on Tuesday morning—the baby's heart rate was up and down, around 100 most of the day on Monday and also, by this time, the baby had severe massive intercranial hemorrhage—it started to be 90, 85, 80, 75. I said, "The baby's going to die soon. If you want to see the baby again, you should come in, and you can hold the baby," and he said, "Okay, we'll be in," and then, when they showed up two hours later, the baby was dead. So, when they arrived and understood that the baby was dead, they told us they weren't allowed to see the baby after the baby's dead; it's part of their religion. I didn't know that. It's bizarre in the sense that I can't remember the last time I let a baby die on a ventilator until their heart rate was zero. If this wasn't a religious thing, I would've said, "Look, I can't do this. You're going to have to find somebody else to take care of your baby," but it would have to have been one of my partners and none of them wanted to do it either.

18:1. This was a very difficult case for us because what were we supposed to do? These parents wanted us to do everything we could, but we knew there was nothing we could do. We didn't want to tell them we were going to do everything we could and then sort of cheat and not give the baby good care and allow the baby to die. I would have even re-intubated this baby, if the tube came out, because that wasn't going to be a natural cause of death. But the residents were sitting there every day wondering, "What do we do?" They asked me, "Do we check blood gases?" and I said, "Yeah, check blood gases and adjust the ventilator as much as you can, because if you're not going to continue to give the baby optimal care, then you shouldn't be telling parents that you are." But optimal care wasn't going to do any good and we're with 56 other babies—we've got beds for 43—and this baby was consuming a fair amount of space and time. It made you wonder that this was not a good use of resources.

Story 19

This is a story about a 2½-month-old child admitted with left ventricular heart failure who suddenly and unexpectedly died from cardiac arrest while waiting for treatment.

19:3. Simone had had a febrile episode early in the morning and was a little bit irritable later in the morning. I had inquired with mother how she was acting, and then, throughout the day, I came in intermittently to either examine her or just eyeball Simone to see how she was doing. Throughout the day, I had general concerns because this was a 2½-month-old female with aortic insufficiency that was very severe and had led to a distended heart and there was some amount of mitral valve regurgitation as well [the mitral valve in the heart does not shut fully and there is backflow]. She had been on a dobutamine drip [IV medication to raise blood pressure due to the heart not pumping properly] for 2 weeks, since she was on the floor. That in and of itself meant that you had a child who was relatively tenuous; a 2½-month-old with a bad heart who had been febrile and there was no source on exam so we made sure she got the appropriate antibiotics. Then she was tachycardic [heart beating faster than normal] throughout the day, intermittently and usually in association with fever. She spiked another temperature in the middle of the day, and she was quite tachycardic, but she was also febrile at 102 degrees. She would have periods of being quiet, but then, as soon as you disturbed her, she would start crying and it would take a while to console her and calm her down. I had some sense all day that there was something that wasn't completely right; that she was sicker than she looked, sicker than what the numbers were showing. Later in the day, I'd gotten an EKG and we'd gotten another chest X ray. I reviewed the EKG with the fellow. Other than this tachycardia, her blood pressures were within normal range and she was perfusing [blood being supplied to tissues] and I could palpate pulses and she wasn't in any sign of respiratory distress. She didn't have any increase in her tube requirements. She was on nasal-gastric feeds, so those were unchanged because she wasn't vomiting and she wasn't having diarrhea, so there was nothing there that was concerning me. At about 7:00 that evening, the nurse who had been taking care of her came in and told me that Simone seemed to be breathing a little bit harder and that she was retracting [heavy breathing] a little bit. I examined her, and she was retracting but not significantly, mildly, and her oxygen stats were normal. She wasn't incredibly tachypneic [breathing fast], but her heart rate was a little bit elevated. At 8:00 I examined her again and findings hadn't changed much from the 7:00 exam, but then I became concerned that she just looked a little bit more tired, and that's why I decided to speak with the fellow again about it and we decided to call for respiratory support to come and help us replace a nasal-cannula with a C-pap [both devices to deliver oxygen through the nose, the latter with pressure]. She was not febrile at the time, and again all the vitals were stable. She looked tired and sickly, but she was a sickly looking baby at baseline. I was helping the respiratory therapist with the C-pap. I was holding her, and he took the nasal-cannula off and put the C-pap on and she was doing fine. Then we decided that the nose-prong was too small for her and we replaced it with a larger one and that's when things suddenly just went downhill. I'm sitting there holding her head and her back upright to make it easier for her and so that I could have better control of her head while he was placing it. Then a lot of things happened at once; it was one of those situations where your brain is filtering multiple things that are happening but they're all happening in sequence in the same amount of time so, in your mind, you're like, "This can't be happening." We had the nasal C-pap on and she just postured that strange posture and I thought that she was starting to have a seizure and then her eyes flew wide open and she just stared and then stopped. There was no respiratory effort, and at that point, I flew into action. I dropped the head of the bed down, and I called for nursing to come in the room. The respiratory therapist got the mask on and started bagging her [manually pumping oxygen into the mouth]. I grabbed a stethoscope and listened to the chest, but I didn't hear anything, and then I felt for pulses, and I couldn't feel anything; by this time, she was becoming white. Now that I think back on it, the strangest thing was that I was watching the stat monitor the entire time we were switching off the nasal-cannula tube to C-pap because I wanted to see how long she was maintaining her saturations [level of oxygen in the blood] and she maintained her saturations in the 90s for quite a long time before drifting down into the 80s, which was where I would have expected her to probably be normally off of the nasal-cannula or C-pap. But then, when all of this happened, the stat monitor stopped; it went right to zero—she must have had no pulse—it wasn't picking up anything, and I didn't feel anything and that's when I yelled, "Call code," and started doing chest compressions and told the nurse to get the cardiology fellow. The fellow took a look at her and I said, "I think she might be seizing"; I couldn't tell what was happening. Then the fellow said, "I'm going to go look at the telemetry" [a collection of patient monitoring devices including heart rate and electocardiogram] and walked out of the room. She had wanted to see if she was having any arrhythmia. That's when I put my hand on her chest and realized that there was nothing and called the code and started chest compressions. The fellow came back in the room and said, "Why are you calling a code?" and I said,

"There's nothing happening here, nothing. There's no heartbeat" and the fellow said, "Yes there is; there's a heartbeat on telemetry," and I said, "No, there is nothing," and the baby was white and she wasn't breathing. So I think her heart was beating potentially, but it was not beating with enough function to provide any type of profusion to her body. The rhythm that you see on the machine doesn't tell you the quality of contraction, and so you can have a perfectly normal electrical rhythm without necessarily having myocardial contraction.

19:1. She was in full cardiac arrest, so we intubated her and continued to try to resuscitate her, but we couldn't get her back; it was a failed resuscitation. They had gotten back a rhythm for a short time, so we thought that she was going to be unstable but stable enough to bring to the ICU so that we could then try to continue the resuscitative efforts. We continued to try to resuscitate, including medicines and ventilation, but no response. Given the type of cardiac defect that the child had, I wanted to see, by echocardiography, whether there was any kind of function, so we asked for the echo machine to be brought in and they echoed and there was no contraction of the heart at all. Things were unfortunate in the way they went, but they went as well as an emergency situation could have—the kid died and we could not get her back. . . . This was a child who was neurologically relatively normal and who just needed something fixed in her heart, and we were waiting to get that thing fixed. Had that thing been fixed, sure this kid probably would have had some other problems down the road and probably would have needed other surgeries, but she would have had a pretty good chance at leading a relatively normal life.

19:1. I sat with the mother and family and told them. It wasn't pleasant, and it would have been much nicer having the people who knew them better there and who had some sort of relationship with the mom, but it was Sunday night and it was so sudden. It was the first time that I had met the family, so I started off letting the cardiology fellow, who I thought may have known them better, tell them the bad news. She kind of told them but was not being very direct and using words that I didn't think the mom understood very well so, then, I basically just told her that her daughter had died and she broke down and started crying. It was unfortunate that the baby died on a Sunday night, at 10:00, when most of the people who may have had a relationship with the mom weren't around. If this would have taken place at 12 noon, for example, the outcome would have been the same, but, at least, more familiar faces to the mom would have been present, even if she wouldn't have taken it any better. We didn't even have the social worker that normally would see them available. I guess dying on the weekend is not a good thing.

Story 20

This story is about a fertility-assisted premature delivery of triplets, two of whom developed severe intraventricular hemorrhage and succumbed, on the third day, soon after having been removed, with the parents' consent, from ventilator support.

20:1. The two infants were the male boy twins of a triplet pregnancy who were delivered at 24 weeks and 3 days, which is the threshold of viability in terms of the likelihood that they would survive unscathed through the neonatal and perinatal periods. I was there from the first day of life, and I physically removed them from life support and watched as they struggled with the premature issues relating to breathing and control of metabolic issues. Ultimately, the reason they were removed from support was the presence of severe intraventricular hemorrhage which predicted a very poor neurological outcome. I had discussed the likelihood of this happening with the parents in great detail on the days prior to the death of the children and was in agreement with their decision to remove them. They had a surviving baby who was the female of this triplet pregnancy who, statistically and clinically, was doing better and, hopefully, would continue to thrive. She was stabilizing, to a degree, and her parents' hopes were bonded with her. They had really had a bad time, a horrendous few days, so our goal was to help them maintain a cautious optimism about the surviving triplet's course and keep them fully informed. They said they wanted a very simple funeral for the two boys with just immediate family and mom didn't want to be away from the hospital that much because she was conscious that the surviving child would be here for a long time. Mom found her ease with how much time she needed to be here hovering and how much time she rested at home over the course of the next week or so.

Our goal was to help her adjust to surviving parenthood. They were a great couple, a superb couple, and they had a sound relationship. I had no qualms that these people would make it through and, hopefully, they'd take their baby home with them.

20:4. I was there in the transitional nursery when they were first born and getting intubated. For a while, it looked like they would be okay, and then it started not to look so good for them. When I came back on service in the morning, one was on the oscillator [breathing machine]—that's not a good sign once a child comes out and was intubated and on a vent and then goes to the oscillator. It means they're doing worse than they were before. As a first-year resident, I was prepared that there would be a lot of acute things to do with them, as far as watching electrolytes, watching their respiratory status, watching their blood gases, that kind of thing. If we could get them through this day, then it would be again watching them through the night knowing that things could change acutely and we would need to do things acutely. I wasn't focused on "they're not going to make it," but on staying on top of all the parameters that I could. Of the three, there was one boy and one girl that were doing not as badly as the other one, so I was preparing for one being a lot more acute than the other two. But they all were very premature and in a fragile state, so I was expecting all three of them to have a lot of things to get done. That morning, I had been assigned to six patients, so I knew it was going to be a busy day and then I'd be on call that night and I knew I was going to be called to come back to take care of them during the night—I was prepared for them in terms of learning as much as I could that morning about how they were doing.

20:1. I told them that we could leave the situation overnight, if they wanted to have family members come in and see the children or if they wanted to have a priest come. We are moving toward acknowledging that bereavement is a real part of our nursery and that we need to extend all of the courtesies and benefits to parents who go through this. And there was no reason to stop support immediately, so if they wanted to do that, we would agree with them. We've had families who brought in extended family and had a service or had a time where everybody could meet and be with the parents. But these parents were very mature and quietly sure that they were doing the right thing and that they should be the ones to make the decision and be with the children. They both held the children while they died. The priest came to give them last rites, and it happened to be the same priest who had baptized the children a couple of days earlier, which was very good for the parents. He stayed and spoke very nicely with them. The two boys were taken off support together and died within a half an hour of each other in their parents' arms. I find that grandparents will grieve as much for their own children as for the loss of the babies of their children, but these parents felt it was unnecessary to bring in anybody else; they felt they had each other, so it was their decision not to complicate their grief and their immediate sense of what they needed to do by having anyone else around.

Whether or not parents choose to hold their infant when he comes off support and is dying depends on religious and social differences. Generally, we encourage it. We have thought through this process and found that, if the parents can stay with the baby and acknowledge that this is a transition and, as much as it is difficult to watch color changes and babies breathe with some difficulty and not run away from the situation, they can look back with a sense of pride later because they stood by their child through this time. We have a bereavement memory box that we give to the parents as a memento that contains a lock of hair, foot prints, and hand prints made from little clay imprints; and we have pictures that can be taken. Some religious or social groups will acknowledge that death is a part of life and accept it as a memory, and there are others who choose to bury quickly and have a certain group that will take care of death and dying. They are repulsed by the physical interaction with the dead person. We are very aware that, in this very heterogeneous culture that we live in, we have to acknowledge these social and cultural differences. It's generally a matter of offering what we do and seeing what they might accept. So, in terms of supporting families, I think we're getting better.

We have a quiet grieving room where parents can be brought. It was unusual to have two babies removed at the same time. We happened to have had a very high census of babies, so these twins were separated in different rooms, and they were brought in and then brought together. The parents went into the room where we would bring the babies, so they didn't actually see the whole process of removal from the support. Their babies were brought to them wrapped in blankets and with all the IVs clamped so they wouldn't bleed. We asked them if they preferred to be alone or have someone stay with them; many parents like to be alone. The priest stayed with them for a short period of time and I stayed with them; then I said I would leave them alone and I would come back at intervals and listen to the heartbeats and that is what happened. I went in at 10-, 15-minute intervals and would listen to the heartbeat. I pronounced one child and they kept holding him, and I pronounced the other child about a half an hour later. We asked them if they would like anything—tissues, water is usually supplied, if they'd like to call anyone, if they'd like anyone to be with them. I think it was done in a very reasonable manner, but it was still fearsome for them and a difficult time. They had barely seen what a premature baby looked like and suddenly they were holding their two dead boys.

20:8. We explain to the parents what's going to happen when we're going to take a baby off the ventilator. We tell them that he may have a little bit of color change, he might start to get a little cold, and, if the baby seems to be uncomfortable, we may give them something to make them more comfortable so that they're not struggling to breathe because that makes the parents very uncomfortable. Sometimes, when you're explaining this to parents, it becomes too overwhelming for them to hear it and you have to repeat it again and maybe word it a little differently. As you're handing the baby over, you're still explaining what's going to happen, and some parents are ready and some parents are just too emotional; they really don't hear it. We go back frequently to check on the baby, and sometimes you go in and they'll say, "Oh my God, the baby's turning blue" because they really weren't listening. But that's okay, we just repeat it again and explain why it's happening. Most parents, when given the chance, want to hold their babies when they are dying.

Withholding and Withdrawing | 4
Curative Treatments

> This is a tough lesson for me
> and doctors like me trained
> in a medical model that posited
> a cure as the only acceptable
> goal and death as a failure.
> — FRED EPSTEIN,
> *If I Get to Five: What Children Can*
> *Teach Us About Courage and Character*

When Is Enough Enough?

Palliative care for children can never be a simple extension (or dumbing down) of adult palliative care. The continuation of aggressive medical procedures, even when there is little realistic hope of a cure, is much more likely to occur for children than it is for adults.[1] Too often, however, this stronger incentive to continue aggressive care means that less attention is given to controlling children's painful symptoms and less time is available for patients, family, and caregivers to address emotions about death and grieving. Along these same lines, in our culture, a greater sense of failure is attached to medicine when it involves the death of a child compared to the death of an adult; this, too, contributes to continuing aggressive treatments in pediatrics that may create a barrier to effective palliation. Facing the loss of hope for a cure for a child poses the greatest ordeal for the pediatrician, and it is for this reason that many primary care pediatricians choose to forgo pediatric subspecialties such as oncology, cardiology, and transplantation.[2]

Children dying in hospitals challenge the caregiver's relationship with parents in myriad ways. Families and medical staff become increasingly intertwined, especially when questions arise concerning the futility of continuing heroic and life-sustaining treatments. Such questions are so emotionally and biologically complicated that they give rise to conflicting opinions within families, between families and treatment teams, and among members of treatment teams. Although it is the physician's responsibility, when appropriate, to explain the futility of further treatments to parents and children, whether to continue or to withhold curative care is never clearcut. Often, physicians' explanations of what is happening medically unwittingly determine whether aggressive interventions for cure will be continued, despite the physician's self-professed obligation to adhere to the principle of patient autonomy. Sometimes, physicians' perceptions of the parents' suffering pushes the decision to suspend care. More often, parents, being in denial or unable to accept the horror of losing their child, insist on treatments that physicians and other caregivers know will tragically prolong pain and suffering for the dying child. At times, too, decisions to prolong aggressive curative care are seen by hospital administrators as a poor use of institutional resources. Further problems are created when there are conflicting concerns, biases, and theoretical ideologies among different medical subspecialists (often between pediatric intensivists in the ICU and specialists treating the presenting diagnoses), as well as among the professional interests in treatment teams: residents, attendings, fellows, social workers, child-life specialists, psychologists, and nurses. Complicating the picture even more are the families' cultural and religious beliefs. For example, some orthodox religious practices forbid ever withholding or withdrawing care; given the kinds of medical technologies available today, this has become an increasingly difficult situation for staff.

Reflections on how medical decisions are made during the course of treatment inevitably are different when they lead to a cure versus when they lead to a death. In cases of cure, physicians are often portrayed as having beseeched parents to allow them to move forward in uncharted territories. In cases of death, physicians do not readily acknowledge their role as the guiding force in making the decisions; instead, they are more likely to emphasize how they carefully and systematically advised parents as to the relative risks and benefits of the more aggressive and experimental therapies. What comes across is that parents hardly ever are able to make such heart-rending decisions on their own. Despite all principles of informed consent and patient autonomy, they often unwittingly collude with the physician in obtaining the most optimistic prognosis for their child. As a result, the option chosen is the heroic effort rather than "die in comfort" palliative care. This is not to say that physicians are always in collusion with parents. Indeed, many parents push physicians beyond reason to seek experimental protocols and to use invasive tests and procedures, in hopes of a cure (or a "miracle").[3] In some clinical scenarios, the push for heroics has led to survival and children expected to die are alive and well today.

Discontinuing Life-sustaining Treatments

The purpose of discontinuing life-sustaining treatments is to allow incurably ill patients to die free of needless suffering. Today, philosophers, medical ethicists, theologians, physicians, and attorneys have reached consensus that it is ethically permissible to withdraw or withhold treatment or even to forgo extensive, invasive, and burdensome diagnostic procedures if the burdens of continuing them exceed their benefits to the patient.[4] Special considerations arise, however, when the discontinuation of life-sustaining treatments involves children. Decisions to discontinue treatment once it has begun are tougher than decisions to withhold treatment. It is hardly ever clear when to discontinue treatment because (and much more so in the care of children than adults), "each child's case, while sharing some similarities with others, represents a unique composite of medical, developmental, psychosocial, and familial factors integral to making such determinations. The evaluation of these factors is complicated by clinical scenarios which are often technically complex and always emotionally charged."[5] When there is a reasonable option to initiate life-sustaining treatment some have found it ethically advisable to provisionally start a time-limited trial using clearly defined and well-adhered-to criteria for stopping, should treatment prove ineffectual or unacceptably burdensome.[6] During the last month of life, the majority of children who die from chronic conditions receive some kind of therapy in hopes of effecting a cure or prolonging life. One study in a major medical center, for example, found that 56 percent of children with cancer were receiving cancer-directed therapies (beyond palliative chemotherapies) during the last month of their lives.[7]

DNR

An issue closely tied to withdrawing care is the decision whether to resuscitate patients once they are no longer able to support themselves. A DNR order means do not do cardiac massage, chest compressions, electric shock, or use medications to attempt to restart the heart, nor put in a breathing tube. Intubation is sometimes referred to as a DNI (do not intubate), but, for practical purposes, a DNR refers to both cardiac and pulmonary arrests. In the United States, the law mandates that unless otherwise directed, hospital patients must be resuscitated. However, at the end of life, when there is no realistic chance of cure, resuscitation might not only prolong dying but might needlessly burden a patient with undue pain and suffering. When the patient is a child, consent for not resuscitating is obtained from the parents and is documented in the medical chart. Many studies document the myriad problems that medical caregivers have encountered in discussing DNR orders with patients and their families.[8] Some of these problems involve when to ask for it, how to approach the subject, and how to proceed when the staff finds a DNR order to be in the best interests of a dying child but the parents do not. One study of pediatric end-of-life care reported that the median time from DNR to death was less than 1 day and that acuity of care, for most children, was very high prior to death.[9] Pediatric oncologists, for example, reported that their most troublesome problems in end-of-life care were the families' unrealistic expectations for cure and their reluctance to consent to a DNR.[10]

Patient Autonomy in Pediatrics

The principle of autonomy in medicine refers to a patient's right to choose or refuse treatment. It is warranted by the practice of informed consent and, in the case of children, informed assent.[11] Informed consent requires that patients be afforded the right to agree or disagree to medical practices with full knowledge of the risk/benefit ratios. In the case of children, it requires that they be so informed (even if they do not have the right to agree or disagree) in a developmentally appropriate way. However, it is not clear at what stage of development and under what conditions children have functional competencies to (1) rationally consider multiple factors in predicting future consequences; (2) comprehend medical information regarding relations between treatment, symptoms, and outcome probabilities; (3) be free from the coercion of others to make a medical decision; and (4) fully appreciate the immediacy and permanence of their choices.[12] Even adults often are confused by subtle yet complex distinctions between being incurably ill and imminently dying.[13] A study found that 43 of 44 parents of children with end-stage cancer agreed that children older than 5 years of age have the capacity to make decisions about experimental treatments and ought to be included in "final-stage conferences" with physicians. These investigators further speculated (without empirical evidence), that "children's emotional and conceptual development seemed to exceed that expected for chronological age, as if the physical and psychological stress of the disease accelerated their emotional maturation."[14] In practice, however, parents aren't so willing to consider their children's preferences about medical treatment when they contradict their own desires. This is understandable because even though we like to think that children in these situations have a seemingly precocious understanding of what is going on, we know very little about what it means for children to consent to initiate or withdraw heroic and life-sustaining measures. Therefore, how much autonomy they ought to be given in such cases is a matter of debate.

Although ideally parents always will make judgments and act in the interests and welfare of their children, that is not necessarily the case. Biases inherent in parent-child relations preclude this kind of judgment. Sometimes, parents' interests are separate from those of their children, perhaps involving their own needs or those of their spouses, a child's siblings, or other family members. Therefore, it is the pediatrician rather then the parents who is ethically and legally bound to function as the agent of children in medical situations. In this regard, there is consensus that life-sustaining treatment should be offered to children despite their parents' protests (or even the protests of the child patient). There is consensus, too, that life-sustaining treatment should be forgone if the competent child patient does not want it and, conversely, that it should not be withheld if the child patient believes it will be beneficial, even in cases where parents refuse it. Medical ethicists have proposed that "if a minor has experienced an illness for some time, understands it and the benefits and burdens of its treatment, has the ability to reason about it, has previously been involved in decision making about it, and has a comprehension of death that recognizes its personal significance and finality, then that person, irrespective of age, is competent to consent to forgoing life-sustaining treatment."[15] On the other hand, there are some ethicists who believe that the premise of patient autonomy is a bioethical paradox that places unwanted and debilitating burdens on patients who put their hopes in the physicians they find competent and trustworthy.[16]

Ethical Principles and Ethical Practices

There is a world of difference between practice guidelines derived from abstract conceptual frameworks and their application in the press of pediatric practice. No decision in medicine has greater consequences, is subject to more emotional biases, and so directly captures ethical concerns than decisions about whether to withhold or withdraw treatment. Guidelines concerning such decisions have been clearly and consistently stated.[17] Those deciding to withhold or withdraw treatment need to weigh the benefits of treatment against levels of harm (e.g., pain, suffering, and quality of life) to the patient. In practice, however, the boundaries between what is beneficial and not beneficial often are blurred and produce scenarios in which the benefits are marginal or uncertain. Similarly, the boundaries between levels of harm are not dichotomized in simple high/low (yes/no) terms. Levels of pain and suffering are subjective, culturally understood, and very difficult to measure. Hence, the quality of life standard is difficult to apply and rests on a range of subjective judgments regarding the benefits and burdens of life, disability, and death. This standard is further complicated because quality of life needs to be judged according to each patient's perspective. Such judgments require the collaboration of the family, the child (when possible), and health care practitioners.[18] Hence, providers and families are faced with decisions when beneficial outcomes are uncertain and possibilities of harm are considerable. Parents have reported that the three principal factors, in descending order of importance, guiding their end-of-life decisions about withholding care from their children were (1) their sense of their child's quality of life, (2) the chances of their child getting better, and (3) their child's amount of pain or discomfort. Factors such as "what I believe my child would have wanted," religious/spiritual beliefs, advice of hospital staff, and financial costs were not critical factors for them.[19]

When to Stop

A survey questioned what percentage of benefit would lead someone to agree to have chemotherapy for cancer. The difference between cancer patients and oncologists (treating adults) was dramatic: patients were willing to accept a 10 percent chance of improvement (not cure) compared to 50 percent for oncologists.[20] Is this because oncologists are more aware of the toxicities of chemotherapy and have seen too many suffering patients being treated for too long for too little benefit, or does it reflect adults' overwhelming fear of dying? But what of the case of children? To what extent do medical decisions reflect parents' fears of losing their child? In pediatrics much more than in adult and geriatric medicine, decisions about when, how, and why to withhold or withdraw therapies intended to cure capture the pivotal issue in end-of-life care. Issues regarding who makes these kinds of decisions, why they are chosen, and how they are presented among medical staff, children, and families are the leading theme of this book, and the narratives in this chapter describe this process.

For many pediatricians who deal with life-threatening diseases, the decision to continue aggressive and invasive treatment in the hope of a cure is a "win-win" situation. The idea of children dying in their care is so difficult for them to accept that they will pursue procedures (e.g., complex micro-neurosurgeries, bone marrow transplants) that hold little hope for recovery but that, without them, leave no hope.[21] A pediatric neurosurgeon described it this way: "Standing by and doing nothing while a child dies was not an option for me. I resolved never to give up on a kid without fighting for as long and hard as the child and his parents were willing."[22] Often these physicians feel that, even if they lose a child to the procedure, they will learn things that will benefit other patients down the road.

Palliative care is said to begin upon the diagnosis of a life-threatening medical condition, its aim being to comfort patients by providing adequate pain management and maintaining quality of life. In practice, however, aggressive and invasive treatment protocols are pursued in hopes of a cure, and parents resist aggressive pain management for their child because it might compromise the child's biological reaction to disease-modifying agents. Health care providers often are reluctant to talk about this sensitive issue, especially when the risk/benefit ratio becomes blurred, as it so often does, when the hope of cure diminishes.

1:1. Generally speaking, whenever we get somebody that seems to be doing really badly and the chances of recovery become slimmer and slimmer, you usually hear two different and sometimes diametrically opposite reactions. There are members of the staff who feel that, "Ok, we've lost this person so anything we do beyond this point is just a meaningless exercise in futility." And there are other people who feel that "We've got to do everything we can until the person gives up, literally; we should not stop." There really is no battle. It's not specific individuals who feel this or that way, nor is it specific professions because, if it were, the nurses who wanted to go on are, at other times, the nurses who want to stop and, other times, there are the physicians who see things differently.

1:8. They keep going and keep going so that, when a patient dies, they can say, "We did everything we could" as a personal philosophy as opposed to taking a stance to help the child die. I'm not so much like that, and I think you'll find a lot of nurses across the country in ICUs who think that way because we're the ones that are left at the bedside. We've been there a lot. You help them live, but then there comes a time when you have to help them to die; to die in peace. It's the physicians who are the ones that pull the strings. They're the ones who write the orders, they decide how far you're going to go in management and when you are going to stop giving the volume to keep the blood pressure up. You can talk to them and give them your opinion, and I felt that they did listen when I said, "Don't do that to her." They heard me.

1:8. In the last couple of years, we've had a few attendings who were much more liberal, much more open-minded than compared to years ago. Ten years ago, we had a couple who were much more at ease with death, but that's not so much the case now. They're very aggressive and hold on much too long. They push too long and too hard.

2:1. The transplant attending showed me the survival curves, and basically the survival was nil in that situation. So we had chosen to go on to transplant him, even though he was not in what I would call a very good position to be transplanted and it was a lot of toxicity with perhaps no benefit. I even thought it was debatable, but transplant attending said, "No, we're going to go through with it." I might have even given the parents an option, but I said to the attending, "If this is the way you want to go, I'm going to let you talk to the family." The transplant attending was writing a protocol for an allo-transplant, which is completely experimental. Then the family asked me, "What do you think?"and I said—I'm trying to remember exactly what I told them because, I feel pretty guilty about this— they said to me, "Is there anything else? Do we have any other options?" and I said to them, "Well, I can't tell you what this transplant is going to be like because it's purely experimental and Devon would be the first one here to have it but, from what the experts are telling me, the toxicity may be less but the benefit may be greater." But this protocol was out of the context of a study. This was sort of compassionate use but it was untried—there is a Phase 1 pilot study now that's through the IRB [Institutional Review Board] that has to approve all experimental Treatment Protocals but at the time he was ready, it was not through the IRB, so was it experimental? No, in that the data was not going to be part of a published paper, and it was untried territory in our woods and I had difficulty with that, I've always had difficulty with that. It's part of why I left transplant medicine, but I respected the transplant attending and part of the reason we work together is because we have a different take and we balance each other out. He says, "You know, we're not doing a good job. Thirty-five percent survival is lousy, and we need to do something else and if we don't try to do something else, we'll never figure out what that something else is." I understand that mentality, and there have to be people who are willing to push the envelope, and I don't mind encouraging people to do it and facilitating it, but I'm not a great envelope pusher myself. I'd like to be but I still have problems with the difference between when you should and should not try something new. For example, this transplant was billed as having probably a less then 10 percent risk for acute graft versus host disease, but meanwhile Devon ended up dying from terrible acute graft versus host disease and all of its subsequent complications, and they could never get it under control. There were lots of indications that this was not going in the right direction, but this [second] transplant had been billed to me as a low risk of acute graft versus host disease and I told the family that. So, I felt very guilty because it may still be a low risk of acute graft versus host disease, but Devon just happened to be the 1 out of the 10 that got it. It's very hard, but the transplant attending's position was, "Go for broke, we don't have anything else to offer him and maybe there's a miracle." In the end, I would have gone that way too, but I think that I would have at least presented the data to the family and said, "His chances here are very, very slim. We could go two ways now." I'm a parent, and I probably would have chosen the same thing. If you give someone two options and one is palliation, when you have a kid running around happy as a lark who really doesn't look sick, it doesn't make a whole lot of sense to people, if you can give them any other option, even if you tell them that the chances are infinitely small that it is possibly curative. With adults, it's very different than with children. With children, it's always this "go for broke" mentality.

2:7. The only chance that Devon had, small though it was, was to do this second [bone marrow] transplant. That's how it was presented to mom. I don't think anybody expected the outcome to be as bad as it was. I mean he would have died eventually; he probably would have succumbed to his disease, but he had so much morbidity from the transplant that mom was not prepared for it; neither were we frankly. I primarily take care of transplant patients, and in that arena, where you have a 40 to 50 percent mortality rate, we get all these new drugs which we think are going to be miracle drugs, but they cause complications; they cause morbidity. Sometimes I think, "Why are we bothering?" but if I was in that situation, I would probably want everything thrown at me too—so let's try it. But at the same time, it prolongs somebody's dying without potentially giving some quality of life. It had potential in Devon's case to prolong his life, but to what end when the quality was not there?

3:1. We're finding that we're getting more and more complicated patients. The longer we're in business, the more patients die. That's just the way it goes, and how do we as a group deal with it? As we move on with new treatments, the intervals are prolonged and made more difficult. Devon was a good example because the technology to do what we did and the therapy we gave him didn't exist 10 years ago. There are certain issues that we didn't know back then so, when the patient's neuroblastoma relapsed, it was, "Okay, bye." If it comes back, it comes back and there's nothing we can do, but here and now, we may go through three or four different drugs, so it prolongs the periods of time that we can keep patients alive and there's going to be greater risks and side effects from what we do. So it's become much more complicated, and it's lengthened the time. But the basic emotions are still the same. There's this child dying, and how do you deal with that? How do you deal with a dying patient? How do you know when to put them on the ventilator, how do you know when to start therapy, stop therapy?

2:9. I've been in situations where they were talking about using an experimental drug, and, to make a long story short, it wasn't going to work. It was like this little thing they were dangling out there. I was talking pretty honestly with the mother and she was like, "I don't think this is going to work,"and this nursing attendant walked in and said, "Oh, this is wonderful that they're going to do this." I didn't want to say anything because the child was there too and she goes on, "Don't you remember this other case when we used an experimental drug and they got better?" Well, one had nothing to do with the other. It was offering such false hope, because there was no hope at that point. I think people who do that are probably protecting themselves and really believing it. This nurse really believed that.

2:2. He was getting progressively worse and we doctors were in denial for 80 days and then, on the 81st day, we said, "When do we stop?" but it was really hard not to. We had a kid with a neuroblastoma, and people said that the chances for survival with his condition—the way he had been reacting—was almost zero. But you're pushing, pushing to try, and try and he's alive at one year so maybe he'll be alive at two years, so you're trying very hard to deal with every complication that comes, with the hope that he'll get over it and get better and go home because otherwise you can't do it.

2:1. Choosing when to stop treatment comes up particularly with the patients that I deal with, which are ones with neuroblastomas. You can cure probably a third of the patients, and so you reach a point where you question how aggressive are we going to be. You get it from the parents. Some parents, even though the odds are small or the therapy is very experimental, want to go forward. Other times, they will say, "No." With neuroblastomas, what we consider the standard treatment is chemo and transplant, and, if that doesn't work, we consider moving onto something else. But if the parent told me that they didn't want to do anything else, then I would say it's their choice because patients who fall short of the standard, will die. With Devon, he had had the standard, and we decided to try an alternative transplant to try and treat him. How do you make that decision? It's a mutual decision that you make with the parents and you say that, "Given the status of the disease, this is what we have to offer and these are the risks." Some parents opt to do everything and some parents opt not to. Devon's parents opted to do everything until the end, so we gave him the second transplant. At that point, Devon was in relatively good shape, so it's very hard for a parent to say, "We're not going to do anything" when a child is looking fairly well. He had some symptoms from his disease; he had a little bit of pain, but overall he was in good shape. And the other options weren't going to cure him. Even though there was chemotherapy, it wasn't going to cure him. It was for palliation and, if your choices are for palliation versus trying something which we don't know whether it works or not, some parents will opt to do palliation and some parents will opt to try to do everything possible, and that's what these parents decided to choose. I think that, in some ways, it was courageous on their part.

2:1. Seeing patients go through these aggressive levels of treatment and then die has been an evolution for me. If you talk to this group of fellows, or people who are still close to their training, or are in training, it's very hard.

With time, I've been able to say, "Yes, we need to try certain things." I'm not going to cure every patient and I can't even cure half of them right now, so I know that's not going to happen. But that's also what I do as far as my research and what I want to try to do is push. Devon is another name to my list of my patients who have died, but there's the motivation to keep on trying and keep on finding something different, something that may have some chance at working. So I keep pushing in my research to find something better. Even though he died, we learned a lot from Devon. You have to learn from what you find from each patient—Do we time the radiation differently? Do we do other things differently? Those are things that we learn from this.

2:8. Sometimes you hear from oncologists that it's such a lousy prognosis that, if only we could learn something for experimental treatments instead of just letting the patient go, it will help us cure other kids along the line. I understand the rationale, but I don't agree with it when you know, intuitively, psychically, spiritually, and organically that what you're doing now is causing more suffering for that individual patient than all of the gains that you might make scientifically. Then, you have to step back and say, "You know what? We have an obligation to the science as much as we have an obligation to the patient, and the obligation to the patient, at this point, is much more important than maybe where the next patient might take us." There are ethical issues on both sides. There are some parents who are able to make that decision more easily and just say, "Stop, enough" and there are some parents who are not able to say that and then it's the obligation of the provider who should have the perspective. It's probably the most difficult decision anybody would ever have to make, and I don't think parents can make that decision very well. That's why I'm always humbled by pediatric oncologists. Part of being a pediatric oncologist and doing it well is being able to handle this elegantly and with grace and I'm very humbled when I see it done extraordinarily well. But you have to weigh your commitment to the science with the ethical and moral obligations that you have to the individual patient.

2:1. Whenever you're a patient or your family member is a patient, you are struck by the fact that medicine is imperfect. It's not a perfect science and there aren't any short answers. For example, I just saw one of my colleagues' patients today who chose not to go through a transplant. She was a baby and her parents took her home against medical advice. They were told to have a transplant and they said, "No," for whatever reason. This was a tiny baby and she had terrible toxicity and they said, "No" and this baby is alive today and looks wonderful. So I said to them, "It just goes to show you that medicine doesn't have all the answers. Sometimes we just need a miracle."

2:3. When we offer experimental trials it's hard to say, "Well this is going to help us treat future cases." It's the right thing to do, but I'm sure it feels insensitive; you're saying, "Your child doesn't have a chance, but maybe this will give other kids a chance," or "This probably is not going to work, but we'll see." That's why it's so hard but we need to own up to our own actions, and a lot of times, we don't do that; we give false hope. It's not really an informed consent if the parents aren't given a real choice. Of course, it's an emotional reaction but they need to know this isn't going to cure their child—that it's not really for their child—it's for the advance of medicine. Unless there is a definite cure, people need to see the quality of life as a bigger issue than just letting this child live 5 years longer. For pediatricians, it's really the quality of the life of the child and not the quality of life for the parents. Having a child suffer for 5 years takes a toll on a marriage, it takes a toll on a family, it takes a toll on everything. So I'm not saying to just give up, but there has to be some kind of balance that we need to strike here.

3:10. It took her months to consent to the DNR, and I'm so glad that our doctor worked with her so hard and explained how bad it would be for Elsa to have to be resuscitated. Her ribs would break, and she just would not do well. If the doctor didn't do it the way she did it, I'm sure the mom would've had her resuscitated and everything, and she would end up being one of those kids in a coma for months and her mom wouldn't have anything. So the doctor and I had an incredible relationship with this mom, and we put so much time and energy into processing so that it really worked. If it wasn't for that, the mom would've wanted everything done. I think most people want everything until they hear or see the reality of what everything means. It depends how it's explained to them. Some doctors say, "Oh, it'll save the kid's life," so of course the mother's going to do it, but if the doctor says, "Oh, it's going to be horrible, she'll be breathing on the machine, her ribs will break, it's intrusive." It's all in the presentation, and I've seen it presented both ways. I think it's impossible to be so objective in a situation like this, especially when they're in the life-saving business. It can be very hard for them. It's interesting for me to watch everybody's styles with DNR discussions with families. Different doctors have such different ways of approaching it.

3:1. I got this call one night from the mother saying, "We can't do this at home." I assumed that what she meant by "we can't do this at home" is we couldn't let her die at home. They couldn't stand it, so they called hospice that night and arranged to have them transport her back to the hospital. Then, what ensued was really the most difficult 10 days I've ever had. I thought they understood they were coming in to have her die and we were giving her pain control. She had high fevers, so we agreed to give her a once-daily antibiotic. We gave her hydration. At this point, she was covered with bruises, had a big decubitus ulcer on her bottom—which, fortunately, she couldn't feel. We ended up putting a Foley catheter in her and she was retaining fluid, and the family would do things that I simply didn't understand. She could barely swallow, she was floating in and out of consciousness, but they were feeding her. They'd push, with a syringe, farina into her and make her swallow. . . . They would fight with me about the transfusions and say to me, "Why aren't you checking CBCs [complete blood counts]?" and I'd say, "Because I'm not treating a number" and they'd say, "Well, I'm sure her hemoglobin is fine," and I said, "If you think that it would make her feel better to give her some blood, I will give her blood, based on those criteria. I know her number is not good. If you're telling me that you think that she needs blood, and she will feel better, then I will give her some blood." And periodically I would transfuse her a unit, at which point they would say to me, "Why are you only giving her one unit? You used to give her two," and I said, "Well, you know, she's retaining fluid, she's not peeing, and if I give her too much, it's going to fill up her lungs, and I've heard that drowning like that is the worst possible feeling that you could have so I'm not going to do that," and they'd say, "Well, look at all these bruises, why aren't you giving her platelets?" and I'd say, "If she's actively bleeding from her mouth, I would give her platelets, but if she's not actively bleeding, I can't give her platelets," and they'd say, "But I'm sure her number is seven," and I'd say, "But I'm not treating her number. I'm treating the patient." . . . Finally, the night before she died, it was incessant. "You are doing nothing for her," and I'd say, "No, I'm giving her what she needs. I'm doing whatever it takes to keep her comfortable." I would have to barter with them. I'd say, "Okay, I'll give her the blood"—they'd move her around in the bed, they'd change her diaper, they'd manipulate her, and she would scream, her groaning would get to a very high pitch—"but you have to promise me that, if you're going to manipulate her, you need to give her some pain medication before you manipulate her, because it hurts her so much." It got to the point where nurses who loved her and had taken care for her for 2 years were starting to refuse the assignment. We were all getting angry with the family. . . . Elsa wasn't mad at me. She may have been mad at me for not telling her the truth, but I respected the family. She was 12 and they had never told her all along, so who was I to tell her in frank words? But toward the end, I started calling her my angel and told her that she was like my baby now because she'd gotten this soft, downy hair and she knew I had a baby and was very excited about the baby, so I said, "Your hair is just like my baby's," and I called her angel. I'd just come in and stroke her hair and talk to her and hold her hand for a while, and I had no problems with Elsa. I used that kind of imagery with her, but I never, never said anything directly to her. When she was in this moribund state the night before she died and I was next to the bed and felt really terrible, her mother said to me, "Why aren't you giving her platelets? Look at all these bruises." I said, "Platelets aren't going to take away these bruises," and she said, "Well what about in the future? What about if she bleeds somewhere else? What if she bleeds into her head? What if she bleeds into her stomach?" and I said, "We're not talking about the future. We're doing what's good now." That was as blunt as I think I said anything in front of Elsa. She kept saying to me, "In our religion, it's our belief, it's our culture, it's our religion that we do everything and then only God can say when it's time," and I said to her, with all due respect, "You've asked me to cross a line which I'm not comfortable with because you're asking me to be God. This is unnatural. This is indecent. The body is weak, the spirit is strong and you're asking me to support a body that can no longer support itself. We need to let her body go and let her spirit be free." It was just constant and really got to the point where everyone was angry. I said, "The real issue is, if you want to do what's important for Elsa, you'll treat her pain," and they wouldn't; they wouldn't, and it was just so hard.

3:9. We have a lot of families who don't want their child to die at home. The push is always to get them out, as if everybody wants to die at home. Well, everybody doesn't want to die at home, and it's wrong to always put that burden on families because it makes the mother feel like she's not doing what's best for her kid or what's right for her child. A lot of families are afraid, especially if they have other children at home, that they have to sort of live with that ghost in their house. And then there's always that need to be heroic. There's that feeling of, "Did I really try absolutely everything?" I've had families go home with DNR orders, with the intent to let their kid die peacefully at home, and they ended up calling 911 and calling us when they got to another hospital and having to have to go there to stop the machines and things. Part of that is how you explain to the families what a DNR is and when do you explain the DNR. With pediatric patients, it's not always done with enough time because people are just so afraid to bring it up. A lot of times it's done so close that there's not enough time to stabilize to get the kid home and get home care involved or for that family to have enough time to adjust to the idea of hospice. We need to do a better job of addressing those issues because if we could get families home and give them the support networks and mechanisms that they need in time to develop the relationships with the hospice care company and the hospice nurse so that, when the time comes, they already have that relationship, it would be so much easier for them. But it's too much to suddenly ask people, at the most critical time of their lives, to no longer rely on us, who are the ones that they've relied on for the last, often many years and to switch to somebody new who they don't know and don't trust and, in a short amount of time, develop a trusting relationship with them. When parents hear DNR, they think it's a death sentence. I had a Spanish mother say to me about her daughter who'd been sick for 7 or 8 years now—and we were talking about going on a DNR—"What's the difference between that and doing everything?" and I said, "Well, do you also mean intubation?" "Oh, no, no, no; I don't mean that," she said, "But if there's a treatment, I'll do it," and I said, "All right, but you know, sometimes the treatment can be worse than actually dying," and she said, "Well, I'm not like those white people. I don't let my child die." This was all in the context—believe it or not—of a somewhat light-hearted kind of conversation, so I responded with, "I think I've just been insulted." But it's that feeling that you have to do absolutely everything, but everything doesn't mean resuscitation and that would be where the line is drawn. So for each family, the line is drawn someplace different.

4:3. You really want to be careful not to judge. You'd hear people talking, "Well, why doesn't she just let him go?" and "This is so mean and selfish, blah-blah-blah." But you really can't put yourself in that position. So you have to work to not say things like that because that's how we all felt. The question is, when does the point come when you say, "Enough." We always talk about limited resources in our hospital, but you never appreciate that because we can pretty much give whatever we want to give—all the medications and stuff and the cost of an ICU bed for however many months he was in there. When do you say, "Enough is enough"? As providers, we have to ask that because resources are limited, and how many times did we need to transfer someone to another place because we needed that bed in the unit that he was taking up? But when do you say to a parent, "We're going to take this ability away from you"? I don't know. Some attendings talked about taking this case to the ethics committee, and some were like, "No. I would never do that." Some thought we should have medical power of attorney taken away from the mother. But I don't know because she would feel like people were against her and telling her that she's doing wrong. But it's got to come to a point because he could have lived an indefinite amount of time, costing a lot of money and knowing he was not going to get better. That's a hard decision to make, to say when is enough enough. It would have been good to bring it before the ethics committee, even if not to push for power of attorney, but just to talk about things like when do you decide.

4:3. In this kind of case, it wouldn't have hurt to get more input because you get stuck in the day-to-day of it and you feel like nobody's stepping back. We needed some people who would approach it fresh. We'd be like, "Well, enough is enough. Let's just let it end already." But somebody else would be able to come in and have a different spin on it because you get jaded and you get bitter. I spent the whole month I was in there taking care of him and knowing that what I was doing wasn't going to get anywhere and that there was no chance he was going to get better. On rounds, we would be like, "Oh, we don't want to spend too much time on him. All right, who's next?" You look at yourself, and you hate acting that way because that's still somebody's child. But it's normal and I guess every provider would have that run through his mind, but it's like you have to take an active role to fight that way of thinking and you don't like yourself when you realize that you've been thinking like that. But what are you going to do? You have to think about why and how you're going to deal with it because you can't let it affect the care you give. You get pissed off when you get paged at 4:00 in the morning when you finally got to sleep and it was about him and you knew that, whatever it was, it wasn't that important in the big scheme of things. You couldn't let yourself act that way, but we all found ourselves doing it.

4:8. If parents want care to continue and they don't want things withdrawn, we must provide that care. For example, if you draw blood and the results show that something is wrong, once you have that result, you cannot not act on it; you don't have that choice. Also, you can't decide not ever to draw labs on a kid who's being cared for in the ICU. You have to intervene and treat it until we're no longer providing care; it's a legal obligation. Even if you know that replacing that potassium isn't going to make a difference in the big picture, if the potassium's low, you've got to give them potassium. You're either providing medical care or you're not.

5:1. The difficult aspect of this case was that the primary problem with the patient was cured and the remainder of physical difficulties were surmountable, or nearly surmountable, and the patient died anyway. There was a lot of kidney damage, a lot of liver damage, lung damage, and questionable neurologic injury. His primary disease, his leukemia, was presumably cured and none of the organ system damage was necessarily irreversible, though he was going to be very sick for a very long time. The other bone marrow transplant physician who was involved that weekend had trouble with Ricardo's parents' request to remove life support because there was potential for reversibility. He may have ended up with no renal functioning; that would be a bad thing, but people do live on dialysis. It wasn't possible to determine if there was any neurologic injury. There was a chance that there was, but also there was a chance that he could come through this with no neurologic injury whatsoever. Those would be probably the two worst things he could have had. He probably could have survived his lung injury, and his liver failure was not that bad; he probably could have survived that too. So it was tough when the disease was probably cured, and, as for the other stuff, you've seen worse cases. On the other hand, we spoke to each other quite frankly, and neither one of us was going to stand in the way of these parents that, in their valid opinion, their child was no longer really their child. . . . I was with the family when we withdrew treatment. No matter how prepared, nothing ever prepares parents, families, people for going through this. There were a lot of tears. I had to leave him on the ventilator for a while, so I think that they just watched the monitors for a while. We had a service and actually had him baptized just before discontinuing things. The priest came, said some prayers with the family, and baptized the child and then we took off the medications. I had to leave him on the ventilator, so I turned down the oxygen and it took probably another a half an hour; mom got more distressed as time went on. All in all, compared to most people, they were more prepared than not. Withdrawal of support doesn't absolutely equate with death. That is one thing you learn as you do this for a long time. Two days later you might still be going in there and seeing the family's anguish. There are so many times that I never tell people that it will; I never guarantee that it will. On a couple of occasions I have been asked to do what essentially is euthanasia, which I won't do.

6:7. The other day, the hospital PR people were here making a video about what we do, and they asked one of the attending oncologists to say how sick the children are and then "how you take them to the brink of death and then bring them back." That's a dramatic way of looking at it, but, in essence, that's what we do. Sometimes you are caring for a dying child and some of them are so sick, it would be a miracle if they lived, and some pull through when you don't think they will. That's an amazing thing to see.

5:2. This was one of the most amazing families I've seen because they were more realistic than the physicians. They really never expected a miracle—if their kid would have done fine, they would have said that that was a miracle. They never thought that I'm going to save their kid and he's going to do fine, and that was amazing because I come from a different country and a different medical system where attempts to save somebody are not as aggressive as they are here. So many times I have the feeling that we are pushing, pushing a lot, and I think that's because we get too close to the child. When we realize that there is nothing to do, we try to find something because there's got to be something we can do—if not cure him or save him, at least we can prolong his life. When things go bad, we still think we have a lot of options in terms of interventions. It's high medicine here, so we always think we can do something; we can somehow reverse the situation; we can get it better, without realizing that the child already had three organs that were failing and there was no way this child was going to live. Sometimes, we kind of miss this, but this family said, "We want a DNR," and we were like, "A DNR? We're not at that point yet." But then you take a look at the child; he was intubated, the lungs were failing, the liver had failed, the renal had failed, and he needed a DNR. This child was not going to make it. It was interesting that the parents were the ones to say, "You need to stop care now. I don't think he's going to make it." They were amazingly realistic without being too detached or superficial. They had, in their mind, already realized their 6-year-old child had been sick since he was 8 months old, so they already had the time to digest, to understand, what was going to happen. When we told them that he had a 90 percent chance of not making it, in our minds, it was the 10 percent chance of making it that counted. Instead, they were able to say, "Ninety percent chance means that he is not going to make it." Usually, at the end, when things go bad, families become angry. They are angry at whatever happened to their child, but they project the anger toward us. This family never did that, so for us the job was much easier.

5:1. I've had parents push us doctors to do things beyond what turned out to be worth doing. We had a great story about a kid who came in and had a serious infection in her blood and had a cardiac arrest. She then had five cardiac arrests in a row in our outpatient clinic and was resuscitated, resuscitated, and resuscitated. Finally, the attending said to the mother, "This child has just arrested again, and we really think it makes sense to just say, 'This is it.' " The mother said, "Nope," and this kid survived and was okay. So yes, sometimes the parents are right about being heroic, but I've never seen a kid with all the organs failing, where the parents were right about being heroic. I've seen scenarios where kids who've relapsed and you say the chances that we can pull this one out of the fire are really slim and you would rather say just take your kid home and let them die peacefully and the parent says, "No," and 2 years later the kid's still chugging along—but not when all the organs are failing.

7:1. She had palliative chemo at home. What I meant by palliative chemo was that there was no intention to cure but to stabilize the disease, perhaps to regress—but mostly to stabilize it. So, even though it didn't look like she was going to make it, she had tolerated chemo fairly well and had gotten clinical benefit from it, if not curative benefit. Then she went for the surgery and, while the surgery didn't do her in, the period that it took for her to recuperate from the surgery actually did do her in because, had we continued on with the chemotherapy, she may have lived longer. The chemotherapy was keeping things in check, and in the interval between chemotherapies, the tumor was growing. What I told the parents post-op was that, if I do the risk/benefit analysis, it was not ethical to continue to treat their child with the kind of intense chemotherapy that we had been giving her before because that chemotherapy is given only with the intent to cure. One does not give that kind of chemotherapy just to prolong life. What we do is to switch to a chemotherapy that keeps you out of the hospital and that doesn't open the door to risks of overwhelming sepsis and other infections. We just give what we think would have the best chance of being effective in the short term but not with intent to cure. That's what I meant with palliative. In the end, I said, "I'll give her a try with this; I've had very good results with it, and it tends to be well tolerated." But I was clear with them that I would give it once and see how things went. So, in the end, I feel okay about this case because I walked the line as aggressively as I could—as aggressively as I would have wanted to be for my own child—to sustain this child for as long as possible.

8:10. The mom was told that if we don't try a second transplant William won't live for very long. The first transplant was so difficult that he was on the edge of death. We had the alarm go off on the first transplant, and then, in the mom's mind, a miracle occurred and he was saved. But what options did the mom have regarding a second transplant? She had the choice to either have a second transplant or not. I have several families who have opted to not have a second transplant. If they make an educated decision, based on the relevant issues, not to have a second transplant, then it won't happen. If a second transplant guarantees life, then we consider it medical neglect, but there is never a guarantee. It's not that concrete. The more that I stay in this business, I realize that there isn't a cure for cancer. We do the best that we can to either suppress the disease or take away the tumor with all these blasting medications that we give these children, but we cannot tell the parents that after 2 years your child will be cured. We tell the parents after 5 years if you don't relapse then the disease is gone.

9:1. What John and his parents wanted was not to get any more chemotherapy but to look for alternative medicines. Mom was going to go to a nutritionist with the idea that she didn't want to give up hope, and she felt that chemotherapy had nothing more to offer John. I had to agree with her in the sense that, although I would have been more than willing to try experimental medicines, I didn't think that there was a likelihood that they would work. So the fact that she and John and her husband had decided that they didn't want to give him classic chemotherapy anymore was really appropriate and fine with me. I know that I have more to give in terms of symptom relief and caring for the family, but in some funny way, I sometimes feel relieved when the family turns to alternative medicines when I know that I don't have treatment that's truly curative. When I know that I can't cure someone, my goal is for the family and child to be as comfortable as possible. If it were a situation where I felt that there was a promising new medication and the family was irrationally refusing to consider it or giving up at a point that was inappropriate, it would be different, but it's actually kind of comforting that I can say to them, "Well, from my expertise, I have not seen these alternative medications to be curative, but they might be helpful." We have a nutrition person here who's involved with some of them about this issue—it's called complementary medical care. She works with the families to make sure they don't get in the hands of someone who's going to rip them off for a lot of money or do things that are dangerous, someone who's selling snake oil.

10:10. When Sarah was transferred to the ICU, the parents said things that led the staff to think that they thought that the radiotherapy she was receiving was to bring about a cure and that it wasn't palliative. That was what they wanted to believe and they didn't want to accept the idea that she was dying and, as long as it didn't interfere with the care of the child, you didn't have to bang it into their head, if they were not ready to hear it. If someone's not ready to hear it and it's not getting in the way of treatment, we don't have to ride in on our white horses and tell them everything and be so righteous and rub it in their face, if they're not ready for it.

10:1. The most difficult part of taking care of her was the parents' misunderstanding, or lack of understanding, or lack of acceptance of her terminal condition. A few days after she came down to the ICU, we were talking about the plan of care, and I came out and told the parents that she was going to die. It seemed as if they had not heard it, or they heard it before but never really listened to what was being told to them. When you continued to talk with them, they continued to ask about therapies that we knew were not going to work, and my impression, from talking with the oncologist, was that the therapy that she was getting at that point was palliative but they were talking as if it was curative treatment. This is very common among families, but a lot of it depends on the type of patient that you have. Oncology patients are more difficult because their course of illness is longer than most of the other kids that we get that end up dying in the ICU. When you compare the oncology patients to, for example, a bad trauma patient or a patient who has just come down with acute myocarditis or acute renal failure, you see that the families know that, with the acute exacerbation, there isn't much time and therefore they are already shocked and the death or the course of the illness just plays out. The oncology patient is difficult, from the intensivist's standpoint, in that the predominance of their care is done outside of the ICU and therefore the intensivist doesn't get as much of a chance to form a relationship with the family. We're then asked to take care of this patient at the sickest point of their disease process without having formed as deep or as important a relationship with the family as we probably should have. It's always tough to tell a family that their child's condition is terminal, but as long as I have the facts and I don't have any kind of contradictory input, I can do that well. So when the oncologist told me this was a terminal disease, I felt perfectly fine being able to sit with the family and talk about that. I have a difficult time being told that it is a terminal disease and it has not been presented to the parents in that way because we are not really helping prepare them; we are just continuing to give them false hopes. In this situation, I didn't think the parents were flat-out told what the reality was and they were the type of people who really needed to be told black and white, not in ways in which more hope was given. I sat down with them and answered a lot of questions, so I eased them into it, but I felt that I basically confrontationally blurted out that she was going to die. I felt guilty because that's not the way I would typically tell somebody and something that I would consider being too abrupt and not sensitive enough. But their hopes were so high that, unless you flat-out told them that the radiation therapy that she was getting was only to slow the tumor growth down, not to cure it, they didn't understand. Their perception was that the radiation therapy was an attempt to cure. . . . I had the opportunity of overhearing conversations by Sarah's primary oncologist with Sarah's parents. The statement that was most difficult was, "Well, we are going to try this and then we will see." If a patient is going to die, saying that "we are going try this and then we will see" gives the impression that we will try this therapy, and, depending on how this therapy works, we will maybe try another therapy and "we'll see" gives the impression that there is hope for a cure.

———

12:1. The parents came to realize that there was little hope of recovery as the settings on the ventilator were getting worse instead of better. That was about 2 weeks into her being intubated. I was preparing myself and I was trying to drop hints but it was really going against the grain of everybody else. I was talking to some of the staff about planning to tell them that it was getting less likely that she was going to get off the ventilator. Two days before she died we had an end-of-life meeting. We had gotten a scare the night before because she became hypertensive, and there had been an earlier episode as well. So we had a couple of warnings, but this was like when older people have heart attacks and they think they can have heart attacks forever and then eventually one of them gets them. She came through these episodes every time. The family would think things were all right, but people were trying to say, "Well, things could happen," but I don't think they really believed that. The ICU staff was getting more uncomfortable with the situation by the weekend so, on Sunday, we had an end-of-life meeting with the family. The people in the meeting, besides myself and the parents, were the ICU attending, the ICU resident, the BMT attending, two of Alice's sisters, and a friend of the parents. The ICU attending was saying that her settings were on maximum and that we could increase the settings, but that might cause other problems and that there was very little place to go with those settings. He said that, as far as he was concerned, she was being resuscitated now and he asked the family if they wanted to think about it. They got very upset then. The father started stuttering and the mother was getting very emotional and they were hugging each other. Then the mother shouted out, "We were in this situation 22 years ago!"—she had a younger brother who had been in a motorcycle accident, and the mom had to make the decision to withdraw support at that time. I said, "Nobody ever said that we wanted you to withdraw support. Where did you get that idea from?" The ICU attending kept saying explicitly, "We are not asking you to withdraw life support," but that was the message they got. The others left the meeting first and I stayed with them and tried telling them it was not time to withdraw support, but again that's not what they heard. Later that evening they requested that Alice be taken off of the jet oscillator-type ventilator and put on the conventional ventilator so that they could hold her, which they couldn't do on the other ventilator, so that she could die in their arms.

That wasn't a totally unreasonable thing at the time, but the staff wasn't quite there yet, but they were there—they weren't and they were. You could have decided that, at any point, because she wasn't getting any better, she was getting worse. What happened next was that the chief of the transplant unit said, "Oh no, she's not ready to have support withdrawn. We don't want to do that right now," and he sent a strong message that that was not to be done. So the family was told that we weren't saying that but we were and weren't at the same time. I was trying to support the family through the decision that they had made, thinking it wasn't a totally unreasonable decision, where we were, and now they were getting this new message. By Monday we saw some mini-improvement. On Tuesday, we had a conference in the bone marrow transplant unit, and the chief was very clear that he wanted to push on the drug that might burn her kidneys and that he wanted to lower the immunosupression medication that she was on to give her lungs a chance to heal. I am not a very quiet person, so I said, "Well, in your experience, how many times have you seen somebody after transplant who has been on the ventilator this long come off the ventilator?" He said, "Well, it's a hard question to answer," and he walked away. So, I would say, fortunately, things started to go sour that night. She started to become hypotensive and the oxygen saturations went down.

12:1. The family experienced me as somebody who felt obliged to tell them the truth about what was going on, and so, when we got to the bad point, I wasn't saying there's no hope, by any shape, but this was a really serious situation and she was critically ill. She very quickly started doing worse, and the ICU attendings and I spent a lot of time speaking with the family about Alice's condition. It was very interesting because I only had one other case like this before—where the family starts running ahead of you and saying they are ready to start withdrawing support before you're actually ready to go there. We met with the family on Sunday because she had a deterioration Saturday night and was much sicker Sunday morning. Although the ICU attending didn't say it explicitly, the issue at hand was whether they wanted to make her DNR and not do chest compressions and stuff like that because she was on very high support and, if her heart stopped, there was nothing we were going to be able to do to get her back. We wondered how ugly they wanted to have it and thought we should begin to address the question so that, if something were to happen, we could say to the family, "This is what we talked about," instead of having to have that conversation in the midst of an emergency. I said, "I don't think we are ready to withdraw support. I'm not ready to say this is medically futile, but you have to know that things are worse. And we don't have to explicitly ask about DNR now, but we need to talk about it." Prior to this meeting, the ICU attending and I had agreed that we needed to talk to them about what would happen if she got sicker and we also needed to let them know that we were getting to the point of maximal support—we were pretty much there. We wanted them to realize this so that they could begin to think about how they wanted their daughter's life to end. It was just a general thing, but then, when the ICU attending had this conversation with them, he painted a gloomier picture than what I thought we were going in there to paint. He didn't say she's definitely going to die or anything like that, but it led the father to say, "Can we take her home to die?" So the attending said, "No," and that he was sort of thinking down the road; like if we switched her from the oscillator to the conventional ventilator, the parents might be able to hold her and interact with her more. We ultimately left the room, but the ICU attending left first so I had a chance to tell them alone that we were not saying that it was time to stop doing things for her, to stop fighting. I told them, "I'm a fight-to-the-finish kind of person, but she's your daughter and, if this doesn't start turning around in the right direction and things get worse, there are going to be decisions that you may want to be a part of and it is only fair to let you start thinking about those issues." The next thing I knew, when I returned to the ICU 3 hours later, the parents were asking to have support withdrawn and the ICU attending was saying, "Well, I can support that," and I said, "Wait a second, time out. I can't support that. I don't think that's where we are." I then learned from the oncology attending that apparently 22 years ago the mom's brother had been in a motorcycle accident and was declared brain dead and they had to make a lot of end-of-life decisions. So I think they went down that road that they'd been down before, which wasn't where their daughter was. So that evening, I met the mother and father and said, "I know where you've gone, but I don't feel comfortable going there yet because I don't think Alice is brain-dead, and blah, blah, blah." So I bargained with them for another 18 hours or so to see how things were, and we agreed that we weren't going to escalate support, which made complete sense. The next day a new ICU attending came on-service and he was not, in any way, saying to withdraw support. He was saying, "I can't say this is medically futile yet and very clearly it may be, but I just don't know it so I'm not there yet," because the only thing was her lungs—nothing else was a problem. So we went through this rather difficult dance with the family, and it was kind of excruciating with all of the other members of the family around. What happened over the next couple of days, after talking to us, the parents realized that we weren't likely to salvage the situation, but we weren't willing to throw in the towel completely until things were clearer. But it was weird because I think they had decided that the child was dying, and then they all started to get into this dying child mode. I guess, in a way, it was good because, when it finally happened, everybody was on the same page.

12:1. The next day the ICU attending suggested switching the ventilator she was on and the father said, "Well, if we switch and she doesn't do well, then I don't want her to go back on the one she's on now." This was difficult for me because he was willing to accept it, and I said, "Well, if you're saying you don't know that it's medically futile, if we switch to ventilator x and it doesn't work, we are obliged to switch back to one that is working." I had to say this to the parents, and that was difficult—not so much the emotions about the kid dying, but having to negotiate through this morass, knowing, in my heart of hearts, and conveying to the family that I thought it was a very real chance this kid was not going to pull out of it and, at the same time, considering the medical, legal, and larger ramifications of, what if I'm taking a kid to her death that isn't there yet. I felt that it was a very remote possibility that the kid was going to survive and, even though I was uncomfortable saying we are going to withdraw support, if the family had insisted, I would have been hard pressed to say, "No."

12:1. When different subspecialties become involved, conflicts arise as to what direction care should take. When it involves the transplant team and the ICU, the transplant team usually is asking for more aggressive care and the ICU attending is saying it's time to be less aggressive, and so it becomes a question of "Whose patient is it?" It didn't surprise me that this happened pretty much to pattern. What very often happens is that the ICU people, in the middle of the night, decide what to do. You can talk to a lot of people, but that is my impression, as I have seen it with my own patients and with other patients. They try to be sensitive to where the family is at and prepare the family for it. I wasn't surprised that the doctor said, "Okay, this is the time that we are going to do it [withdraw treatment]" because the family was pretty much there and was starting to have unrealistic hopes, and you don't want to continue that piece of it. The head of the transplant unit apparently was very angry because the ICU decided that he did not need to be informed at 3:30 in the morning that they were withdrawing treatment; that it could wait until 6:00 or 7:00. I am not sure what he would have done differently.

14:1. Our fellow was asking, "When do we decide to stop resuscitation if there's no DNR in place?" I think, with HIV, it's different than with other diseases. He had AIDS. There was no coming back. He was never going to have quality of life. He would never have any functioning. He had a virus that was progressively eating away his brain—not even HIV virus. People with AIDS are different because we had nothing to offer. Even if we brought him back, we have nothing. We have no medicines. We have nothing that's ever going to make him better. Compare that to a kid who has a bacterial infection and arrests. I would do everything possible to bring that kid back. But you have to make a judgment call. In some cases, you know what is going to be the quality of life for a kid but, in other cases, you wonder if it is going to be worth it. You sometimes have to make a judgment call, because there's nothing written on that. There's more to it than what it appears to be. Part of it too is how emotionally attached you can be to life and the process of living. It seems to me that some of the oncologists are very like that. They will do anything to prolong life, anything. I'm not so into pain and suffering. Three months ago, I had this kid that I was caring for for 8 years. She had AIDS and it got to the point when there was nothing I could do for her; I couldn't treat her anymore. We took her off the Bi-Pap [oxygen delivered under pressure through the nose], and she died in 10 minutes. Her mom was ready to do it, and so we didn't code her. I guess we're not supposed to have that kind of power as physicians, right? We're not in charge of making judgments about what's going to be a good quality of life for somebody. But we do that anyway. Then also there's the family and I think about what kind of torture is it going to be for them?

14:3. There are issues of how far therapy should have gone for him because all the doctors knew that he was close to dying, but there was sort of a slippery slope in terms of how much we were doing for him. Initially, he was on C-Pap, and we would say that that's all we'll do for him; we can give him oxygen and morphine to make him comfortable, but then he was on G-tube [gastric] feeds [directly into the stomach] but he wasn't tolerating

136

that. We thought he had aspiration pneumonia so we got a chest X ray and started antibiotics for that as well as getting blood cultures. Because he wasn't tolerating G-tube feeds, we discussed whether TPN [total parenteral nutrition, which is nutrition provided through a broviac or port] should be started. I felt that it was not an heroic measure so he was started on TPN but then we had to get TPN labs for him on a semiregular basis. Then there was the issue of trying to bring him back to G-feeds so we converted a G-tube to a GJ-tube [gastro-jejunal tube]. So, for someone who really should have had minimal interventions, we slowly did a lot more for him. But these decisions were coming from the infectious disease attendings who were bringing in other services as well—TPN was involved, GI was involved. The residents only had a chance to discuss these interventions after the fact. When the decision was made and we asked them why, they'd give us the reason, but it didn't feel like we were very involved in the actual decision-making process. They'd make a decision, then tell us, and eventually we'd get an explanation. But there was a sort of luxury of not being so involved in making the final decisions of really how far we should intervene because I'm not very well versed in terms of the ethical issues about what is considered heroic and what's not. So I was glad to defer to the attendings; it made my decisions easier.

15:7. Sometimes death is very sudden but sometimes there are interventions that you can do that can extend life, which enables the family to have more time to decide what they want to do and how they want to react. For example, at the end, George was on bi-pap. Had he not been on it, he probably would have died much sooner. It is hard to say because it was more time for the family but it may have been more time for George, suffering because it is not pleasant to have air forced into your face. So how do you make the decision? We want to save the children, and so it becomes a question of whether we are doing the right thing for the patient and the right thing for the family, or are we pushing things too far?

14:1. I knew that he would never get well enough to receive experimental drugs. I would love to have been proven wrong and that he got better, but it was pretty clear to me that this was going to be the time that he would die. So I found myself, during this last admission, working for his comfort. Whenever anybody wanted to do anything aggressive, I saw myself as trying to tone it down a little. For example, I was not even in favor of the first time they tapped his chest. Although I would say ultimately it was the right thing to do because it gave mom the message that we really, really did try everything. But then it was discussed by some people on rounds that we should do it again, or maybe we should put some kind of corrosive medicine into the chest fluid to sort of coalesce it so it doesn't expand as much. Different suggestions were made for ways to make him comfortable, which I thought would not make him comfortable and wouldn't meaningfully prolong his life. But it's right for the younger people to constantly be thinking of what can be done, as long as it doesn't get out of hand. But here, we're talking about aggressive ways of providing comfort, not cure, and a lot of young residents don't see that. They don't think that putting tubes in people the day before they die is necessarily aggressive. Let me explain it. Palliative care and end-of-life care involve trying to reduce suffering, and sometimes palliative care could even involve palliative chemotherapy or even experimental chemotherapy because it will raise hope and decrease pain, even if the end result is going to be the same. I have never, ever, objected to that if it wouldn't cause that child harm. In this scenario, there was some talk of using phase I experimental medicine. Phase I experimental medicine is different because it involves, first of all, the potential for unknown risks to the child; that is why it is phase I. Two, there is no known benefit; that is what phase I is. And three, it requires ongoing pharmokinetic studies, which means there has to be a lot of blood monitoring and urine monitoring. So even if the child were stable enough to go on one of those phase I trials, it definitely doesn't fit what I consider good palliative care. It is good care for someone who has enough of a life expectancy to possibly benefit from it. I think people in our group sometimes misuse phase I treatment. Because, by definition, to be eligible for a phase I trial, you are supposed to have a 2-month life expectancy, which means that your overall state of being is not so bad but bad enough that the tumor is growing. When someone has reached the point where they can't breathe without oxygen or outside support, you can't say that they have a 2-month life expectancy, so to offer a phase I trial in that situation isn't appropriate.

15:1. George wound up with this apparatus in his nose. It is called continuous positive airway pressure [CPAP]. It is not intubation and it leaves the mouth open and you can still talk and stuff, but it's fairly uncomfortable for a child to have this huge appliance on their head. It happened because one night, in the middle of the night, there were low saturations, meaning he wasn't getting good oxygen supply, and the resident who was on-call happened to be a very good resident but one of the more aggressive residents, and he put him on the CPAP. When I came in the next morning on rounds, I raised the issue that maybe this shouldn't have been done, that good medical care doesn't necessarily mean doing everything exactly by the book. But he was adamant that he had to do that because if he didn't, something could have happened way too rapidly and couldn't have been controlled. Ultimately, I have to admit, I gave him the credit because I wasn't there, I didn't see how George looked, I didn't have the burden of that moment and he did what he thought was right at that time. Maybe even for the mom, it was the right thing to do because it probably fit into her sense of not giving up too early. So, even though it is not my style— when someone is clearly dying, I would not so easily put them on this thing—it was done and he wound up staying on that until he died.

15:6. Mom was very much on top of everything—what's going on, what are we doing, why are we doing it. Even toward the end of life, it took a lot of convincing, on my part and on the part of the anesthesiologist, to let mom have us give George medication to make him comfortable with this incredible air hunger that he had had for the last week of his life. She was afraid that we were going to give him so much medication that it would stop him from breathing, and we had to frame it that the medication was making him comfortable. She was smart, and she knew that some of those medications that make you comfortable also make you sleep and, when you sleep, you don't breathe as well. She knew damn well that George was not breathing well and that the only thing that was keeping him alive was his drive to breathe. She knew we could have hastened his demise by taking the bi-pap off, but she would not allow it. She wouldn't let us do anything to hasten his death but she allowed us to do things to make him comfortable.

17:1. One day I was sitting in the room with her aunt and Christianna, and I was trying, in the gentlest way, to explain to Christianna that things weren't going as we wished and that she needed to think about what she wanted to do. I started by saying something to the effect of, "You know, the last treatment you got, which was intensive treatment, didn't work exactly as we'd like it to." I didn't even get specific; I didn't say she had lung metastases because the aunt didn't want her to know that because her mother had died of lung metastases. I just said, which was obvious, "Christianna, as you can see, the tumor on your leg hasn't gotten any smaller." I couldn't think of a more gentle way to say it. It was almost humorous that I'm sitting on this couch next to the aunt and she's kicking me as I'm trying to talk and I looked at the aunt and I looked at Christianna and I said, "I know you really don't want me to talk about this, but I think it's really important that we just think about different possibilities." And I said something to the effect of, "Christianna, one of the things you might want to think about is whether you want to go home." I spoke to her the way I would speak to most 15-year-olds, and the aunt was sitting there getting angrier and angrier. But what was more amazing to me was that Christianna got herself up in her bed, sitting erect, shoulders square, and looked at me and said, "I know I'm going to get better. I know I'm going to get cured" and completely cut off my conversation. I'll never know whether that was because the aunt was giving her signals—because the aunt was certainly giving me signals by kicking me—or whether it was entirely Christianna's own being. But I'm always telling people that, if a teenager doesn't want to hear something, they're going to tell you, and this was about as clear a message as I could get to back off. So although I was willing to push a little through the aunt's denial, I allowed Christianna her denial and I stopped.

18:2. It was distressing for me because the baby was dying and it had gotten to the point where you say, "When is enough enough?" How do you deal with the situation when you have a severe premature baby who isn't doing well and in this particular situation, where for religious reason, the parents wanted to do everything and anything? I started asking myself when do I stop being the physician and when am I starting to play God? I'm having a hard time with this whole thing of saying, "When's enough' enough?" I guess even for my own religious beliefs I question all this; doing everything for this baby goes against my own beliefs. I was brought up Catholic—pro-life, everything. I've never been for abortion or anything. That's one of the things that's always drawn me to this field—the life issue. But the gray zone has always been the hard issue and, for the most part, I morally or even scientifically have come to the conclusion that this was a baby who wouldn't survive. There come times when you can keep any baby alive with pressors and management to a point where eventually they survive, but then they end up with all of these horrible complications like cerebral palsy or lung disease so that 6,

7, 8 months later they end up dying anyway. I can't guess how a child would do, but sometimes you know, when a kid has had such a horrible start, that they're going to have awful problems, and it's hard to have to deal with the parents and tell them this. They always want concrete answers, and you can't give them that and that's a very frustrating feeling. In this situation, we left the decision to the parents and they wanted everything done and I felt, as a physician, I was being forced to keep ventilating a baby whom I knew was dying. I sometimes felt that we are more humane to animals than we are to humans. Then, on the reverse side, you have these parents who want nothing done on a baby that I don't think is that bad and I think will survive. I don't like being put in this situation either, and I always remind myself that I'm always going to do what's best for the child; I've always played it safe that way. We're humans, mistakes and all and things happen, and ultimately we can't dictate whether the child's going to be alive and be healthy or dead. If the parents want it, you can't withdraw support without going through a whole spiel and then you have to go through courts and who knows if it would even work. Over the past few years, I've seen that there's a lot of distrust of physicians and medicine. It almost feels like it's out of our hands and so sometimes I wonder if we're practicing medicine or practicing what the parents want. Sometimes, I get the sense that parents think we're withholding something from them, or like maybe we just don't want to work extra hard. In some situations, I sense this by the constant questioning of something. Sometimes you think, "Well maybe they just didn't understand," but there's other times when you know they understand but they don't want to hear it. I don't know, maybe it's my misunderstanding of the grieving process of what parents are going through. I think it's probably the most frustrating situation because I think there's grieving on both sides. From the parents' point of view and even as a physician because, as a physician, I know you can't save everyone, but I still, in some ways, feel like a failure.

18:8. It's okay for them to hope but, even when some of these infants survive, you don't know what's the long-term consequences and you have to tell the parents that. Most of the statistics are not good; there might be retardation or something. When parents ask, "What will happen?" we always tell them—mostly it's the physicians who tell them—that the possibility is very high that there will be complications and that they have to think about this. Recently, we had parents who didn't want their baby because of all the care that it would need. A lot of the nurses didn't feel that way and felt that the parents should not be saying that to the doctors or reach that kind of decision. We had a meeting with our director to discuss the decision of the parents to discontinue the support. Even though the baby was on a ventilator and could not be weaned off or extubated and he had a bleed also, he was very alert, very active. So most of the nurses were upset about the parents' decision to take the baby off the ventilator. Speaking for myself, I think the parents have the right to decide what to do because they're the ones who are going to be taking care of the baby after they leave here.

20:1. With advances in neonatology, you realize, unfortunately, that the technology that one can use to support life may not be the best to optimize or continue survival. My experience, coming from a more junior time, where I have children who still stay in touch or families who stay in touch and who have profoundly handicapped children as a result of severe intraventricular hemorrhage, has made me more conscious about informing parents, as fully as I can, about the potential for neurological deficits in the presence of grade IV intraventricular hemorrhage. We can never predict absolutely, but there are national statistics that we can quote. But then, there are also children we have seen, although as incidental cases, that surprise us in how well they're doing based on their perinatal findings. But this was an at-risk triplet pregnancy where the mom was admitted at 23 weeks and crossed over to the legal 24 weeks, but that didn't affect the continuum of life for these fetuses that were at risk. I shared that with the parents and I was putting myself in the teaching role of helping them through the decision. I wanted to protect them from sending at least two severely handicapped children into the world, and that was a part of my conversation. The parents wanted to know what kinds of development problems there would be, "How would my baby be affected?" One of the babies had a far more horrendous course than the other and it was clear that this baby was unlikely to survive and it would only be a matter of time when we would remove him from support; that's what I told them, but I also said, "There is absolutely no hurry in removing him from support. We can wait overnight if you want a second neonatal doctor to speak with you. That would be fine." I discussed it with three of my colleagues, in case they would like somebody else to come down. With the third baby, it was categorical that this baby was unlikely to survive and that it would be a matter of time and they could choose to stop now, or we could continue and keep a DNR order in place so that, if the baby's heart rate stopped, we would not provide any more intervention methods than we were currently doing. We were actively providing complete resuscitation to the baby at the time. With the second baby, the hemorrhage was severe but not catastrophic, but it was likely that this baby would have learning problems and certain motor problems, and would need assisted living; it depended on what happens. But I could tell the parents, without hesitation, that it was more than likely there would be some neurological deficits in this baby. It was their decision but I would be in agreement, if they chose to stop, and I would've continued to the point where it was utterly useless, if they didn't. So it was a timing issue. I also shared with them that we occasionally support children to a time when it is inappropriate to remove life support; when the children recover vital functions that will keep them in a manner that they will breathe and sustain themselves but that the parents would still have a neurologically impaired baby but then it would be inappropriate to remove them from care that was sustaining them. . . . Generally, babies don't present neurological deficits until they are in the first or second year of life, so that even the profoundly affected baby in our nursery may end up doing what we ask of them, which is to nipple feed, to breathe, to poop and pee, all the things that we like babies to do. They may have some limitations or some possible clues to neurological deficits, but they don't manifest them until the times when the neuro-developmental milestones are not being met and it becomes clear, with successive months and years, that the children are not at the level of other children. Some parents accept it, but it certainly can be a depressing sense of ongoing loss as your child does not achieve what other children are achieving and you're accepting the gravity that this child will need extra help. The parents of these children specifically said, "Who would care for them when we are gone?" and I think that's every parent's worry; if they had profoundly handicapped children and if something happened to them, they would be leaving a legacy to somebody else to take care of their children. I told them, on the day the children were born—and they died on the third day of life—that this is a time to sit as parents and discuss with each other if and when they would choose to stop support. I've seen times when we delay withdrawal because one or the other parent is not at the same level as the other. These parents indeed had very meaningful conversations with each other and, when I left them alone to talk among themselves after telling them the bad news of the grade IV hemorrhages on the third day, within the hour they had come to this conclusion, and within 4 hours the children were dead. It was a situation that they had been thinking about evidently for at least a week, since she went into preterm labor but clearly, once the children were born it became a lot more critical.

20:2. Previously, doctors didn't notify parents about the option of withholding support—I'm talking from my experience. In the literature, there are so many cases like that, and in many places it depends on the physician himself. Some are more willing to talk to the parents and give them the option to withhold support, especially in grade IV intraventricular hemorraging. Some doctors encourage parents to keep the baby alive no matter what the consequences in terms of quality of life but that's more likely in grade III. When we have grade III, and sometimes it progresses, sometimes it stabilizes, many people do not approach the parents. I also might do the same, because with grade III there is still some chance, although it's a slim chance, of near normal. So it's not a routine thing that, with grade III, we approach the parents about withdrawing support. But here it is discussed on many levels and we don't depend on one ultrasound; we repeat the ultrasounds and discuss it with the attending on call, and with the radiologist and with the neurologist who's always here. Also, we have ethics meetings where we discuss some of the cases.

20:3. I want to give children as much of an opportunity to do whatever they want with their lives so, for me, they have their whole lives in front of them, if I can get them through this point. I don't really think of what they will not be able to do once they finish their NICU course; I think of what they will be able to do if we get them out of this acute stage. I look at all the children here as potentials for the future and realize that amazing stories could be written about all of them. That's how I look at it; they have potential to do lots of things with their lives. But once the neurological data is in and you have evidence that neurologically this child is going to be devastated and the quality of life for him in the future is going to be devastated—if you have data to support that—then I think it is the parents' decision whether or not they want to continue. If they choose to do that, then, as a physician, we have to support life, but I don't like making decisions based on possibilities, because I always think the possibility of them doing good things is greater than the possibility of them living a horrible life. I've heard stories that, once you've been around long enough and have seen some of these babies grown up and how devastated they are, you question if this is best for the child and for the family, but I'm not there yet. My eyes are still bright. I'm not there yet so until I get there, I'm just going to continue to see everything positively.

Pain and Suffering | 5

There are some things
worse than dying.

— PROVERB

Consider the following advice given to parents whose children are dying in hospitals: "If your child has to die, he can die peacefully. You can make sure he is free of pain. You can make sure that everyone has a chance to say good-bye."[1] Offering parents this kind of unconditional assurance overlooks the disturbing realities of what it is like to care for a child, when it becomes increasingly apparent that curative intent is failing and staff begin to question how best to proceed. The complexities and uncertainties of pain management and symptom control often prevent pediatricians from clearly differentiating between curative treatment and the prolonged suffering of a child before an inevitable death.[2] For example, at the end of their lives children commonly have the following, sometimes intractable, symptoms: pain, anorexia, fatigue, dyspnea (gasping for air), constipation, vomiting food and blood (hematemesis), bleeding, seizures, fear, anxiety, and terminal agitation.[3] Children who have cancer experience considerable (moderate to severe) treatment-related pain throughout their treatment protocols.[4] However, as shown in the few pediatric palliative care studies that exist, issues of pain management and symptom control at the end of life do not appear to be so difficult to resolve. These studies promote false ideas that satisfactory end-of-life care is not achieved because of medical mistakes or inadequate staff training and, therefore, children were made to suffer unnecessarily. Such ways of thinking lead bereft parents to feel guilty for not taking greater control of their child's care and for failing to do "the right thing" for their child.

A recent retrospective study of end-of-life care for children dying from cancer at one of the nation's preeminent children's hospitals found that, in their last month of life, parents reported that 89 percent of 103 children suffered a lot or a great deal; they suffered primarily from pain and/or dyspnea. Despite efforts to treat children for specific symptoms, treatments were successful in only 27 percent of children with pain and 16 percent with dyspnea.[5] Similar findings have been reported in adult studies of end-of-life care. One study, for example, found that a third of elderly patients were in "unnecessary" pain during the 24 hours prior to their death and two-thirds had pain in the last month of their lives.[6] Another study found that only one-quarter of adults with prostate cancer were judged, by their physicians (but not by patients and their families), to be either asymptomatic or only slightly limited.[7] Such findings support a widely held belief that dying patients receive less relief from pain and symptoms during end-of-life care than they should and that it is even more pronounced when the dying patients are children.[8] For example, there are reported discrepancies between amounts of postoperative analgesia (as adjusted for body size and weight) administered to adults and children for the same diagnoses and procedures.[9]

Part of the problem is that pediatric staff in tertiary care medical centers do not recognize the extent of children's suffering at end of life because their training emphasizes cure as a goal of aggressive treatments over caring for dying children. This finding is not surprising when one considers that children with cancer account for the largest proportion of deaths from medical causes but for only 4 percent of childhood deaths each year.[10]

In end-of-life care, children experience varieties of pain stemming from invasive procedures, toxic therapies, disease, and psychological factors. More so than adults, the correspondence between trauma and the experience of pain in children is highly unstable and dependent on a variety of situational factors.[11] "Children's perception of pain is defined by their age and cognitive level; their previous pain experiences, against which they evaluate each new pain; the relevance of the pain or disease causing pain; their expectations for obtaining eventual recovery and pain relief; and their ability to control the pain themselves."[12]

When there is no hope for cure, children are provided with whatever can be done to relieve pain, manage symptoms, and provide a decent quality of life. There even is broad agreement that "analgesics may be ethically administered to terminally ill patients at doses risking death due to respiratory depression, provided that lower doses and other means have proven inadequate, that the intention is to relieve pain and not to induce death, and that permission has been obtained with full disclosure of the risk of death."[13] But, with children, for a myriad of reasons that are absent among dying adults, uncertainties always remain about when hope for cure can be abandoned. Also, because levels of pain and suffering are subjective (not purely nociceptive or a direct function of tissue pathology), culturally understood and expressed, pain management always is difficult. Moreover, because pain is particularly difficult to measure in children, whether using physiologic indicators, systematic observations of behavior, or reports by children themselves, medical staff and families are faced with difficult decisions concerning when the uncertainty of beneficial outcomes is outweighed by the probability of harm. The multidimensional aspects of pain include the interaction of cognitive, emotional, socioenvironmental, and nociceptive aspects and therefore suggest a multidisciplinary approach to pain management that goes beyond sensory biological models. Best practices to pharmacologically manage and assess pain in children have been limited owing to the lack of standardized and randomized trials, which often are justly precluded because they raise pragmatic and ethical issues in caring for children.[14] Bridging the gap between our limited knowledge and everyday clinical practice remains "a major difficulty."[15]

Hence, the aim of comforting patients by providing adequate pain management and maintaining quality of life is an elusive one. This is a sensitive issue for health care providers, and they are accordingly reluctant to discuss it. They find it difficult, if not frustrating, to know when to relinquish hope of curative treatment and to provide the palliative means for children to have calm and comfortable deaths. This issue affects parents as much as the medical staff. Despite parents' avowed primary concern with maintaining their child's quality of life in the absence of pain and discomfort[16] and recognizing their children's fear of pain from medical trauma,[17] when considering end-of-life decisions, parents will often press for increasingly more aggressive care for their child, even when it significantly compromises quality of life and pain management.

Issues surrounding pain management at the end of a child's life are captured in the following narratives. The first one is from a registered nurse who is a distinguished member of a pediatric pain team. She talks about caring for a 5-year-old who, in spite of his caregivers' heroic efforts to achieve a cure, died suffering in intractable pain. Her narrative raises a range of personal and professional issues that, in the end, exemplify how, in practice, principles of palliative care and comfort come up against the pressing and immediate need to find ways to save a child's life.

2:8. One of the things that is very humbling about the business that we're in is that we realize that there are a lot of things that we can do that make a difference but, also, there are many things for which we can't make a concrete, recognized medical difference. And when it was vis-à-vis the issue of pain with Devon—which was an important aspect of his care—we were not able to make a measurable difference no matter what we did, and it became very frustrating because it was very sad. You felt that you were failing. Devon's suffering was part of the physiologic triggers of pain, what we know must be going on physiologically, chemically, and biologically, but this was different from what his perception was of his suffering. Pain is really a perception of one's suffering, and the way that one perceives pain may actually have to do not only with the actual stimulus or trigger but also with the way that that's interpreted and the way that that's expressed. As Devon got sicker and sicker, he got more frustrated, and the way he was able to articulate his pain may even have been more than just the abdominal pain that we were trying to treat but a kind of ongoing suffering. So we weren't just treating the pain itself, we were treating the subjective perception of his suffering as well. There were times when we were unclear how much of it was pain and how much of it was that he had gotten used to being able to reference his belly and he was actually able, on some level, to translate a lot of what he was feeling into his belly. There were times when we thought that, "My belly hurts, my belly, my belly, my belly" was a mantra that he may have developed. But it was kind of hard to take apart what you could treat with medication and what were other things that needed to be treated in other ways. Our desire was to make more of a difference. If the goal of care for him had been comfort, then we would have been able to treat his pain differently, because when you define the goal of care as comfort, you're willing to deal with the side effects of sedation. That is, you might give a dosage of pain medicine that might put your child at risk for something else, like increasing respiratory compromise. If the attending says that the goal of treatment is to make the child comfortable and that you can use the narcotics and the medicine to make the child comfortable, then you are able to use them with more latitude than we were actually using them with Devon. We probably would have pushed them up higher, but, in his case, the overall goal was to get him cured—so, would we have used higher doses otherwise? Probably.

The morning that I found out that Devon died—I saw him that last day in the ICU after he had been transferred—it became clear to me that the level of suffering in this kid was so visible and so palpable that I thought that this was an exercise in medical futility. We needed to take a step back, because somewhere we had lost the perspective. We were dealing with him one organ system at a time. We were dealing with a child that we had divided into arms and legs, livers and lungs, heart and kidneys, and what was going on in his head, but we had lost perspective on what was going on with the child and how we could really be of service for him at this point. I said to the attending, "This little boy needs permission to die, and we need to start redefining our goal of care for this kid." If our goal of care had been, "Let's relieve his suffering," and then, if he sleeps because we're relieving his suffering, then we've relieved his suffering. If you give enough narcotic, eventually you may get to the point where the child is sedated so the question is, "Is it ok to have this child sedated?" Well, with Devon, the goal was to keep him alive, so the answer would be "No," because, then he would probably need help with his breathing; he wouldn't be able to use his lungs properly. The question I had was whether the dialogue was ever had with the family that, if we're going to give him narcotics and the goal is still to cure him, how much narcotic are you willing to give him vis-à-vis having him awake for you versus asleep and comfortable? Because if you compromise respiratory function, you get into a whole bunch of other bad outcomes as they relate to the ability to move that child toward a healthy cure. The idea to transplant this child was a last-ditch attempt to offer some salvage therapy, not curative therapy. We didn't see this as a cure for him, but as another opportunity to treat, with an eye toward hopefully giving him that very slim chance of getting ahead of the disease. But I never saw this transplant as a real option in terms of curative therapy for him and so, when weighing the checks and balances of that, when it comes to children, it's very hard to withdraw therapy. It's also very hard to have conversations with families where you really present options. I'm not an oncologist, but were the options truly presented without giving the parents a false sense of hope for a therapy that may not give them the outcome that they were truly looking for? We never moved to a palliative care mode in this child.

In describing the role of the pain service in this institution, our mandate is to treat pain, but our obligation is also to look at pain as a continuum of care. We are very interested in evolving that aspect of what our true mandate is—to treat pain along a continuum. To treat pain but also to treat at the end stages of life when you shift your goals of care and goals of cure to not just treating the pain but redefining the goals and treating the suffering and helping the family toward those later stages of the disease which are somehow defined differently. So, when does salvage therapy end and palliative care begin? Ultimately, I think it's the oncologist's decision and the family's decision, but I think that the way that information is presented is critical to families. Families will hear what they want to hear because of how information is presented and if you've developed a relationship that is trusting and truly valuable with the family, then you can be there for them as they move to the realization that their child has cancer, to the fact that the first therapy failed, to the valiant attempts to get ahead of the disease, toward realizing that we've lost some ground, to then reaching for straws and pulling at opportunities that might make a difference, and get to the point where you can say, "We have tried and tried and tried. We've done our best. Let's talk about where we are now and about what's important," and be able to talk about death and dying as it relates to a child's illness and disease. I think that's a place where we don't do so well, and it's interesting because I watched some of the oncologists here and I'm very impressed with the way that they move toward that, but I wonder where those decisions are made and why, sometimes, they're not made or made too late. In this child's case, I'm not sure that anybody ever had that conversation with the family, except maybe moments or hours or just days before. Did they ask us if things were working or why they weren't working? No. Did they tell us that his pain was not well controlled? Yes. One of the things that we have to come to terms with is our communication with the oncology service around this issue. When do we [the pain service team] have the privilege to begin to use that language or those words that begin to make dying a part of the dialogue of care? I think that part of the care of any child who has cancer is to know that the end result may be that the child dies. So how can we as a team really work with that, to have all the players involved on board as we move toward this continuum? To do this, we need to meet more as a group. We need to be more involved in multidisciplinary meetings, and we have been, in some difficult cases, but we never met for Devon, which was interesting to me. Although everybody knew that he was dying, nobody ever came together to address the fact that he was dying and what were we doing for this child, what where we doing for his family, what were we doing for ourselves? So, in a sense, we failed him here. He was transferred to the ICU hours before he died. When you're transferred to the ICU, it's usually not to let somebody die quietly.

I heard it said once that the role for the pain service really starts at the time of diagnosis when you can develop a relationship with the family and with the oncologist, who is the key point person. But that's not feasible. It's not possible for us to get involved with all the children who have cancer in this institution, because we don't have the resources and manpower to do that. We've got many fingers in so many pies and, given the extraordinary demands that are put on the service right now, we just don't have the resources to be able to be a consistent presence. But it's still important to have more of a dialogue around the issues and talk about a part of a child's life that's often very difficult to talk about because children are not comfortable with dying and providers are not comfortable with dying children. Losing a child is a big deal for the physicians, the nurses, and for the family. So it's not an easy thing to talk about. The dialogue for death needs to happen a lot sooner than the moment of crisis and if with Devon it didn't happen sooner than the moment of crisis when he died in the ICU, then it should have. But for the attendings in pediatric oncology, I think ego gets involved and they lose perspective. They have good intentions and they really, truly want to serve the patient, but sometimes you think that you can do anything despite the odds, so they'll push forward and take the very long or broader view that their mission is to advance the science of treating children with cancer. And yes, that is something I think that everyone should be committed to, because the way we treated 30 years ago is not the way that we treat today, and the way that we will treat 30 years from now is not the way that we're treating today. But that's different than having your perspective on the child, even if it's not for the sake of the science. I hope they've learned something from Devon. Devon told different providers that he couldn't do this anymore, and I'm not really sure, at 5 years, what he was saying, but it saddened me to have heard those words. I think children can tell you, along the way, what they can do and what they can hear and what they can handle. I don't know the mind of a 5-year-old and I certainly didn't know the mind of Devon, but I was very struck with the fact that he could use those words, "I can't do this anymore." I was very struck with the fact that he could hold his Teddy and find comfort in that. I was very struck with the fact that he could cry out to Jesus and, on some level, in whatever way, was able to find comfort. I also was very struck by the impression that one of his attendings shared with me, which was that moments after he died she saw again the child that was not riddled with suffering and distress. That the look on his face was one of quiet peace and resolution. I remember that child's hands trembling. We did not succeed with that kid; we failed him. I have this vision of the last time I saw him. He was trembling and he was shaking, his brow was furrowed, he was agitated, his hands were shaking. It was just horrible, horrible, horrible, horrible, horrible, and here we were pumping pints into him and sending him for MRIs. Maybe it was his way of saying, "You know what? It's over, done, time out." It's not every child that you're struck by, but he was one of those. Yes, everything that you do in this business impacts on you, but not everything impacts to the same degree, in the same way. This was one of those children that really touched me and that really had an impact on me. It's hard to do this work.

The next narrative considers how the physiologic experience of pain can differ from anxiety, distress, and suffering. Although, at one point, Devon was clinically getting better, his pain was getting worse. It led the staff to question, "What are you actually treating here?"

2:8. He got a narcotic in more than one form. We were escalating doses of methadone. Before that he was on a continuous infusion of narcotic. So we needed to give him, or somebody, the ability to rescue him when he had these episodes. So that was what the [PCA, patient controlled analgesic] button was for.[18] Then the background pain and the tolerance and dependency he developed on narcotics was treated with either the continuous infusion, Fentanyl or methadone. We knew that Devon's pain was probably not going to get better and we anticipated that it was probably going to get worse. What we kept being told by the primary service was that his pain wasn't in proportion to what was going on with him clinically; that there were clinical signs that he was getting better but his pain was getting worse, which made me wonder how much of what Devon was going through was actually experiencing pain versus experiencing suffering. The suffering was more about being sick for so long, being hospitalized for so long, feeling bad for so long, and how that all translated into, "My belly hurts." All of these measures that they were using were pointing to the fact that he was getting better, but Devon was expressing more and more distress. It makes you wonder how reliable the measures were, but you make decisions based on objective indicators. So that's where the element of suffering comes in and leads you to wonder, "What are you actually treating here?" You would expect, if somebody's feeling better, that they would require less drugs to feel comfortable all the time. That never happened for Devon. There was never a trend where he was using less medication, which reflected the fact that clinically he might be improving; that never went hand-in-hand with him saying, "My belly hurts less," and demonstrating this by using less drugs. So I wonder how much of what we were treating was pain versus his perception of his pain and suffering as it translated into, "My belly hurts." That's why I think this kid was suffering for a lot longer than we ever knew.

2:2. He would always say, "My belly hurts, my belly hurts" and the last week he was like, "I can't take this pain anymore. It's hurting too much. I can't stand the pain anymore," and Devon was not a kid to complain. He would be sick but he would never complain, and the main thing was the belly pain, "Rub my belly, rub my belly." Toward the end, he was like, "Oh, it's hurting too much. I can't stand the pain. I can't stand this pain anymore. I can't take it any more. It's hurting too much, it's hurting too much," and it's hard to say what he meant. When you think back, and now that he's dead and I've had time to sit back and think about all that has happened, maybe what he was saying was he didn't want to go on living but we just didn't know; we didn't understand how a 4- or 5-year-old kid tells you that he doesn't want you to keep him alive anymore—the last couple of days, he said it to a lot of people, to the attending on service, to me, to his mom, to his grandma, and his mom even commented on his dying. She said that he was tired and the pain was too much and he didn't want it anymore. And I would tell him, "Devon, I'm sorry. I would, if I could, make the pain go away. I'm going to rub your belly." After a while he didn't want to push his PCA button anymore. When you think about it, maybe he didn't want it. He was on a PCA and he wasn't pushing it as much as he could. I asked him once, and he said he didn't want to push it. He didn't tell me why. He would tell me he wanted me to rub his belly, and I took that as he thought that would be more relief than the medicine. We knew the medicine wasn't working like it was supposed to be working.

2:10. For the last 3 months, he just talked about his pain and how he wanted somebody to help him control his pain. He was really good at verbalizing his pain, his frustration, and his anxiety. So we would try to do different things to cope with it. We would do breathing techniques, or we would talk about how maybe thinking about different things that make him happy can help him cope a little bit, but he was definitely frustrated. One of the things that really helped him and that made him smile, even toward the end, was talking about all the support that he had from different people. He loved to talk about all the people that were in his life. He would name all those people. He would name his grandparents, he would name mom and dad, he would name his younger brother, he would name his doctors—everyone by name. He memorized the names of everyone that came into his room and what they did, and liked to go over that again and again. That really seemed to comfort him. Also, his faith really helped him cope better. Whenever his tummy hurt, he would always pray and he would say, "Jesus take my pain away." He was so eloquent in his prayers. And he had this teddy bear that had angel wings and it played this gospel hymn, "Jesus loves me, this I know," and he kept singing that over and over again. That was definitely comforting to him.

Other narrative accounts about how difficult it was to manage pain and control suffering, for different reasons and in different cases, include the following:

8:1. They have medicine that will paralyze a patient because you have them on a ventilator and sedated and you don't want them to move or fight or fight too much, even though they are not in pain, they may move and fight just because they don't like where they are and then it can damage their lungs but isn't necessarily preventing them from feeling any pain. So you don't know from examining them or looking at them if they are really feeling pain underneath because they are not responding to anything. William was so sick and his lungs were so bad that he needed to be paralyzed and sedated, but you give an amount of pain medication also. They go through periods where they lift those medicines so as to not mask the exam and, then, they can monitor their heart, their response to vital signs, to know if they seem to be having any discomfort. That is how they decided to dial up the pain medication, and they were doing that with him. You always are telling families that you are making them comfortable, but you wonder, "Are you really?" I haven't had patients that have been that sick and have come out to say that they remember having a lot of pain.

16:6. He was in a lot of abdominal pain. He was unable to urinate. He had, from the onset of his disease, not just a central line, like most of our patients, but also two drains coming out of his back because of the complications of his disease. He had a drain put in in an attempt to free up his liver, being bright yellow all the time, wasting away from up here but having his entire lower body swell up like a balloon. The pain that came with his disease at the end was because it was obstructing anything and everything in his abdomen. We had to give him ridiculous doses of narcotics to make him comfortable. Then, the very last thing was when he had a pleural effusion [water accumulating between the two membranes covering the lungs], and it became difficult for him to breathe. There is nothing more distressing to a human being than the sensation of not being able to catch your breath, especially if you're awake. If you're asleep or comatose, then it doesn't make a difference, but he was fully awake the entire time, and that's suffering and not something that you want to have happen. He didn't really talk about his pain so much, but you could tell if he was in direct pain or uncomfortable because he wouldn't get up out of bed. When he was feeling okay, even in these last days, he would get up and walk around the floor chatting with people, and when he wasn't feeling okay, he stayed in his room in bed. So that was how you could tell, but if you would ask him directly, he'd tell you what was hurting, what wasn't. If you asked him, "Is the pain medication enough?" he would say "Yes" or "No," depending on what the situation was, but he wouldn't volunteer the information, but you could tell just from the comport of his body and whether he was up and walking around or not. He was narcotized most of the time, but at the end, he was not having pain—or at least no pain that he would relate to us—and he was able to get up and walk around. But at the end with the respiratory distress, we had to give him benzodiazapines to prevent him from feeling that he couldn't catch his breath. We controlled that sensation, but then that made him basically just sleep; there's only so much you can do when you're not going to take any further drastic measures. In a sense, we were putting him to sleep to allow him to die peacefully.

16:2. His pain was being managed by the pain service but he still had been in pain from the regimens that they had him on, and one of the primary reasons for admitting him was to get his pain under control. He was on so many pain meds that it wasn't from lack of trying that he was still having pain. It was frustrating that we couldn't eventually get a comfortable level.

Sometimes it is pediatricians who are reluctant to accept medical futility and shift from curative intent to palliative care and comfort. However, most times when pediatricians and parents are not on the same page, it is the parents who are unable to accept when enough is enough and, consequently, resist appropriate palliative care and sedation.

1:1. At times, she was too conscious for her own good. The family wanted to have the feeling that they could talk to her and hold her hand and pat her and touch her and all of these things, which are clearly very understandable. However, when you are so critically ill, a lot of times the stimulation, no matter what the intention is, can be counterproductive. There were instances when we wanted to sedate her and the family was refusing to let her be sedated. It's a problem because overstimulation translates into physiologic changes. Your heart rate goes up, your blood pressure goes up, and it may go up to points that clearly become harmful, really dangerous in some cases. Also, there were a lot of instances when she was trying to breathe on her own and you counteract the ventilator then; you work and expend energy that you should use for more vital functions. There is a wide spectrum of all of these things, but there were definitely times that she seemed to be very anxious. I don't think that it was a pain issue because, by conventional standards at least, I think we were providing good pain control. However, she was very much aware of what was going on around her, and she was trying to communicate; she was trying and she could not do it. There were times that she was communicating. You would ask her a question, and she would make some response. She had tubes in every part of her body, she could not move her neck, she was intubated, so clearly, for any conscious human being, this was extremely unpleasant. It was practically impossible to separate, for any given moment, how much of it was her being conscious and trying to communicate something, or whether it was mental status changes due to her illness, or a combination of the two. Regardless of which one of the two it was, the point is, you had somebody who was actively trying to move around and fight the ventilator, and this was counterproductive. Although, in the parents' eyes, that was a sign of life, medically, it was not. It was not the best thing you can do for the patient. We had to work with the family and try to explain that to them.

3:1. They would not use the morphine PCA because they said that she wasn't feeling any pain—but she was. She was wagging her head back and forth groaning. She was restless and couldn't sleep at night, and I said to the parents, "This is pain. She's in tremendous discomfort" and I'd say, "Elsa, are you having pain?" and she'd say, "No-o-o," and she'd groan. I told them, "She doesn't have the vocabulary to even articulate what it is that she's feeling. I'm sure there are no words for what she's feeling," but they would not give her the rescue doses of morphine because she'd sleep or they were afraid that it would cause respiratory depression—because they were savvy enough to know that—and that would take her from them sooner. They would say, "It's our belief, it's our culture that you don't make things happen before they need to happen and, when she goes, that's God's will and so we're not going to hasten anything by giving her pain medication." I had a real hard time with that because I was watching a young woman suffer incredibly.

15:1. At the end, when George was dying, he was really uncomfortable—he was pulling his tubes out—and so I was pushing to give medication so that he wouldn't suffer, but his mom wouldn't let me do it. She would prefer having him uncomfortable and having him open his eyes and grab her and say bye to everybody rather than end the suffering. I really had to push her. I would say, "He is suffering. He is suffering. I need to give him something. He is not going to go faster, don't worry." I really had to push a lot, which hardly ever happens. Usually parents get so scared that they cannot see their kid suffer so much; they just tell you to make him comfortable. And she was like, "No, no, no, he is not uncomfortable." She just wanted to see him awake, for whatever reasons. And the way he looked was also quite scary. He would look at me like he was asking for some kind of help. Kind of staring at me like, "What are you doing?" or "Why aren't you doing anything?" That was the way I was perceiving it. Maybe she was perceiving him as wanting to be with her. Obviously, we were seeing him in a different way because, to me, he had the look of somebody who was scared, who needed something.

Parents are not the only ones who resist the staff's attempts to administer adequate pain management. Sometimes adolescent patients are afraid of pain management:

9:8. He had a horrible night and needed to go lie in a bed when he arrived. He was here all day and was in a lot of pain and uncomfortable, which was hard for me to see. He had been on pain medicine, but John is the type of kid who does what he wants to do, so his oncologist and I negotiated with him to get him to really understand what we were trying to tell him would help him. I explained to him everything that I was doing, and he knew that he was getting fluids and blood and more blood. He said he had pain, and he was fighting me that he didn't want to take pain meds because he was itchy. I said, "Well, I'll give you Benadryl in the IV" and we negotiated that and he said, "Okay" but then said, "I don't need the pain medicine." I said, "John, we had a deal" and he said, "Alright, you're right" and then he agreed to take it.

7:8. She had a lot of pain and was seen by the pain team. She was on pain medication, including methadone and oxycodone. You could tell she was in pain by her grimacing and moaning. Sometimes there's crying, and although I don't remember Carol being a real crier, there was a lot of grunting with her movement and restlessness. Was it pain versus air-hunger?—I don't know—but if you then give her methadone or give her an oxycodone and it makes a difference, then who cares whether the narcotic is acting as an analgesic or as a respiratory depressant? At least, if overtly, she's somehow looking calmer and more peaceful, it's accomplishing something. You don't want them to be somnolent; you don't want them to be asleep but maybe, sometimes, it comes to a point where you have to. You can tell pain and it doesn't matter the age. Babies don't have to tell you; you can tell, and especially with a baby that we've worked with almost everyday for months. We know what she looks like when she's happy.

Trying to manage the pain and suffering of preverbal infants presents particular challenges for the staff and raises issues of infants' awareness and capacity to express their sense of pain and anxiety.

9:8. When you're treating a child who doesn't speak, you got to look at the vital signs to treat pain. When the blood pressure is sky high and the heart rate is sky high and if he has a fever and that is the reason his heart rate is so high, you give him something for the fever, that should take care of that. If his blood pressure is still sky high and you have eliminated all possibilities by giving him medication, then it's a sign of pain. You look at the vital signs because usually that is the only clue you have. You expect the pain meds to bring the heart rate and the blood pressure back to normal levels. We put them on morphine drips. We are very pro pain management here, and we put them on drips and we make sure that we are not denying pain; that they are sufficiently sedated. We give them morphine for the pain, and we want them to be sedated, nice and mellow, calm, so that they don't feel anything. Sometimes, we paralyze them, but a lot of times they are so sick that they can't even move so they don't even need to be paralyzed. The morphine and the sedation take care of that, and they don't feel the pain. That is what you hope for because that would be the worst thing. Families question that, if you sedate the child, the less opportunity you have to allow the heroic interventions to work, but if you give them too much, the blood pressure drops. So you put them on medication to bring the blood pressure up and you give them fluid or whatever med to correct that problem, but you also have them well sedated and in a pain free state. . . . If I gave him 15 milligrams of morphine at one time, he would be dead, but if I gave him 15 milligrams in the course of 24 hours, it is a whole different ball game. When they arrive in the ICU, you start them on the lowest dose and, then they get used to it, so you have to keep going up, and going up, and going up. You get to a point where you are in max, and you are like, "Oh my God, I am giving enough to kill a horse and the kid is like a wild man." So it all depends. We know how much to give and know the balance so that they are pain free, sedated, and we can take care of their physical needs without jeopardizing their situation.

12:1. One of the things that we do well in the ICU is help people die, regardless of whether somebody is "do not resuscitate," "do not intubate," whatever. We can make them more comfortable by giving them more sedatives and narcotics for comfort and pain resolution than the other divisions are able to do. So one of the reasons patients are transferred to the ICU is if there is a question about how we can make them more comfortable. It is difficult to tell parents that you are going to give their child as much pain medicine as it takes to make her comfortable and that the downside of giving all this medicine is that it will stop their child from breathing and make her die—it is a difficult situation. If the parents understand that and have accepted the fact that their kid is going to die, then we can talk about not wanting her to die in pain and so, if it means that they die 3 days sooner but free of pain, that is okay. At that point, pretty much anybody, from a nurse, intern, resident, fellow, attending in whatever subspecialty, can manage that patient's pain because there was no limit to how high you can go and no worrying about what the consequence were because the patient was going to die.

Staff Reacting | 6

We flee from logic and order
because they remind us that we
must die, while illogic and disorder
soothe us by proving that nothing
makes sense, that nothing is
certain, not even death.

— HAROLD BRODKEY
Stories in an Almost Classical Mode

How the staff reacts to participating in pediatric end-of-life care raises issues across a continuum of professional and personal concerns. Along the continuum, four themes arise from the narrative segments in this chapter: (1) staff communicating with patients and families, (2) staff relating with one another, (3) staff coping and moving on, and (4) staff expressing the need for education and training in end-of-life care.

Communicating with Patients and Families

The first theme, communicating with patients and families, is the nexus of appropriate end-of-life care. Together with symptom management, it captures what families find to be the central component of their dependency on the staff to assure themselves that they are doing all that they can for their child. As hopes for a cure increasingly diminish, communication becomes more difficult and conflicting messages, both between what a caregiver tells a parent and what the parent is able to discern, as well as different messages between different caregivers to a parent, become paramount. It becomes as difficult for the staff to break the bad news as it becomes for the family to hear it.[1] This is understandable because, with diminishing hope, we look for it anywhere we might find it, no matter how elusive, uncertain, and indirect.

1:1. We had problems with how we were all communicating with the family, especially in the 2 or 3 days when things started getting worse. Although medically all of us understood exactly what was going on and understood each other's opinions on the matter, the family was getting totally mixed messages. Not necessarily because the physicians told them something wrong or something that was not true, but how they presented the issues. To give you an example, it was the day before she passed away, and that day she had a number of complications and things were clearly not going well at all; she clearly was going in the wrong direction. I talked to the mother just before I left, and her understanding after talking to the liver service was, "We may have to postpone the extubation for 1 or 2 days." Well, as life proved, in less than 24 hours, this could not be any further from the truth. Then, talking to the liver service, I learned that they did not put it in those words, but they left slightly more optimism than what should be allowed by the circumstances. This was always a problem with critical inpatients. You don't want to take away hope, you don't want to be the voice of doom, but there is a very fine line and, unless everybody talks to the family at the same moment, in the same room, there is a very fair probability that some people may present a more rosy picture and other people present a much worse picture while still telling the truth.

1:1. They were extremely angry because I don't think we adequately prepared them that things can go wrong. You tell them the percentages and the percentages are there, but the percentage for the individual is 0 to 100. She's going to survive and do great or she's going to die, but I can only give them what our track record's been.

1:8. It got very frustrating toward the end taking care of her because the philosophy behind taking care of children who are hem-onc patients is that you've got to be optimistic till the very end—you're fighting for this miracle. In the meantime, you have nurses who are at the bedside 12, 13 hours a day, nonstop, and we see what is going on and we see the deterioration. People will stop in briefly for their 17 minutes or so and say, "She looks much better. Her numbers are much better," and then they leave and mom is given a glimmer of hope, but then she continues to see how her daughter deteriorates. . . . We realized she was dying the weekend before, and the other team members continued to stop by briefly and looked at the numbers, scanned the numbers on the flow sheet, and would see that a couple of numbers were a little bit better than the previous numbers and proceeded to tell mom, "Oh, she's doing much better," and we would think, "What are you saying?" On the one hand, you didn't want to be too pessimistic, but on the other hand, they kept painting this upbeat picture when it wasn't true. Mom was told the weekend before she passed away that they were going to extubate her on Tuesday. Now, why someone told her that—she was very critical, her pulmonary status was horrible, and someone on a Saturday said, "Oh, she should be extubated by Tuesday." All these different team members would come in and there was no consistent communication. . . . The liver team was always very optimistic; 2 minutes from arrest and they're very optimistic. I guess to be in this field of medicine you always have to hope. But nurses quite often see the other side.

1:1. Having a family meeting is a mixed blessing a lot of times. I have seen it, for example, work in exactly the opposite way because, when everybody shows up, it's very intimidating for the family. Unless we have some really good news to tell them, a lot of families think, "Okay, this is it. They all came up here so they can tell us that there is nothing that can be done." Regardless of what you say, psychologically, it works a lot of times this way. In other ways, the family meeting, with all the services involved, becomes the equivalent of when they say in an organization or government that, when you don't know what to do or you don't want to do something, you create a committee. So the family meeting a lot of times serves like, "Let's have a meeting where everybody else is so, until then, we don't need to make any decisions." In reality, what really makes sense and a difference for the patient's care is whether the services communicate with each other about the practical issues about what is going to be said to the family, who's going to say it, and how we're going to say it. Is it better to hear it from five attendings talking at the same time to the family? I don't think it's necessarily the best way.

1:3. I walked in to sit down with her and I remember the father just looking at me very intensely and being like, "Is she better? How is she?" My first reaction, which I regretted later, was, "I don't know." I felt this intensity when I said "I don't know." He looked crushed, absolutely crushed. I couldn't tell him—and this is hindsight, when I say this now—I couldn't tell him "better." I couldn't say "better." I didn't even want to say "stable." I didn't want to say all these kind of euphemisms because I felt like I'd be lying to him. The intensity of his look was very easy to feel and so I said, "I don't know," and he was just so crushed. I was rattling my brains about this; I went home and I kept thinking, "Should I have not said, 'I don't know'?" I thought, I just can't say "better," even though I knew that's what he wanted me to say, but I just can't say that because I didn't know her at all really. I hadn't examined her in 2 days [resident just coming on-service]. I can't say anything and I was confused about saying the truth. . . . Another day he asked me, and that's when I started to realize the intensity of this case, "Is her tube going to come out today?" I must have looked aghast because there was just no way that was going to happen. I didn't even know where he had got that idea. I just said, "No," and he looked stunned and then he said, "What about tomorrow?" and I said, "Well, I don't think it'll be today or tomorrow, maybe after that because we have to go very slow." But I had no idea what was going on then—how could he even have thought that? Then Monday, when I came in, slowly the pieces were emerging. I think the nurse had talked to someone that had said that that's what the liver team had told the parents, that she would be extubated by Monday and that she was doing really well. That's when I started to hear that the optimism was coming from the liver team. I was in shock because, at my level, I knew she wasn't going to get extubated, so I didn't understand at all how anyone thought she was going to get extubated or could have told the parents that.

2:9. We try to protect everybody, the patient, the parents, the siblings, and we're doing more harm by doing that. I don't mean to be morose about it, but you can find ways to bring them into doing things for the child and things that are healing for the parents too, instead of being the secret keeper all the time; you become part of the conspiracy about how "They're okay. They're getting better" when they're not . . . I was at this family meeting one day and we were talking about talking to one of the older children and I had been talking to her basically about dying. Now, of course, I didn't say, "Are you ready to die right now?" but we were talking about dying in a lot of interesting ways. The mother had opened the door for that and I had permission from her, but the doctor said, "You can't talk to her about dying." He was horrified, and I was like, "What do you think she thinks is going on here? What do you think? There might be some things that she wants to do." People have ideas on what they want to do before they go. Some people like to plan things, some people have wishes and a lot of other things.

Often, a critical barrier to communication between the staff and families occurs when a patient is transferred from the primary service, where the staff has established and familiar relations with a family, to the ICU where the staff is new and unfamiliar. Many families now feel alone and abandoned at a time when they most need medical support.

3:1. When the child gets transplanted and then deteriorates and ends up dying in ICU, the families are very much alone. They haven't established a relationship with the staff there, they don't fully understand the situation, and they're very angry. This was a bone marrow transplant child and, although this child had had a long-standing relationship with a number of the physicians in the bone marrow transplant group, it wasn't the same in ICU. He died of complications of the transplant, not complications of the disease, and that led the mother to be very angry.

7:8. Often, families ask me what I would do, and I usually say, "I don't know what I would have done in your shoes. I don't know." Some parents have asked me—they become very close to you—"Do you think this is the time to stop?" and, then, I will say, "Yes." I will be honest with them and I will say, "Yes," and that he is not suffering.

The need to communicate with a dying infant is as important as it is to communicate with any child at end of life.

7:9. You can't help but approach a situation differently when you care for an infant that's dying compared to a toddler or a preschooler. Although you use touch and maybe play and you talk with each child, your intonation is different and you use touch in a different way and you use some songs. Songs are something that I use a lot with infants. We all sing to the babies all the time, and it's very soothing to be able to do that. You see the difference in them when you deal with them that way. I still tend to sing to them and stroke them because you need to communicate using something else.

10:5. As a fourth-year medical student, it was extremely difficult for a number of reasons. First of all, I started my care of Sarah toward the very end of her disease process. When I came onto the ICU, she was not doing very well and I came into this family's life and Sarah's life too, and I initially felt like I was an intruder in what was a very sensitive and emotional time for them. It took a while for me to feel like I was becoming a part of Sarah's life. I was there every day looking in on her and making sure the family was okay, but I was never not quite sure what my role was, in terms of what I was responsible for telling them. I tried to alleviate that by arranging for meetings with the attendings and other people because I didn't feel like it was my responsibility. I would have liked to tell them everything I knew, but it was very sensitive. They would say, "When do you think she's going to stop breathing?" or "Why do you think she's not responding?" These were questions that I really didn't feel I was qualified to answer. I felt myself in a strange role wanting to tell them what my ideas were but not wanting to give them any misleading information. It became difficult for another reason. I took on this role of just being there to talk to them about stories of Sarah. Toward the end, we had gotten to the point where there were occasions when I would just be in their room with them as they had come to grips with what was going to happen and they just needed someone to talk to. At that point, I had been at all the family meetings, so I fell into that role of hearing how Sarah had been when she was feeling well. It was difficult because it was extremely sad for me to see the family going through this and to see Sarah when she wasn't responding or having any interaction with her family.

10:7. People are afraid to talk about death because, when you start talking about it with families, it leads you to think about your own limited life span and about your feelings regarding death. So a lot of times, people don't want to get too involved. It's easier to do the medical management part of it and not get emotionally involved. It becomes like, "We'll just wait now. My work here is done." But it has to go beyond giving drugs and ordering therapies.

——

12:1. That afternoon we got into a little bit of a dynamic where the family started asking questions over the bed of this kid who was intubated emergently and on very high pressors. Another attending had come by and had been somewhat reassuring that we could pull her out of this. So then, when I went in, they asked me some questions about how sick she was. I said, "Well she's very sick," and the aunt said, "Would you describe her condition as critical?" and I said, "Yeah, she's critical." Then the father got very angry and said, "Everybody is telling us something different." That was my first time interacting with the father and he had this wild anger at me. I said, "I think that it is perfectly normal for you to be feeling angry and I can only imagine, if it were me in the bed and my father was standing over me, his level of rage at what was happening." Then I said, "Well, you can be angry at Him [looking up]. You can be angry at the situation. You can be angry at us, honest. If you are angry at us, that's okay. We can take it. That's part of our job, if you're angry at medicine." He said, "No, no. I thank you. This is a bad situation and I'm angry but I'm okay; I promise, I'm okay." I don't think my father would have been quite as rational as he was, if it was me in that bed. So I think that was a piece of it and I realized, when I said, "I could only imagine my father," that that's exactly who he reminded me of. He reminded me tremendously of my father. So the father and I had this initial like, phew, kind of meeting and it was hard for me. I can understand that anger and you get used to it; it comes with the territory. I've learned that when you diagnose a kid with cancer there is always something you say to the family, and then you have to have the Kleenex box right there because, for example, you say, "There is nothing that you did. It wasn't that you went out in the rain without your shoes on. It wasn't the cold that you had for a month and it wouldn't go away. There was nothing that you did that caused this to happen." You say that, and you don't realize what a powerful thing you are getting into until you do it once or twice and the family gets hysterical. So you come to learn that that's what they are carrying as their baggage, from the first moment. You learn over the years that you never know what will make the family angry or cry or whatever, but then one day you say something like, "The sky is blue" and the father starts yelling at you. I didn't think the father was angry at me personally, I just thought he walked into his child's room and saw her on a ventilator. He wasn't there that much, and whenever a parent isn't there that much, it's harder for them, whether it's guilt or whatever, it's just harder. When you're in the middle of it, it's easier than when you walk into it and he wasn't around that much. Somebody gave him hope that things were going to be okay and then I came back with what sounded less hopeful and he just lost it, but in the end it was fine.

15:1. I didn't know what to tell these people and so every time I knew I had to go and see them, part of me did not want to go because it was so horrible to see and I didn't even know what to say to them, so delay and delay and delay. Then I'd start to feel guilty because I haven't seen them, so then I'd go. It was especially difficult in front of a child who was playful and was running around to say, "Oh, don't worry. I will make sure that he goes with no suffering," because that wasn't even the right time to say it because he was fine. The only thing the mom would say is, "What do we do now? What do we do next?" In the end, I didn't know. Before, we could say, "Well, we can try another drug or we could try some radiotherapy," but I can only say, "I don't think there is anything else we can do now. We have tried everything and nothing is working. It is really a matter of waiting." I wondered how she would feel once she didn't have these kids anymore.

18:2. I remember it being a little more of a pleasant experience, even though it was tragic—the baby died. But I had a sense of this closeness with the parents. I actually felt like the parents knew that I was on their side; I was their friend, and I wasn't just there as a physician. They had the sense that we did what we could and that we were there for them, despite the death. I think that's what made the whole experience pleasant. There's a trust issue, for parents, with physicians, and I think there's also a trust issue for physicians with parents. You want to feel their trust for you. I want them to feel that I'm doing the best for their child, and if I don't even know them, they're never going to know that and I'm not going to know if they knew I did what I could. Not that it was like, "Your kid's just another baby through the line." But that's getting harder to do these days. Physicians are not clinicians any longer; they're technicians.

Staff Relating with One Another

The increasing complexity of end-of-life decisions in pediatrics is reflected in the involvement of a growing number of treatment teams across medical subspecialties. For example, one of our cases, a patient with postkidney transplant lymphoproliferative disease, involved nine different subspecialty teams in end-of-life care: renal, oncology, PCIU, nephrology, cardiology, plastic surgery, neurology, ophthalmology, and infectious diseases (see Table 2.1 for other examples). The involvement of so many subspecialties is compounded by the different levels of training, experience, and responsibilities among team members (e.g., attendings, fellows, and residents) and the hierarchical lines of management and administration involved in the hospital-based care of children. Coordinating care among so many providers can be daunting. At its best, everyone is on the same page, and there is clear and due recognition of the role and contribution of each team member and open lines of communication among them. At its worst, disciplinary boundaries become blurred, and questions arise about "whose patient is it?" One could argue that it is more essential that staff communicate well with each other than with families. It is inevitable that medical staff will have, at different times in treatment, different and sometimes conflicting perspectives, and these become exacerbated as hope for a cure diminishes. What then becomes important, in terms of quality of end-of-life care, is how well the staff is able to express themselves to achieve a reasonable consensus in decision making that allows everyone (including the families) to feel that they are all on the same page, share common concerns, and have mutual respect for each other and for the patient and family.

1:1. One of the things that is disturbing is that, toward the end, when she's in the ICU, I'm not there and she's got a whole other level of physicians who are there all the time and constantly making decisions. I'm not there, nor can I physically be there for every decision. Some things were run by me, others were not, which frustrates me because I'm usually completely in charge of my patients' care, especially out of the ICU. But in the ICU things are happening so fast, and a lot of decisions need to be made.

1:1. It varies tremendously. A lot of times in the ICU you take over completely, regardless of who was the referring physician or service, at other times, you cooperate, and other times, you relinquish your service under the premise of—regardless of what I think, this is what your physician wants. I'm here to assist and provide this kind of care, and it's a whether I-like-it-or-not kind of thing. But generally speaking, most of the time, we tend to take over the patient simply because the ICU staff, by definition, are going 24 hours a day. The referring service is making rounds with us, making some recommendations, that type of thing, but you take over a very significant portion of the care. How involved you become depends on the case, on the patient, who is the ICU attending, and who is the referring attending. Over the years, I have seen every possible variation from complete cooperation, the best possible, to the other extreme, diametrically opposite opinions on what could or should be done and infighting about how things should proceed.

1:3. The mother called me and said that the liver attending wanted to talk to me. The liver attending starts screaming at me on the phone. Apparently, they had switched antibiotics that morning at rounds, and he didn't know about it. He's like, "No, don't do that. I don't agree with that," so I tell the PICU attending, "He doesn't want this," but earlier in the day, at morning rounds, when we had switched antibiotics, I had been told that the infectious disease team had come and said that if she were to be clinically worse, we would switch antibiotics. That's all I was told. I have no idea who asked for the ID [infectious disease] consult, so in the morning it was like, "Okay" and then the attending was like, "Well, this is clinically worse. I think we should switch this now." How much sicker do you have to get? Apparently, we switched to this antibiotic that is in the same family as an antibiotic that she once had an allergic reaction to. The pharmacy had called and told me this during the day. I told the attending. The attending told me to call ID. I called ID, and they told me that they were fully aware of this and not only that, but the ID fellow had been on call when she had the allergic reaction and it's nothing to worry about; they approved it. Then we go ahead, and I don't know if the mom found out about that, but by this time I decided that I'm not telling the parents about every single change we make anymore. And I overheard the same liver transplant person telling the family, "You can't go by each and every number. You don't need to know each and every number." I overheard this, and that's when I decided that I'm not telling them every little thing. So I didn't. I don't know if she found out about it from the nurse. I don't even know what happened, but the liver attending started yelling at me that we made this switch in the morning and "You didn't tell me." There's this whole thing on the floor with the residents and the liver team. On the floors, when the residents have liver patients, we round up the liver team, they tell us what to do and if we want to do anything, we ask the liver team. In the ICU, the ICU is in charge. There's no like, if we do something, we have to tell liver; there's none of that. It's the ICU attending's decision and that's that, but he was yelling at me, "How would you like it if we did something and we didn't tell you?" I definitely got the impression that the mom must have gotten mad about something and spoken to him. My theory was that she found out that an antibiotic had been changed and she was angry about it, so that made him take it out on me. So I was so upset that I had been yelled at and she's doing so much worse and then, to top it all off, the nurse tells me and the fellow to be prepared that the mother's just hysterical. She's in there talking with someone and that she's making a list of all her grievances with the PICU. She doesn't trust the PICU, she doesn't trust anyone in the PICU. She thinks, the nurse is telling us, that we're not doing what the liver team wants.

1:3. The liver attending didn't think it was sepsis, which was part of his whole lecture to me about why he didn't want the antibiotics because he didn't think she was septic. He thought we were drying her out; that we were removing too much fluid from the dialysis, and then she had bled and we weren't giving her enough fluid. That morning I said to the PICU attending, "Well, the liver attending doesn't think it was sepsis," and now the PICU attending was like, "Well, then, what does he think it is? He says he doesn't want this, he doesn't want that, but what does he want? What does he think it is?" By this time, the liver team finally came to rounds. After all this time, they've never come to rounds with us before.

1:1. I tried to mend some fences with the ICU people because, in a way, you're angry at them because you question why didn't the patient survive under their care? But at the same time, I tried to talk to them. Some people felt that they may not have done the right thing, but if you can get it out in the open and you can discuss it in an M and M [mortality and morbidity meeting] kind of forum, then you get over it. You don't win by pointing fingers or by insulting people. I could definitely see some relationships getting worse. Among the nurses, who I know were in there and doing everything, it's like now every time they see me, there's a big smile. Even though the result wasn't good, there's obviously a bonding among us.

We survived the war together, even though we didn't win the battle; we survived the war and there's that appreciation.

1:1. When my partners saw things were getting close to futile and not going well, they backed off. Everybody had a nice opinion when things were going fine about how to micromanage things, but when people are really sick, then they say, "Well, she's in good hands. Do what you can." They say those kinds of things and back off. That's a natural reaction, but it puts the burden on you.

1:1. The family was getting input from multiple physicians, and while that could be beneficial to some patients, in other ways, it was devastating for this family. Our consult physicians from the infectious disease service were coming in making comments to the family regarding her prognosis, "Oh she's much worse now. We're going to have to really broaden out her coverage," rather than saying, "We're making adjustments and we're recommending them to your main doctor and the ICU staff." I could see the emotional impact on the parents. One time the mother begged me, "I don't want all the doctors to come in here and tell me that," so I met with the staff and I said, "Listen, I want things to go through me." I tried, but then there's the fellow who tries to be empathetic, an intern who thinks she's established rapport with the patient and goes in there and says things. I'm still finding out that maybe one of the interns, who was not even on the service, is still calling the family. They're saying things that are probably inaccurate, so it opens us up to medical legal implications.

1:8. We had the PICU team, we had the liver team, and we had the surgeons. Quite often they would come in at different times and speak to mom with different information, points of view. Some were very optimistic, and others were not so optimistic. It really created a tremendous amount of stress and anxiety in mom. At one point she even sensed that there was turmoil within the team taking care of her child. She would give me different examples of conversations that went on between physicians, things that they were saying when they would come into the room and things they wouldn't say. She right away picked up on the fact that there was not very good communication among the treatment teams. A lot of physicians would come in and would brainstorm in front of the mother, so she saw that kind of bantering back and forth, trying to figure out what was happening. But that goes on, especially in an academic university setting, and so I tried to reassure mom that that's what's good about being in an academic institution, that you have these people coming from different directions and brainstorming. But I think that created a lot of anxiety for her because she interpreted it that people didn't agree with each other and mistakes were being made. It really peaked 2 days before Karen died. I told the mom that I was going to try and clear the air. We pulled in someone from the liver team and someone from the PICU team and made it very clear to mom that we had a definite plan. That seemed to help a little bit, but Karen was so critical and unstable at that point that mom was very distraught.

1:8. You need to have one central person in charge all through and talking to the family and not have the resident, the fellow, and the intern all coming in from different directions and giving her [mom] information that wasn't always accurate. Like someone came in one morning and took her pleuravac off suction; just completely took it off suction, and then the surgical fellow came in and said to mom, "Oh my God! Who did this? She could collapse her lungs." Mom told me after this that "I have a daughter in high school at home that we're very worried about but," she said. "Quite frankly, I'm not going home. I don't trust anybody here." That's what's so stressful—not all the medications, not the ventilator or the CPPH; it was trying to deal with the mom—trying to explain that this is what he really meant when he said that and that and you need to pick one attending that you can talk to, that you can really trust and talk to.

1:8. It's always the hardest for the nursing staff, especially for the primary nurses, because they literally spend the entire 12 hours of their shift at the bedside. For a critically ill patient who's not doing well, they spend 12 hours on their feet without time even for the most basic things, like drinking a glass of water; even going to the bathroom becomes an issue. They are also the ones who develop the closest possible relationship with the patient and with the family, which always makes it harder. They serve on 12-hour shifts, but under the circumstances 12 hours sometimes is the emotional equivalent of months or years. You feel that you get closest to somebody and that you know them better than other people who knew them for a lifetime. We keep seeing that over and over again for all of us.

We tend to develop both positive and negative feelings toward somebody in our care in an extremely short period of time. The last days, especially the last 2 days, were extremely tough, especially for the primary nurse who was clearly very stressed by the fact that she was fighting a losing battle. This was one of the most senior people who has seen many, many, times similar situations but, unfortunately, that did not make it any easier because, for every person, it's always like you're seeing it for the first time.

2:3. The problem is that we're [residents] always on night call so there's days when we're not there, and then there's days when we're in clinic, so we have to be proactive in voicing our opinions. It's not just about whether the attendings are letting us participate when they have family meetings, but you have to be proactive and present at these family meetings and be vocal about what you think. This happens in the NICU all the time where there's family meetings and either you don't know about them or you're not proactive enough. But definitely for residents, if we feel strongly about something, we should definitely be proactive about it. But, at the same time, it depends on where one is. Like most of the oncologists have a closer relationship with the patients and the families than we do because they're seeing them in clinic all the time. But for those residents who are constantly taking care of them, I think it's important that they show up to these family meetings. Like with oncology, there's a lot of things that are so intricate that that's really the attending's job to talk about stuff like the adverse side effects. But when it comes to talking about day-to-day care, there needs to be more interaction between the attending and the residents about where is this kid going, so that everyone is on the same kind of foundation. A lot of times, some of the residents may think this kid's doing well and the attending's thinking this kid's really terrible. That's where some of the things get mixed up, when communicating with the parents. A lot of times you walk in and the parents will say, "Well, the attending told me this," and you'll be like, "Oh, I didn't even know about that."

4:2. There were numerous services involved, and it was a very long hospital stay. We had several services and each service had attendings that would keep changing. So every week, every other week, there was a whole new set of people involved. His primary oncologist was the one who was probably the constant person in the picture so he could direct things. But we should have established a situation where, whenever there's a new set of people in the team, we should all have sat down and said, "This is where the other team left off and this is how we're going to continue." Unfortunately, or maybe fortunately, the teams change in a staggered fashion, so we may have the neurology team change on Thursdays, and the oncology team on Fridays. We should have acted in a more concerted way and sat down together more frequently.

5:7. I'm able to segue and willingly give up the responsibility of caring for the patient [when they're transported to the ICU] and to just deal, on a consultative level, with either the staff or the family. In a way, it's a relief because you're not responsible for curing the suffering on a daily and minute-by-minute basis. Someone else might find it difficult, but I'm relieved that I don't have to be in charge of it. But then our team, when things go wrong, asks, "Whose patient is it?" That's always an issue when we send a child to the ICU, and it's an issue for them too. For example, the ICU nurse said, "Well, I don't know anything about cancer," and I'm like, "Get a life! You've been in the unit for 2 years, so what have you been doing?" But you know that their heart is in the right place. This particular nurse is very good—she just has a personality flaw. So you just have to look by it and accept it and know that this kid's going to get what he needs. I was very fortunate to have a resident that I could report to and relate to. But some of the attendings and nurse practitioners treat us like dirt. So I was very glad I didn't have to talk to the PICU attendings. Some are fine, if you've known them for a long while. It's like, once you've built up a reputation with somebody, they know you on a one-on-one basis and then they'll be nice to you.

5:7. The ICU unit doesn't like our patients; they only like the cardiology patients, because they think that all our patients die and they don't want to deal with patients that are going to die. They're not familiar with how oncology patients die, and to die from leukemia is not pleasant. If we hadn't sent him to the ICU and eased his suffering from breathing, he would've suffocated in a very uncomfortable way for several days with his family in agony. It's not *Love Story*, dying in those rooms. For some families that can cope with the anxiety of watching their child be uncomfortable and to whom you can adequately communicate and do the best you can to keep them comfortable, the oncology unit is absolutely the place to be. If you can't keep them comfortable and you think there's a shot at making them better, then the ICU is the place to be. But the ICU staff, across the board, doesn't perceive itself as oncology educated, and they're not. It's a different institutional culture in the ICU. They think a lot of what we do is futile, and, if it's futile, then why are we doing it?

6:2. Doctors and nurses always have very different impressions of the family. Nurses are at the bedside, and they deal with them much more longitudinally than we do. We're in there for a brief moment. Nurses probably have a much better sense of the family dynamics than we ever do because they're there in the room more consistently, and often, with the really chronically ill children, they get drawn into the family, for better or for worse. That's probably why there's always that tension between doctors and nurses, meaning that they always see us kind of come in, go out, come in, go out, and not really get what's going on in the room. But we take care of 20 or more patients, so that's just the way things work, unfortunately.

6:2. I'm new at this, so a lot of the questions they were asking me were extraordinarily difficult for me to answer. I didn't fully even understand the questions that they were asking. The obvious one was the prognosis, "Is he going to make it?" and I didn't know the answer. But also they were asking me details about how to declare somebody brain-dead and what that meant and organ transplantation and all this. Those are issues that I'm sure I'll have to deal with multiple times and get used to, but I was starting out and I didn't know how to go about answering them. And they would ask me details about the neurological exam that we were doing and what that would mean for him. That was also something that I was unfamiliar with, in terms of what that would mean for him. When I don't know the answers, my response is to always be honest. Having done this job for only 3 years, I find, almost every time, that, if you withhold even a small amount of information, you always end up getting yourself in trouble. It just snowballs from there because they'll ask some sort of followup question or something else will come up, so it's better often to just say what you know and what you don't know. When I don't know, I'll tell them what my function is here and I can tell them who would know and I can obviously ask that person to come and speak to the parents about it. Every parent always asks everybody involved what their opinion is because they're searching for a better answer—meaning more acceptable for them.

They'd rather hear some better news, and if they are always asking some-body for better news they think that they'll find it, which is another reason why I always tell them what I know and don't know because often it's a re-peat question from somebody else that they're asking you.

7:1. We have had some patient situations where the bedside nurses felt that the doctors were asking that too much be done or that treatment be continued beyond some reasonable point. Or maybe they felt that the parents weren't exactly tuned into how negative the outcome was appearing and the nurses were frustrated that this wasn't being communicated by the entire team. We sort of are visitors when we go to the ICU because they have their own com-plete staff, but they are dealing with a family whose idea of what is happening has still got a lot of input from us. If we have one or two of our patients in the ICU, they immediately become a priority for me and so I go straight there and try to find the ICU team. Maybe I can do this because of seniority, but I'm saying to them, "Here I am. We got to see this patient; this is going to be your next patient to round on." It is very important that people in the ICU know the expectations. Sometimes I will say, "The outcome for second trans-plants is half or two-thirds the outcome for the first transplant, so now we are talking about 20 percent or something like that." And they will say, "Oh re-ally?" Otherwise, the ICU staff don't differentiate between a newly diagnosed child with a temporary air obstruction from a lymphoma who is going to be curable versus these complex immunodeficient transplant patients that have many problems and are more likely not to survive than survive. So it helps very much to explain how we came to do this transplant and tell them that we have talked to the parents and they still want everything done or not. The ICU nurses generally join us in these discussions. They leave the patients' rooms, so most of them are willing to speak up, if they think, for example, that this mom just doesn't seem to get it at all or whatever their comments may be. So these kinds of discussions among staff are really critical to our function because otherwise you get into this with people looking at it in different ways and that interferes with the consistency of care.

7:8. The biggest conflict we have in the ICU is between the ICU nurses and physicians. We [nurses] come to terms with it much quicker then they do, and we get very upset with them because their oath is first do no harm and do whatever it takes. We are educated so differently. We are educated to take care of the whole family, from the beginning to the end, and when the end happens and it is okay to happen, we just need to be there and support them all along and give them all of our best. Physicians are not trained that way. They are not trained for death. That is not in their vocabulary. We feel that they should be more open with the families and say, "This is all we can do." But no, they say, "What if we try this CVVH [continous veno-veno hemofiltration, a form of kidney dialysis]? That is going to do it," and we are like "What are you doing?" The nurses here were very angry when they put this child on CVVH. A common reaction by the nurses was, "Can't they just let her have death with dignity? What is the problem with a child dying with dignity?" They were falsely reassuring the family, and, meanwhile, it was torturing this child. But I can't go to the mother and say, "Listen, I think they're just practicing on your kid." Instead, what I do is try to bring the family back to the original problem and tell them, "This is another complication on top of all the other complications, and the physician has decided to try CVVH and give it a go and see if it will help. This may or may not work," and leave it like that. . . . If they ask me, "Do you think if we put her on CVVH it is going to make any difference? Is it going to make her get better?" I will tell them the truth and say, "No, it will not make her any better. It may bring her a little time so that you can spend some time with her, but it will not make her better." Sometimes that gets me into trouble with the physicians and we sit down and we hack it out. We have gone into these big pow-wows, with the nurses on one side and the physicians on the other, and we are at each others' throats. They have to listen to us because we are part of the health care team and we are the ones who are there 24 hours, 7 days a week. We are the ones who get attached to the parents. They are there for the 5-minute doctor visits and then out the door, and I am the one who is left answering all their questions and I am the one who is taking care of the child and seeing the changes in this child. Pediatric nurses are very territorial. We speak as, "My patient this," "My patient that." "My." "My." She becomes my child essentially, and it is my family and it becomes part of us. For them, it is a patient and then a diagnosis. We are patient advocates.

8:2. The social worker was unbelievable; she was unbelievable. She was the one person that the mom could talk to, and the mom knew that she understood her and she would be able to tell us exactly what she wanted. I thought mom trusted her so much and that whatever the social worker told us, it was what mom wanted us to hear. The social worker also understood, from our point, what we wanted from the mom and was able to express it to the mom without antagonizing her about the medical aspect of it. So it really worked beautifully. It was just perfect. She did a great job. It was really good because sometimes you get very frustrated when you don't speak Spanish or you don't speak whatever language the family speaks. Even if you did speak it, some parents don't trust you. So the mom looked at the social worker as her advocate. I was able to tell the social worker, "This is what I want. This is what my fears are," and she would meet with the mom, without us, so that way the mom didn't feel threatened, like, "Oh, the doctors are here again trying to tell me x, y, z, and all the bad things that are happening to my son." Having the social worker going to meet her in the room later, away from us, allowed mom to talk about what were her concerns—"What is it that you want me to tell them? What is it that you are uncomfortable with?"

11:2. One good thing that came out of this night was—sometimes it's easy to say, "Oh, the nurses are terrible," but they did a great job. For the shock that they went through, they did a tremendous job. I wasn't even there when she coded, and I was shocked when I arrived. The resident too; she was awesome, totally awesome. I really appreciated her because you have a floor of kids who are sick all the time, and you needed somebody who could act quickly. Fine, the outcome was death anyway, but can you imagine, if it took 5 minutes for somebody to get there and do anything about it? She had prompt attention. The code was called right away, and the people who needed to be there were there. Sometimes you say that this floor is so horrible, nothing works, but in this situation, when it really mattered, it worked—it was like clockwork. You would almost think that they had expected something bad to happen. They were all ready. I've seen places where you're calling a code—I was bagging [giving oxygen to] the kid for 5 minutes and there was no anesthesiologist, no ICU; I was there by myself with no IV, no pulse, and no suctioning. That's a horrible situation. They really did a good job, and they rallied together. They tried to support each other and help each other through the night. Everybody was getting me food to eat, asking if I wanted something to drink. It was very tight and it was very comforting. Yes, it was really good and it spilled over to the morning shift. The night nurses were gone and the tone for the day was very somber and very sad, but they did a great job.

17:10. She came from abroad and didn't have a support system here and that made it extremely difficult because the family often relied on me. They had no money, and they were not eligible for a lot of the charity organizations that have very strict requirements regarding either citizenship or residency. She was alone in this country with her aunt, and for the 3 months they were here, the aunt never left her bedside; never left the building. They didn't have any family members here and they didn't have any friends here, and basically there was nothing that I could really offer them. The staff got very upset, and the aunt obviously was very angry and all the staff on the floor, including the nursing staff, got overly involved in this case. That, for me, was the most overwhelming thing because often they overstepped their boundaries. For example, one person would say, "I'll pay for this, for them" and would pay out of pocket. That just put me out of that relationship because I didn't plan to do that for one patient if I could not do it for another. It just created a lot of tension. It got to a point where everybody just held such anger and frustration inside that it came out in everything. I did not expect the staff to react that way; I expected more from them, and I was very surprised and disappointed. . . . I felt that there was so much pressure on me from the aunt and pressure from a lot of the staff. I never experienced so much pressure; never in my life. I think some people got in trouble because they were, at times, inappropriate; overstepping their boundaries. There was too much overinvolvement on too many peoples' parts and it brought out the worst in everyone.

20:1. We all are extraordinarily loyal and support each other. As crude as it sounds, often a baby will die, the space will be cleared, and another baby will be there, sometimes within an hour. We do the very best, while these babies are alive, to sustain them and, if they die, there is this acceptance that it's all for the better. But there probably isn't enough done to talk about formal grief support for the staff here. There is a resistance from staff in intensive care areas to talk freely about death and dying because they have this critical front-line approach. You come in and you work to the best of your ability, and if you fail or the baby fails, there is this acceptance and moving on. There is an intense friendship between many of the nurses here who speak freely to each other. What we'd like to do is to pool some of those talks so that we can get feedback from nursing and medical staff so that if there are issues that are affecting all of us in terms of how anyone is handling it or ways of improving what we do in this nursery, we'd like to hear about it. But the time out of a busy day, when you're monitoring sick babies, to come and speak is extremely limited. I don't know when is the right time to try and catch people, and there has to be some give from everybody if we need to get together as a group.

20:2. Usually, it's the nurses who are the ones that actually withdraw support, take the tube out, or disconnect from the ventilator. They are the ones who suffer more than us; we are just observers. You see the emotions in the people around you and you get emotional for them, but you expect it and you say, "This is the best thing for the family."

Staff Coping and Moving On

Grieving always encompasses guilt. Anyone who has grieved the loss of someone has questioned whether there wasn't something that he or she could have done to have prevented it or made it easier. As difficult as it must be to resolve this kind of guilt for parents who have lost a child, it is as difficult, in different ways, for the medical staff who have lost a child in their care. They are trained to expect to save each and every child, and because we find a child's death so unnatural, they question, "How can we have let this happen?" The question typically comes from within them more than from the grieving families who sometimes might blame them for their losses. This is a useful distinction in terms of finding ways of helping the staff cope with the failure of treatment. It raises basic issues about the mission of medicine and how those in practice might move beyond the dichotomy of either cure or failure to more fully appreciate the holistic needs of patients and families, when cure no longer is a reasonable option.

Medical staffs are torn between two conflicting tendencies in how to deal with caring for a dying child and be able to move on to another child. On the one hand, there is the need to provide compassion to the child and family, which leads to greater intimacy and involvement in sharing the child's and family's distress. On the other hand, the tendency is to move away to protect oneself from the pain of involvement and the frustration of failure.[2] This often is reflected in staff's dispassionate analyses and clinical judgments about case management of the dying child (and morbidity and mortality meetings after the death). Although staffs differ considerably in how they are able to maintain control and yet be compassionate when caring for a child who is dying, as the following narratives show, there is no standard or canonical procedure to best assist staff to overcome their sense of loss, failure, and inadequacy. Some, for example, find comfort and closure by attending the child's funeral; others avoid it at all costs. Some need to talk about their grief; others need to distract themselves. Some favor the idea of a focused professional bereavement group for staff; others prefer collegial activities that provide time for staff, at all levels, to come together somewhere outside the hospital to reconnect with each other in terms of who they are outside the context of medicine—spouses, parents, grandparents, athletes (practicing or observing), musicians, film buffs, whatever.

1:1. One of the things that makes this very difficult is that we have an excellent survival rate. When I talk to patients, I tell them we have a 90 to 95 percent 1-year survival, and I truly expect 100 percent survival. Forget that liver transplants are high-risk endeavors. In most cases, people do very well; they survive. If there may be retransplantation, they need a constant adjustment in the medications but I never expect them to die.

1:1. If it's cancer, we'll transplant her; we'll rescue her. But we didn't rescue her; she died. And it's more than frustrating because it was unexpected. It shouldn't have happened, but it did happen so, though I'm not devastated by this, I'm not comfortable with it. The number of patients who died since we started this program [liver transplant] 4 years ago, you can count on one hand, on three fingers, so it's not a lot on the pediatric side. The adults are much sicker; they go in and they die. Our results are better, far better than national averages, and you start to believe your own hype, that we don't lose patients. Well, we do! Maybe there were delays in some of the things that were recognized, while I wasn't here. I'm sort of a detail guy, and so I look for everything. I spot stuff early, and maybe our survival's better because I'm around most of the time. I don't know. You always question then, if I didn't have my vacation and if I was here, would I have caught this early? Maybe I could have. There's multiple places where you probably could have made a concerted effort, and may have stopped the cascade. By the time I got back, the cascade was full blown, and then she bled. When I got back she had a GI bleed. Then, she succumbed to a hemorrhage into her lungs. Those were things I can't fix. . . . You always have to find out what happened so as to prevent another one of these. Just like a postmortem would help you try to figure out what happened, you have to postmortem your entire experience. You hash over it; you go home, you're sitting in bed, you jump up and say, "Wait a second, why did we do that?" That's how you grow, but it's not pleasant.

1:1. I'd been here almost 2 days. I went home and I came back within 4 hours. So at this time, after maybe an hour and a half of sleep over 2 days, I went home knowing she was sick but stable, stable shitty. I don't know what you want to call it, stable but obviously not well. Then, I got four calls in a row [at home], minutes apart, from the doctor taking immediate care of her, saying that they were in there coding her almost continuously now and it didn't look good, and I guess they were preparing me for what was going to happen. I asked about certain things and gave some advice, but I'm not there. I thought about just throwing clothes on and shooting back down there. I have a 25-, 30-minute drive in but I'd just gotten home and I hadn't seen my family. I was tired and I was not the most effective. I was falling asleep driving home. I just didn't feel up to it. So they called me back within about half an hour, 45 minutes, and told me that she had passed. I knew my fellow was in-house, so I called her and asked her to stop by even before she [patient] died. So when I heard that she'd died, I figured, "I don't want to be there when the family's wailing and beating their chests," so I waited about an hour, got dressed, took a shower, came down, and the family was gone. They didn't do any of that chest-beating when she died. They left within a few minutes. So now, instead of having a one-on-one chance to discuss things and have closure for all of us, I had nothing. I talked to the ICU staff and tried to establish some closure with them. I said a small prayer over the child—she was still in the room and not cloaked or anything but visible. Looking at her, she didn't look anything like the kid I started with 4 weeks ago, 7 weeks ago. I checked on a couple of things on some other patients who were sick and then went to the office, got the chart, got the phone number, and called the family. I gave them a chance to get home, and I wasn't sure they were going to want to talk to me. The mom was protected by waves of family members and she eventually got on the phone with me. We talked about things, but she said lines that you hate to hear, "I know you have children and I hope you never outlive your children." She went on, and it was a horrible feeling. . . . I offered her assistance with her husband since he needed to be medicated. I said, "Our relationship is not over, we're here to support you through things," but I didn't feel comfortable asking about a postmortem over the phone. I wanted to know what happened to this kid, what did we do wrong? I had her on everything I could think of, and I should have asked her; I could have said, "You know, I'm required by law to ask." I could have made it so that I can give a reason that I have to ask, but I just didn't feel comfortable at that point. Things just happened too fast. . . . She's been dead now a few days, and it's the only thing that's on my mind. I wish things were done differently. I wish the family and I had more to say. I felt a part of this family, but obviously they didn't feel that. I was still an outsider to the point where, even though I had invested a significant amount of time and energy into this patient, they didn't think it was appropriate for me to say goodbye to her.

1:1. I didn't have a long-lasting relationship with her—we're talking weeks, right? A significant part of the end of our relationship was when she was completely unconscious, intubated on high support. She became—I don't know how you want to put it—sort of reminiscent of the lab dog in school, where you have it intubated. It's not a human at this point now, so you can sort of separate yourself in order to be able to deal with it. Same way a pediatrician can put an IV in a kid who's screaming. When I go home, my wife says, "Don't you hear your daughter calling you?" and, quite frankly, I don't. I mean I've been trained to ignore children. "Daddy, Daddy!" And my wife says, "She's calling you," and I say, "What?" It's funny that you sort of learn not to hear certain things that you don't want to hear and it's the same thing in the ICU setting. You separate yourself from "This is a child who. . . . This is the patient and this is the data." Every once in a while, you walk up and you see her face or you see her parents crying at her bedside holding her hand and you realize this is a patient, while I'm seeing her as systems, as respiratory, infectious disease, cardiovascular, hematology, nutrition. I don't know how anybody chooses to deal with something where they lose a significant percentage of their patients. When I transplant people, they get better. My goal is a normal life, for her to have her children, to get her friends back because, God knows, this kid could have been, should've been an A-plus student.

1:1. The stress for the staff, a lot of times, is almost exactly the opposite of what somebody would expect. One possibility is the one where you clearly get involved both physically and emotionally in the case and you literally try to save somebody's life and that has, a lot of times, a very profound effect. But there are also a lot of other times that you are stressed in an immediate way because you don't feel this way. To put it very bluntly—and, hopefully, in a little exaggerated way—"Why did she have to arrest at 6:30 just 15 minutes before I was ready to go? I'm missing my train, and I have plans to go somewhere with my husband/my date/ my friend/ my whatever, and I stayed 2 more hours last night and I'm sick and tired of staying." Then you feel totally guilty because somebody's clearly dying in front of you; you hear the family and you cannot avoid thinking, "Okay, now either get better or die. Let's not prolong the agony." This is an oversimplification and an exaggeration, but, clearly, for the staff, you cannot expect everybody to be equally involved in every case, definitely not, and we should not, as far as I'm concerned, become emotionally involved to the level that the family is getting involved. Because for this family and many other families this is a lifetime event. They are going to remember it for the rest of their lives, and everything is going to be, from now on, before this event and after this event. For the people in the ICU, in general, it's one more patient that did not make it and we have to do it this way; otherwise none of us would be able to function for more than 1 day; it would drive everybody completely crazy. But you still cannot avoid feeling guilty for not feeling something more about the case. This is what I meant that it was a routine case; one more critical care patient, and some of them make it and some of them don't make it; it's an "Okay, now, let's finish rounds, let's order lunch" kind of thing because there are 30 patients, at any given time, who are very close to these circumstances. This is our job; this is what we do.

1:8. This was good for me. I was so frustrated, and it was good for me to be able to talk about it. Thank you very much.

2:7. At first, it was a pleasure taking care of Devon because he was such a great kid, but as his illness progressed to this chronic, very sick constantly in pain condition, it became pretty stressful for me, almost to the point where I didn't want to take care of him anymore because it was terrible to see him suffering every single day and not making any difference with all our medical things that we were doing with him. I felt helpless often because his grandma and mom would just look at me and say, "Why isn't this working? Why does he feel like this? Why is he in such pain?" My reaction toward the end was that I just wanted to run away from him.

2:1. I try to be as complete a doctor as I can so, for me, I don't know, I may not be able to do it my whole life; I may get burnt out. But when things end like this, I feel it's my last duty, as Devon's physician, to give the family some closure, and to know that I was invested enough to go to the funeral. It also gives me closure, and it gives me tremendous insight because now I know the community he came from and the faith that he came from. I understand better the way his family dealt with things while I was taking care of him. I go over these things a lot, and just because Devon died last week, it doesn't mean that I wouldn't keep thinking about him, so the funeral really helped me. For example, when I lose a patient, I talk to my father, who also is a physician and the only person in my family who can really deal with any of this. My first patient that died, died on his second birthday. I said to my father that to me, that's a sign, and he said, "What do you mean?" and I said, "I don't know. It just seemed so blatant. It's gotta be a sign from God that this child was designed for some other purpose." That she's an angel because to be born and die on the same day is—like, for an adult, I can understand that they're waiting for a certain day and they get there, but for a 2-year-old?—for me it was a sign. He said, "No, it's not. It's random chaos." And you know what? I said, "I can't live like that. I gotta be able to rationalize and give it some kind of meaning because I can't live believing that everything is just random chaos—it doesn't help me. I couldn't get up in the morning and be a physician if I thought that everything was random chaos." With Devon, I stood up and spoke at his funeral. The other reason that I went to his funeral was that it was an act for the child, because I felt that he had spent the majority of his last year in the hospital and all these people came to the funeral and they barely knew him because he spent the year in the hospital. They had kinda like an open-mike prayer meeting thing where they said a few words about Devon. I listened to their language and realized that it meant something to them, if I could say something, having been there, having witnessed—and they're big on witnessing things and testimonials—if I could give them the testimonial that this kid really was an angel on earth because, if you could see his smile, it was extraordinary. So, when I think about Devon and when I think about angels, I'm going to picture him in my mind, and it helps me. It packages it in a way that is accessible to me; random chaos is not accessible to me. It helps me to go the funeral, and I do it out of deference to the family and I do it as my final doctor act.

2:10. I wish we had more of a formal thing when someone passes away in which the whole staff gets together and has a wrap-up session, but because things are so crazy and so busy here, we haven't had that opportunity to do that. Informally, those staff members who were very involved in his care got together and talked about our feelings, and I followed up with them and spoke with them on a one-to-one basis. I've been going to most of the funerals, but, with Devon, I found myself backing away and I purposely didn't go to his burial. His funeral was on Sunday so I told his parents I had my own church that I needed to go to and they understood. But I felt the night that I came in [to the hospital] was good closure for me, and I didn't physically need to be at his funeral; maybe it would have undone the closure.

2:10. He was such a charmer and he was so witty, so incredibly giving. That's the part that I love about this job. I get to meet all these incredible kids and these incredible, inspiring parents. Devon inspired me every day. I would walk into his room and he would say, even though he was in so much pain, "How are you?" He was very concerned about how I was doing, and, for example, one time during Christmas, I asked him what he wanted for Christmas and he said he didn't want anything because he wanted Santa to bring other kids gifts and he didn't want to take away from other kids. Another time he looked at his mother so lovingly, with so much adoration and he took his hand and he held her face like this and looked straight at her and said, "Mommy, you know I love you, right? You know I love you?" And this is coming from a 5-year-old. Her tears started flowing and she couldn't look at him straight, so she turned her head, but he kept turning her face back and saying, "Mommy, you know I love you." This was about 3 weeks before he passed away. The night he passed away, I was driving back to the hospital [to be with the parents], and that's what kept coming through my head. When I met with the parents, I reminded them of that story, and she laughed about it and said, "Yeah, that's how Devon was." Even after that day, I was comforting myself by telling Devon stories to other people, sharing his stories with other people. That's what the parents had been doing with me and with other people, and whenever I speak with the parents over the phone now, we're always swapping stories of when he said this or when he said that. It's been comforting.

2:3. As you go through your residency, you can see the differences in the way people react to death or near death—people who are going toward death. If you look at the interns, they're more emotionally attached and they get hit much harder, even though they don't know the patients as well or don't have as personal a relationship with them. Lots of times, we tell the interns, "I wouldn't get too attached because he's probably going to die." For me, it's more of a numbing experience. In the back of your mind, you're saying, "This patient is probably going to pass away, sooner or later, whether it's now or whether it's a year from now." I think there's more of an acceptance without separating ourselves from the patients.

2:9. I've become a little more comfortable in not running away when I think somebody's going to die because I feel that a lot of people do run away. They hide in their work, and then there's nobody there for the patients and families. We don't have a program that addresses this. We don't ask, "Who's gone in to talk to them about this? Where are they at with it? Are they together with us or not?" Instead, it's fragmented. We're very good at saying, "Okay, what tests are we going to have done?" but not at saying, "What are we going to do for them, for their emotional needs?"

2:9. After a while, I almost feel that they didn't die but that they just sort of went home. I do this a lot. Of course, I know they did, but it's almost easier to think of them in the present than in the past. That's okay, as long as you can keep that, like I can picture Devon's face and his smile, but you don't know how long you can keep that. Sometimes I can keep it longer then other times, and right now it's real vivid for me. I can see his smile, I can hear his voice, I can hear him laughing, his conversations—it's very real. I feel good talking about him now because he was so special. He was just such a unique child, it feels good to talk about him and I wish everybody got to meet him and I wish everybody knew him. Sometimes I cry for a few minutes and just get it out like that.

2:7. I've gone to wrap-up sessions where everyone talks about the patient, but I'm personally not comfortable with that—for some people it works very well. I tried it, and it actually got me more upset than it did good for me. I think everybody has to know their own ways and what might work really well for them—I wish it did for me, but I didn't like doing that at all. I didn't like the fact that there were so many people in the room who were going around and telling these stories. It was almost as, if you didn't say something, you weren't honoring them; that you couldn't just be private about it. I thought it was cold; it was cold and formal, and I don't work well like that. But for some people it really helped so I guess that different people just have different ways of dealing with it.

2:7. I don't really care for the support group environment. We had one of those at the last place I worked when we did debriefings, and I just didn't find them very helpful for me. I just found myself sitting there, and I didn't say a lot. We all just sat around and "How did you feel? Tell me a good experience you had with. . . ." It was pretty stream of consciousness, everybody talking, and I just didn't find that helpful. The informal talks with colleagues and other people who knew him and took care of him help the most.

2:1. When it comes to sending a condolence card to the family, I usually ruminate about it for a week or two and I never say the same thing. It comes from the heart and you can't force it. It comes when it comes, and part of why I actually do it is that I read this *New England Journal of Medicine* editorial, about a year ago, about how they thought it was a lost art—the physician's condolence card. That is part of why I go to funerals because they said that you can't underestimate what that one last act means to the family. It's interesting because when I came back from maternity leave, this patient had died and I went to the funeral the day I came back and this was a family that I was very connected with. It took me about 3 weeks to write the condolence card. Then, I came in one morning, and there's a voice on my answering machine saying, "Hi, it's Susan. We just got your letter, and it was really nice to have it and thank you so much." I kept that message so it's still on my voice mail, and every once in a while, when I'm thinking, "Am I doing the right thing?" I play it back and hear a voice that says, "Thank you, that really meant something." I used to do rough drafts, and, occasionally, if it sounded like something sour, I would copy it over, but I don't do rough drafts any more. It used to be a very, very hard thing for me to do, but it's getting easier.

2:1. How do we help some of the other people, the fellows, the social workers, cope with a patient who is dying? I think it's been very hard on them. As you get older, and have been doing this long enough, you figure out ways to protect yourself, but some of the younger practitioners were very devastated over this and the social worker was very upset. So how do you help people get through these episodes? That's probably the one area that pediatric oncology, as a whole, needs to try and address better. I've had enough patients die that, although it's upsetting still, I know how to protect myself and move on. But how do we help the fellows to deal with that? I'm not sure. When Devon died, I drove the fellow home because she was so upset, and that gave us time to talk about it, to put it into perspective. I don't think I would particularly like a formalized way of dealing with it, like in a staff meeting, because I think everybody deals with it on a very different level. Instead, it should be more one-on-one, and we can't formalize that. It's not enough that the fellows may talk with the other fellows because they don't have the experience among themselves necessary to impart a perspective. I have a perspective because I've done this for a long enough time, but they need to question, when patients die, what are the good things we've done for the patient, the parent? We need to make sure that the fellows have someone watching over them when this happens. Since they're in training, we're obliged to do that. It's a matter of trying to figure out, how do you have the experienced person help the less experienced? People will help, if you ask them, but sometimes it's hard for people to ask, and they're so distressed. If she can ask, "How do you keep doing this, after all these years?" I can tell her how I deal with it. I don't know if there's a formal mechanism to do this, but there is certainly a need for a greater awareness, for people to support one another.

3:1. It had just been so hard for me. It had taken me to the edge and back, and I haven't fully recovered yet. I can still bring myself back there, but at a certain point, I can't because I've got to get on with the next case. But if I have another one, in rapid succession like this, "Whoa, I'm not long for this job." You can only do this every once in a while because you lose a piece of yourself, you really do. I gave a piece of myself and I willingly gave it, but I don't know if I have that many pieces to give, long term. The same day Elsa died, a new standard risk leukemic came in, and even though I wasn't scheduled to have him, I fought my division chief. I told him, "If I only take care of stage 4 neuroblastomas and phase 1 protocols, I'm not going to make it. I need a standard risk leukemic every once in a while.

You've got to understand I need someone who's going to do okay, otherwise, I'm going to get slaughtered. You can't replace one patient with another, but give me somebody who has a good likelihood of doing okay, because it's been three patients in 6 months, all stage 4 neuroblastomas and if that's going to be the bulk of what I do, I won't make it."

3:9. Why do we do what we do? Well, it's an honor to be allowed into these people's lives. When a child dies, or even not, I often thank families for allowing us to get to know their kid because the kid has to have permission from the parents to get to know us; otherwise, that kid is not going to ever develop a relationship with us. So I thank those parents for allowing that because I can't imagine doing anything else. Some people would say I'm insane for doing this kind of work, and it's not that we're gluttons for punishment, but there's something about being a part of this process and watching miracles every day. Miracles come in all shapes and sizes, and it's not always that a child's life is saved. Sometimes, the miracle is that Elsa and her mother got together when they needed to get together or that her physician had the courage to tell this family what was happening so that they could prepare themselves, or that I found the words to explain something that was very difficult to talk about. It's all very amazing to me to be a part of that.

4:1. To find out the transplant didn't work for Danny, in the sense that he died, doesn't mean that any other patient that walked into the door with Wiskott-Aldrich syndrome should not get that treatment. I felt uncomfortable with the outcome, but that's part of what we do in pediatric oncology and particularly in pediatric stem cell transplants. We know that the mortality risk is very significant, it's probably close to 40 or 50 percent, whether you die from the transplant, or the transplant not working and the disease coming back, or from a complication of transplant. So for her other son (who also had Wiskott-Aldrich syndrome), I didn't recommend a transplant because this was a special circumstance in which this woman could end up losing both her children and that was too much, but for any other child that walks in with Wiskott-Aldridge syndrome, it's very clear that a transplant is the only way to try to cure the disease; otherwise, they just die. So this is one of the toughest cases that I've dealt with because whose agent am I? I guess I am an agent of the mother, but, basically, his chances of not making it through a transplant are a flip of a coin and it's hard to flip a coin with someone's life, even though he'll lose eventually. I guess I am an agent for the mother, what can I say? If she says that she wants to try the transplant for her other son we'll go ahead, but if she says, "No, I can't," I don't find it in me to push her to go that route like I did for the other son. I can't force this mother to do that and, in that sense, I am an agent for the mother.

3:1. It takes its toll on you. You take it home with you. There's no doubt about it; it's taken a toll on me. You lose a little bit of hope in what you're doing, and you lose a little bit of hope in your relations with parents who come back to tell you, "I was forced to do this," and when patients threaten that they are going to sue you. I was very disappointed and very angry when I found out that his transplant wasn't working at all. It's taken a pretty big toll and also seeing a child die who, a few months ago, was a happy, active—not completely normal but a relatively intact young boy. It's hard and I feel guilty, to some degree, and I carry it with me.

4:1. I'm sure these things are more significant for the residents. "Why are we wasting all this effort on this patient?" I've just done it too many times to worry about it anymore. There's been some evidence—I'm not that famil- iar with it—that residents who take care of patients in intensive care nurs- eries have, in general, a more pessimistic sense of the likely outcome for the patients than the attending staff do. Their pessimism is not really founded in reality, but they get the severe cases and the poor outcomes be- come overemphasized, in their view, and they don't have the long-term horizon that you need to see the successes in some of these patients. Their whole experience of the episodes in the intensive care unit is very stressful, things going wrong, babies bleeding in the brain, or they have injured lungs and they think, "Oh man, this child is going to be so severely dam- aged." They get very discouraged.

4:3. We have another kid who's just waiting on the floor to die, essentially. She's been here for a liver transplant and is not going to make it. It was just really sad the other day because, when the parents agreed to not push forward with resuscitation efforts, I saw her 9-year-old brother in the hall- way crying. I went up to him and I was like, "What's the matter?" and he was like, "My sister's really sick and my mother says she might go to heaven tonight." I was in tears; I mean it's horrible. People say you can't get too close, but I think that's crap. I think the day that that doesn't get to me—a 9-year-old boy saying goodbye to his 6-month-old sister—then I've got to quit. You can't let it get to you to the point where you can't function, but I have no problem walking away from there with tears in my eyes. What do you expect?

5:1. Sometimes you're very close to the family; like being a privileged close family friend there at the end. Sometimes you're in some kind of tension with the family, but you're there to show them respect and support the physician. I've been in rooms where the family isn't talking to any of the doctors and still you're there saying goodbye to the patient. There's all kinds of convoluted takes on the situation. It's hard because sometimes it can be really awkward because your role is sort of gone; you're the doctor and now the patient's not there anymore. What can you do? You say you're sorry and say goodbye to the patient.

5:1. One of my fellow attendings, who was on when Ricardo was starting to have major problems, was going through a lot of wondering and worrying, "What if we had done this?" and "Should we have done that?" or whatever. Fortunately, I wasn't feeling that way about this case. I didn't think there was anything that fell through the cracks, and I was grateful for that. It's hard enough to lose a patient without worrying and second-guessing yourself about what you did. I've been doing it longer than he has, and this is what happens; these horrible things happen. You lose kids, and I guess it's sort of easy to say that but, in reality, it is pretty awful. A few years ago, when I was a more junior attending and had only done transplants for a year or so, if I was on-service and somebody had a bad outcome or something went bad, I had the same level of second-guessing—not that I don't still do it, but it's a little bit of a growing pain and you come to a place where you realize how to accept it. One of the ex-perienced doctors in the intensive care unit said, when I thanked him for the care he'd given to a patient of mine who I thought had made an almost miraculous recovery—I said, "This is an incredible job and thank you so much," and he said, "Well, I'll take the compliment, but really I think that God makes the decision and we're just the gatekeepers." I think that sounds a little too fatalistic, but that's probably just his way of coping.

5:8. The nurses and doctors knew I had been following him, so they called me at home and that's definitely important because it's pretty difficult coming in, after taking care of a kid, having to work a shift, and then finding out he died when you come back on at 7:00 in the morning. This way, it gives you a little bit of time to focus and deal with grief.

5:7. The hard part about taking care of a child who's dying is that, as you get to know them, you get attached to them and then they leave you—in a self-centered way. Or you get to know a family and understand the importance that the child has in the family and then you see that aspect destroyed—it's a strong word, but it's a strong experience. It's very difficult, and I must be schizophrenic because I have the capacity to block off my feelings. I divorce myself from my own sense of personal sadness, and it's the only way that I can keep doing my job. It's a protective mechanism. I remember the day I sent him to the PICU—they hardly ever come back to us from the unit. He didn't arrest overnight and I'd seen a lot worse situations, so I felt good about the way that was managed.

5:1. A large percentage of our patients, by the time they get to the ICU, are not conscious and so you don't talk to them. I am very used to it, and I actually found it an attractive part of this specialty early on; it relieved me of interacting with some very sick children. On the other hand, the tradeoff is you spend a lot more time and more effort with their parents. I spend a lot of energy, early on, figuring out how not to become too emotionally attached to families in general, so it goes well beyond the patient. I create some artificial barriers so I can do that. I never use anybody's first name except the patient's. I never use the parents' first names, even when we are invited to. I try to have people refer to me as "doctor" and never by my first name, although that doesn't always work. I maintain a certain sense of distance, but that breaks down when the patients die. You hug people, you touch people, but to make the tough decisions sometimes, I have to not do that.

5:7. When this one child died, there was one nurse who practically went into mourning for 3 days. She was more upset than the family. Sometimes some of the physicians seem more upset than the family and are not ready to let go. Some people are just very emotional, and they grieve as if they are a family member and feel the loss very deeply. Those individuals need perhaps a different type of guidance. Everyone has to put their feet in the water and see what it's like and then see how they're going to cope with it.

5:10. My husband always says that every time somebody passes away it chips away at me, and I think he means that it takes part of me away. It chips away at me because I mourn but like I mourn in a constructive manner; that is, I usually get ice cream and I get chocolate all in one night. I get a bottle of wine and I cannot deal with any unhappy thoughts or feelings. So I think that's what he means; my husband needs to make sure that he's encouraging because I don't want to talk about anything heavy duty for that night. I can't handle it emotionally. It just chips away, and those who say it doesn't bother them anymore have just done a really good job at shielding themselves. It's a very sad thing, and we don't have here the mechanisms to process what we're feeling. Somebody dies and you come right back to work the next day and you're at it and then somebody else dies. What saddens me is seeing doctors here who are not dealing with how it has chipped away at their joy. I think it has increased burnout because there isn't a forum where people can say, "I'm really sad about this." I know several physicians, for example—I know because I asked them, "How do you know how is it affecting you?"—who were like, "I'm just freaked out. This is so hard for me." Some have said that they feel guilty, "Did a child die because of something that could have been avoided?" I think that these feelings will increase unless we create a forum where people can talk. Those who have been around longer have identified the tools that have helped them, but not everyone is that mature. I have a director that, every time someone dies, she's like, "Go home," and I go home, running; I don't even have to be convinced. I have a great support system at home so then I talk about what I'm feeling. I'm not afraid to cry or talk or say, "You know what? This is hard." But not everyone can do that.

5:8. Sometimes, I just have to take a day off. Yesterday I totally needed one. I just took a day off, and I was just outside in the sun. I didn't really talk to my friends; I just needed time by myself to think things over. I called my family just to say, "Hi," and it made me appreciate what I have. Today I need a break, so I'm going to take a light assignment, and that's good because everybody looks out for each other and we're able to do that.

5:7. If you're taking care of a child that dies, we all need to take better care of each other so that the person who's taking care of that kid has some private time; has some time to just decompress. Often, it's having other people voluntarily take their patients, if they're stuck on the floor, so the person can just go do her own thing. It's really such an amazing thing that you have to take care of someone that dies and then, the next minute, walk into somebody else's room and be happy, uplifting, and make a joke or just ask, "How are you doing?" That kind of juxtaposition of life and death is too much for anyone. If you're on the floor and a kid dies, it's not a choice, you just keep going with all your other patients.

Many clinicians in end-of-life care in pediatrics are married or have partners who work in the same field, often in the same institutions. This is a common situation in any professional field, but questions inevitably arise about what it is like living with someone who does the same kind of work in such an incredibly stressful field of practice. Does it help them to cope day-by-day, or does it make it worse because they can't so easily leave the disturbing issues in the office and decompress when they go home. Here is how one person talked about her situation:

5:7. We're the same cut; we're pretty much from the same mold. He very rarely talks about that piece of his work, and we have the same sort of warped sense of humor. Some people laugh at it and some people don't, and if you're with someone who doesn't laugh and you want to, you're miserable. If you're with someone who's crying all the time and you can't, you're miserable. I don't cry, so I go to these wakes and funerals and I look around and I don't know how to cry. I never took method acting, so I can't make myself do it; it's like a real problem, but he's the same way. The other thing is that it's the Pollyanna in me. It's such an enriching experience to learn about other people's lives and what they have and how it gives them strength.

We went to a wake in a Baptist church and it was an Afro-American family who'd adopted a Hispanic boy who had AIDS. His parents had AIDS, and he had the bad luck of getting a neuroblastoma. His family were his foster parents, and they adopted him after he was sick. It was just an amazing thing to go to this church and to see all these people supporting this family and then to go up and share a meal with them, upstairs in this very modest room with the chicken. Okay, it was a really horrible dinner and all I wanted to do was go home and I said to my husband, "Can't we just go home and eat spaghetti? It's Friday and it's our day to have spaghetti and drink some wine," and he said, "No. We're going to share with this family." For me, it's very helpful to have someone that's on the same level, and I might have said that to him in a similar situation and drag him through it. It was a great experience having dinner with them, but I was resenting that my time was my Friday night and that's when we both decompress, every Friday night, by eating spaghetti and drinking red wine. It's like, we're getting so compulsive about it that going out to the opera is not the same as going home and having the red wine and spaghetti. So that's like our ritual, spaghetti and red wine on Fridays thing, and we both are ritual-istic so, in that way, we're together; that's what helps us through it.

6:2. It seems so unfortunate that such a small child should lose his life over something that clearly was preventable, a car accident. There's definitely a different response you have when a child dies from an acute trauma com-pared to a chronic condition. For whatever reason, you seem to connect more with the kids who come in for an acute trauma like drowning or heatstroke or something that seems a lot more likely to happen to you or a loved one than say, for example, somebody with some sort of debilitating but unusual chronic illness. You can distance yourself from that kind of scene very easily, and I find that those cases are much easier to take care of.

7:1. The funeral was helpful to me because the priest echoed the words that I'd been telling the family all along, which confirmed that I had done the right thing for them in helping them. The priest said he just used the parents' words and put them in different order, and obviously I think I'd helped them by giving them some vocabulary to better understand this too. I heard back, from the priest, what I had told them, which was helpful because this one was a mind-blower, the whole thing. The priest said to me, "You took very good care of this family and they have the utmost respect for you."

7:8. I learned from my experience of losing my first patient. I had got very, very attached, and it just wasn't healthy. So I learned, in my subconscious, to put up that wall and you don't break that barrier. What I try not to do is to get sucked up into the parents' saying, "What would you do?" and give them my opinion. I try to respond from a medical standpoint rather than my own personal one. That way, they know that there's that wall up between us. That's the way I handle it. So when they ask me, "If this was your child, what would you do?" I say that, "It's not my child so I can't answer that." They don't like that answer, but then I'll say something like, "Well, what are your options? How do you feel the decision should be made?" I reflect it back on them, and I help them problem solve it themselves. So I think I'm helping them, but I'm not giving them my opinion.

7:10. I had a very interesting dynamic because they were a family that I could relate to because they were of the same ethnic background as me, same neighborhood that I live in, and the same kind of socioeconomic level. They were someone that could be my friends, someone in my community. So it was very hard because I became very attached to them, and it was because I connected with them on a different level than I would with somebody else—not a better level, just different because I feel close to patients in other socioeconomic levels and ethnic backgrounds. But it made it a little harder for me than some of the other deaths and then, because my sister has a baby who's that age, I pictured my sister in that situation. I just had all these crazy thoughts, so it was kind of hard to put that professional wall up.

8:10. I am getting tired of grieving. I have had four kids die through my third year, and I am tired of grieving. I have never had anyone die personally in my life, and I am not very effective in keeping people at arms length. If I am going to care for someone, I am going to care for them, obviously in a professional manner, but I am not good at just providing services without having some feeling for them and this has been very difficult for me. . . . I feel like I am growing old very quickly. It is probably why William's death was so difficult for me. It was very painful watching the mom grieve for him. She kept punching William, I mean she was punching the body. It was a very extreme kind of grieving and they had to give her Ativan. It was the first time I had seen someone display grieving in such a dramatic manner, and it freaked me out. . . . Last week, Friday, William had a heart attack and I remember how she clutched one of the doctors, and she is a pretty big woman, and the doctor was not really comfortable with that and didn't know what to do. I was walking by and the mom saw me and so she clutched me; it almost knocked me down because, compared to the doctor, I am super tiny. But it was very painful because she almost fainted; she started hyperventilating and she almost threw up. When he died that Sunday and they paged me and I heard the screaming and I couldn't come, I just felt like I needed to protect myself. And I have somebody else who is going to die and there is only so much I can do. I can, to some degree, talk about my feelings with my colleagues, but you have to understand that we are all trying to protect ourselves, and so there is only so much that we can hear about each other's cases. We are trying to protect our hearts because, when we turn around, we are getting new cases and somebody always is dying. I realized yesterday that I have been coming to work for a week and a half now and every day I just want to cry. I know that is not healthy. Those are symptoms of depression. I come in and no one has done anything to me, but I just want to cry. In this place, there is some kind of stigma if you say that you are grieving, because you are supposed to be able to handle this.

8:2. It always is good advice, when a child is dying, to have the parent say, "It is okay for you to go." It is good for the parents, and it is good for the dying child. But they can hang on forever. I have had kids with agonal breathing for hours; agonal breathing is like they go "huuuuuuu," the arrival of death they call it sometimes, and I can hear them for hours. Some physicians feel uncomfortable doing anything about that. We used to work with an unbelievable physician in this unit that was the best, and we were very sorry she decided ICU was taking too much out of her life. When we had cases like that, she would administer a nice amount of morphine, just slowly, and she would be there with the parents. If there was someone you wanted there, when you die, this was the person. But it took too much out of her. After 15 years, she had to go and she went back to anesthesiology. She is still with patient care, but she doesn't have to deal first-hand with the death and dying. It was just that it really took a big hit out of her because she was such a different physician from all the others. For one thing, she didn't grow up in the United States. She grew up in a Third World country, so her first experience as a physician was watching kids dying of a cold, so death was not a stranger to her.

8:1. For a few years, we had a memorial service, not for families, but for staff. It was in the chapel, and it was meant to be in honor of all the children that had died in that year. The child-life service was involved with organizing it, and the format, as I recall, was that they had little signs with the children's names that you would pin to something on the wall that was a memorial. That was the intent, that it was specifically for the staff. We haven't tried the idea of inviting families. We stopped doing it when the person who was in charge of organizing it left. Like anything else, if you are missing the person that most wanted to organize it, then somebody else has to pick it up. I thought it was very helpful for the staff. If you start from the premise that it is unnatural for a child to die, then, at least in our country, there is that need to come to grips with the fact that you're wanting to help children but you are still losing some.

9:1. I can see myself changing a little bit over the years, but I don't ever want to get to the point where I don't care at all. I guess I have a lot more layers of protection. Part of it is that I work with really great staff so I don't feel like it's all on me. Part of it is a positive thing because there was a time in my life when my need to be the perfect doctor for an individual family was about my ego; in some way it fed a need of mine. I don't think I have to feel needed as much, so when a family gets more of things from other people I work with, I welcome it and feel it as a relief rather than feeling that it all should be on me. A lot of the staff were very close to this family, so there were lots of different ways the family could get cared for. I didn't feel like it had to be me all the time. But there is a little bit less intensity than at earlier points of my life, and some of it is my own pulling back. There's just so much loss you can deal with.

9:10. Toward the last few months of his life, I found myself backing away from the family a little more because I knew this was coming. I knew that he wasn't doing well, so I removed myself a little bit and kept very busy focusing on concrete tasks for the family. I kept very minimal contact with him and I feel a little guilty about that. I was much closer to John when I first met him last year. We had a lot of good talks in the beginning of his diagnosis, when I first met him. He would say, "Why me?" and "It's not fair. It's so annoying," those kinds of talks, but never the possibility that he might die. In my practice, I've avoided it. I used to work in pediatric AIDS, and that's all I would do—talk to the children about their illness.

But now, for some reason, I can't. It's getting so hard that I've remolded my practice, and I don't do that anymore because it's a way to keep my engine going. It's exhausting. I've lost several kids in the past few weeks and the more I lose, the more detached I'm getting from the families, which is not fair to them. But I also love my job and I don't want to leave, but I'm thinking that maybe they should have a social worker who's more hands-on with the kids. But we have child-life specialists who do that, so that gives me some sense of comfort, but I don't give it my all to sit with the kid and talk about serious things because it's getting too hard for me.

9:8. Since I've had a son, I try to save my Saturdays and Sundays for him and my husband. I have made it a rule to try to separate work out. I think that's how I've survived in this business for 24 years. I try to separate it, and on Saturday and Sunday, I give them my time; otherwise I won't be any good to my son or my husband. So when I came in on Monday I found out, and I wasn't completely shocked; I expected it by then. When I got home that Friday, I talked to my husband about it. I got home about 9:00, by the time we finished with John and we finished winding down, and my husband said to me, "Look at you. You're mentally and physically exhausted. Have a glass of wine." We talked for about 10 minutes, and he said, "Try to push it out of your mind for at least 2 days." I have a very good husband who's willing to listen and is very supportive. He doesn't understand how I do this sometimes. He could never do it. He walks into a hospital, and he's like, "Oh the smell," but it's hard for him to see me go through this.

9:1. Going to his house the night he died was an unusual experience for me. In the earlier part of my career, it was not unusual for me to make house calls for palliative care, but they were generally calls during the time when a child was dying at home, not at the time they died. We usually had hospice involved and they would take care of that, but in the case of John, it had accelerated so fast that we didn't have all of the hospice mechanisms in place, so it was important that somebody who knew him and his parents was the person who pronounced him dead and made sure that there were no problems because, to be blunt, funeral homes don't generally pick patients up at houses—they pick them up in hospitals. Theoretically, if someone dies at home, unless it's certified by the treating doctor, they make it a medical examiner's case, and I didn't want anything bad to happen to the family in terms of their emotions about this so I went to the house. . . . His mom called and said he wasn't doing well and could I come. I got there about a minute or two after he died, according to the family. It was very surreal because I've seen any number of children dead in a bed in a hospital, but it's very different to see a child at home in bed, with his colored pillows and, I don't know, just everything that just should've been normal but it wasn't. And then it was weird because, as I arrived in front of the house, the mother was standing out front, which was the last thing I expected. I was shocked to see her there. She hugged me and said she just couldn't stand watching him anymore so she came out. So we went up together and she walked me into a room where everybody was crying and looking teary-eyed and he was lying in the bed with his aunt lying next to him. He looked just like he always looked, except paler and thinner and colder. I listened to his heart for a second, to be official about it. I didn't actually use a stethoscope; I just took his pulse and I kissed him on the forehead, I rubbed his hair, and I said, "Goodbye." It was this weird scene where there was this dead teenager in the next room and life around was touched by it—everybody was crying and upset—yet there was a little kid watching television and people were feeding their kids dinner. It was this mixture of life goes on and there's death. I called the funeral home, and it was annoying because they didn't answer right away. So I stayed there for about an hour and a half with the family waiting for the funeral people to call back because I didn't want to leave them with this dead child in the bedroom without plans made. Ultimately, it was good because it also gave me time to just be with Mom and talk about John with her. She was calm, but when the funeral people came to take him, it all sort of hit her. I guess I should have realized because she had said, "It's okay, he could stay here, if the funeral parlor didn't call back." I didn't really pick up on how much she really just didn't want him to leave. I thought it would have been creepy for her to have him in the house overnight. I never thought that that would be the right thing to do, but she just wasn't ready for him to physically leave.

10:5. I left work Friday afternoon and it was a couple of hours after I left when she passed away. My team had said that they felt badly because they didn't have a way of getting in touch with me, but I didn't think that she would go that weekend. She wasn't doing well, but she had been stable over the previous couple of days so I didn't expect it. I came back to work that Monday, and she just wasn't in her room. There was just no way to prepare for it. I didn't think it would be as hard for me because I didn't actually know Sarah when she was well, but I felt like I got to know her just from hearing her parents' stories about her. I didn't discuss it much with anyone, just a little bit with a friend of mine. Things got really busy—we had a number of patients afterward—and I just never dealt with it directly. But it's definitely still with me. I think about her every day, and I've cried about it. I don't feel like there's been closure because I wasn't there when she died. Ideally, it would have been great to have had someone to talk to about it; if I hadn't sat and talked with you, I never would have used a resource like that because I kept going and felt I could deal with it on my own; if I'm going to be a doctor, I have to learn to deal with this. But I guess it would be nice to have available someone with whom you would want to talk about it.

10:7. Death doesn't particularly bother me. If it did, I couldn't do this kind of work [PICU nurse] full time. I don't really have a problem with it. Of course, it bothers me to see a young child pass away, and I try to be as helpful as possible making sure the child's comfortable and the parents' questions are answered. After about 5 years in PICU, I'm much more comfortable with death, talking about it, being there, witnessing it; much more comfortable but from a practice point of view. When I say that I'm more comfortable, it's not that I distance myself or not feel it so emotionally. I mean that, in the past, I would have been more tempted to stay away because I wouldn't know what to say to the families, other than "I'm sorry." But I'm much more comfortable addressing those feelings and those hard issues now with families than I used to be.

11:1. The first thing that goes through your mind is whether it was something we did, something we gave her, or was it her disease that suddenly killed her? That's your immediate reaction. She was going to die at 3 or 4 years of age with no treatment, but we precipitated this and that's something I'm still having trouble dealing with. Right now, we have a lot of cases that are just harder to go home with. These patients come in with complicated conditions and they're here to get treated and sometimes the treatments we do will precipitate events but it's nothing we did. We can't keep saying we missed something, which is the first thing we think of, and I'm having a hard time trying to learn to realize that I'm not causing all of these awful things to happen. A lot of times, I walk away feeling, "Oh my God, I missed that,"or "How did I not see that that blood pressure was so high?

How could I have done that?" or "Did I cause this infection by doing that procedure?" This guilt or blame I feel, I put on myself. . . . It's hard to reach out to the family when you're thinking, "Oh my God, are they blaming me?"

11:3. Afterward, I sat with the senior resident and was like, "Is there something we missed?" We went over and over it and she said, "It sounded like you did everything right," but when a child dies, there's always something you can't resolve. A code is not commonly seen on the floor. You usually have some warning. You can gather the people involved, transfer the child to the PICU, and whatever happens, at that point, will happen. That's usually what happens so this was unusual. I hadn't been involved in any codes prior to this, so knowing what the steps are, forcing myself to go through the algorithm, was important because it was so scary. You have to try to make yourself step back and think, "What are the steps I need to do here?" The support I got from the staff was amazing. The senior resident was very supportive. She said, "I'm here. Call me anytime." We went over it and she sat with me until the fellow came. When the fellow got here, she took my hand and said, "You did a great job. There's nothing else you could have done." It was the same thing with the attending. The nurses were all very upset. The nurse that was taking care of her was praying over her as this all started, and I was watching her and trying— it's like I'm trying to be very, kind of scientific, to do the logical thing, when, at the same time, it's such an emotional situation and she's praying. I was thinking, as this was occurring, "Where is the mom?" Then I realized that she had already been taken out of the room by someone else, so by the time all this stuff was happening, she was gone so I didn't know how much she actually saw but it was one thing I thought about. It was hard continuing to work that evening, and in an ideal world, when someone has to deal with something like this, it would be nice to get relief for the rest of the night. I was just constantly going back in my mind thinking about what had happened. Even though you're going into a field like pediatrics where you hope to see mostly fairly healthy kids, we see a lot of very sick kids in residency. So it's been hard recently, and then, when this happened, I thought, "What's the world coming to? Why do little kids, 13 months old, have to die? She didn't have a chance." I had all those thoughts in my head but knowing too that I have to do what I have to do right now. So doing it, seeing the other patients on the floor but, in between, thinking about these things. The other families pretty much acted like everything was okay, asking me their own questions about their kids like, "My child has a light headache. My child's feeling nauseous." These are things that we deal with all the time, but that night I felt like, "Yeah, okay, that's not a big deal compared to what I just saw." But you have to force yourself to take those things seriously because they're affecting the life of that child in the moment. I was fortunate enough to not be on-call again for almost a week. It was hard for me to go on my first call back on the floor after that. I was not looking forward to going back to the same place, knowing full well that the call would probably be fine and that this kind of thing was not likely to happen again, but there was something, a reminder, that it was the same place and it was some of the same staff and I knew people would probably still be talking about it. But when I showed up, it was business as usual. There were a lot of things to do, and the day just kind of went by.

12:2. I found it difficult to see a vibrant child totally unresponsive. It happened over a very long time, so it gave you a chance to prepare emotionally for the fact that she was not going to be responsive. That was difficult. In the first few days, when I saw that, I thought, "Well maybe she is going to recover," but by the time it became more than a week, it was difficult to go in there day by day. I've been talking to a couple of people about this. We are very well defended, we doctor types, probably nurses as well, and so it allowed the defenses to go up and for us to be very fortified. You can see how I am talking very calmly, pretty much unemotionally because I am still very well defended right now. I started telling myself that she was going to die, probably 2 weeks ago. That will slip at a certain point but not quite yet. That's what I was talking to people about, about how the defenses go and then they drop, when you're not looking. What happens is that at some point, when you're not looking and when you're thinking about something altogether different, something is going to trigger you and you have no idea what it is. It is usually when I am driving in the car because then I am all alone and I can let it pour out and it all happens.

14:3. An important issue is how the interns and residents deal with having a person die that's under their care. The intern who was present when he passed away was very emotional and was crying. I talked with her, making sure that she was okay but she didn't want to talk about it. She said she was fine and I didn't pursue it any further, but this was the first patient that she had under her care that passed away, so I'm sure that there are emotions and issues that probably need to be or should be talked about. I'm thinking back about the first patient that I had that died. My senior pulled me aside and we sat in a room and he asked me what feelings were going through my mind and how did I feel? It was an opportunity to express how I felt and for him to reassure me that everything was done right, whatever my feelings were, and that these are issues and feelings that you will have to deal with as a doctor. I thought that that was really beneficial to be able to express how I felt then so that's why I asked to talk with the intern about Roberto dying, but she didn't want to and I didn't push her.

15:7. When the stress level increases on the floor, people become more irritable and angry. This floor [oncology service] always seems to have a high stress level so it's hard for me to tell, but when people's stress levels are increased, they are just not as patient with other people and it leads to bad morale in general. For me, the best way of handling it is massage therapy, honestly. I don't think that a lot of people would feel comfortable having a group session and just kind of airing their feelings. I feel like a lot of people, even though they are very emotional, try to block it out and just move on, or they will go in the bathroom and they'll cry. You can't really show your emotions here, so sometimes you need something private, like a massage. It is something where you are relieving your stress and you have some time to be on your own and decompress a little bit. The few times that the massage therapist has been here and I've felt particularly stressed and I've gone to her, it just really brought me back down. If we were going to get together as a group, it would be better to do it outside the hospital and not to focus just on our stress and grief and stuff but instead just help people to relate to each other. I had a dinner party a couple of nights ago and had the nurses over to my house. It was very nice to be out of the hospital setting because, in the past, we had done it in the clinic. The other thing is that we all share a very special bond in that we care for these very sick children and you can't talk about it with other people because they can't deal with it. I've tried. Yesterday, I told my mom that it was just a terrible, terrible, terrible day at work. She was like, "Oh really, why?" and I said, "It was just so unbelievably sad. It was just the saddest situation that you could ever imagine, and there are so many sad situations, but this just beats all." She was just kind of like, "Wow." I get that response from people a lot, so I feel like I can only share with the people that I work with because they know what it's like.

15:6. We could go on and on talking about the tragedy of this family and we can all come together and talk about our sense of grief and our feelings for them, but there is also another way of grieving. We can all go out for some beers and burgers and connect to one another as good friends and colleagues working together. This isn't the "good grief" model; it's the Irish-way model, and I'm a big fan of the Irish-way model. Last night was the departmental Christmas party that I went to with all the residents who knew George, and we toasted George because he was a great little kid. And we did that for Joey back when he passed away. A bunch of us residents went out with some of the nurse practitioners, and we had a couple of beers and some burgers and just sat around and talked and kind of hung out together and got to know each other better.

16:1. The thing that is hardest for me is figuring out how to give condolences to the family because it's so much a time when the family gathers inward and it's hard not to feel like you're intruding on a very private time. Jose died in the middle of the night, and I purposely chose not to come in because the last time I came into the hospital after I lost a patient it was such a tough experience. I had this horrible sense of coming in and intruding when the family was in their own grief. So I had called a few hours later, but then I felt bad because the mother said, "Oh, you weren't here." She said, "We're very, very grateful," but she also said, "You weren't here when he left us." I felt terribly guilty. It's not that she felt that there's anything I could have done differently. My real issue is that I still don't know what's the right way to say farewell to the families.

16:6. This was the hardest case I've had so far. I usually don't shed tears about dealing with death. I'm usually able to distance my emotions from my responsibilities and make whatever treatment decisions that need to be made, but I could not do that this time. In this case, I found myself crying. Even though I was prepared for it, this was the hardest one I've had to deal with because Jose was beyond a patient; he was a friend. I knew him from camp [a special camp for kids with cancer] in a nonmedical setting, and that made a big difference for me. With the other children I've taken care of, there's only been a connection on a patient-to-doctor basis; it never crossed the line. But 2 years ago when I was at camp, I was one of the counselors in Jose's group, and then, this past year, I saw him in camp. We would talk about things like sports and all the crazy stuff that people who have similar interests talk about, not just doctor-patient things. . . . I think everybody should make their own personal choices about how involved they'd like to get with a patient and be willing to accept the consequences. I knew full well from the first time that I knew Jose that he should have been dead a long time ago and the fact that he wasn't was a miracle. But that didn't stop me from establishing a relationship with him. It was because he was a likeable, friendly guy and just very easy to become friends with. I know that I'm still able to take a step back and step into the doctor role and do what I need to do to give them the best care that they deserve while still being able to then turn back into a friend again.

16:10. This was a family I was not very connected to, and I did that on purpose. I made sure their needs were met concrete-wise, but I had a hard time getting close to them because I needed to protect myself, and I said to myself, "Well, they're connected to child-life, they're connected to their attending, to psychology; they have tons of support so I'm going to give myself a little break." And that's what I did with this family. I didn't get too close because he was such a sweet kid, and I knew he was going to die soon because of his cancer; it was an aggressive, horrible cancer. So, knowing that from the onset, I kept a huge distance, probably too much of a professional distance. I should have pushed through it more and been there more. I popped my head in the room, I touched base with the family, but I didn't sit down and try to engage him and draw him out. I connected better with the parents because I knew I wouldn't be losing them. I took care of their concrete needs, like paying for things and getting a medication covered. I got involved in very task-oriented ways. I didn't deal with the bereavement piece because it was too hard for me and I knew it was getting addressed in other ways; if it wasn't, I would have made myself more involved. That's one of the ways that I've learned how to survive here; that you don't have to get intensely close with every patient because you can't. So I'm not hard on myself for it, but I am a little bit. I felt like I should have been there a little more, but I did what I could to help myself.

16:11. This was the first patient of mine who's passed away. While I wanted to be there for them, I was aware of not wanting to lean too far in, get really crushed or hurt or sad, and then start pulling back and retreating from other patients in the future. So I tried to establish some kind of boundaries and distance that I felt comfortable with, that I could maintain beyond this patient. I'm still figuring it out for myself. Like, when I went to Jose's room one time, there was a man walking out of the room that I never saw in my life; never met him. I didn't know what it was about the moment, but I just reached out to hug him and we embraced each other for like a solid 60, 70 seconds, firmly embracing. He went off, and it was such a powerful moment—I didn't know what it was, I just reached out and grabbed and hugged him. Not a word was spoken. I turned to the psychiatry fellow in the room—I was really horrified because I didn't know who that was, and it turned out that it was Jose's father. That opened up something between us for the future, and when I ran into him again, the second time, I hugged him and he was saying, "I love you, I love you." Mom and I had been quite distant and I hugged her a few times toward the end, but it was very powerful with him and it stuck in my mind. It just happened and I can't explain it.

18:2. This is nice to be able to talk about these things one-on-one. There haven't been times in my career that I've tried talking like this. Most of the time, I find that people don't talk about their feelings and they get shoved aside and that's been a hard thing for me. It's something that needs to be addressed because there's times when you just want to say, "I'm angry about it or frustrated," not that I want to do anything more; it would just help clear my head out, and we don't do that a lot in this field and I don't think that's healthy. Sometimes I've talked to my wife, she's a child-life specialist, so she's somewhat understanding, but if I try to talk to any one of her family, they don't have any insight so, to them, it's always too horrible. I've tried bringing it up, and then, all of a sudden, you start thinking about how horrible they may think it is rather than that I just want to talk about it with someone. It would be nice if there were some sort of service where physicians can deal with it because they don't. What happens is that, over time, you become a little bit more callous to the situation and you see how people change; some just say, "This baby's going to die," and you see other physicians who are trying to save every baby, no matter what, and they have him on every pressor and they're torturing him. I've seen these two extremes—one who's done overkill and the other who was like, "Just let it go" and that's frustrating. So thanks; it helped for me just to talk about this.

19:3. For the last week, every day, I've been thinking, "What did I not do? What did I do? What should I have done? Should I have advocated more for this? Should I have pushed the fellow more on this? Was there something about the physiology that I didn't understand; that I should've been aware of; that I missed throughout the day? She was one of three babies on that service that day who were considered sick and who needed to be watched. She was not placed on the top of the list by anyone, except by myself, in my mind, in the beginning of the day. So she was the one for whom I consistently went into the room or checked vitals or at least asked the nurse how she was doing. The ward senior who was with me during the code was a really good friend of mine, so she and I talked all night, pretty much. Then I went home and managed to fall asleep but not for very long. Then my friend and I talked again that night for like an hour and went over everything and pieced everything apart, everything that happened—what could it have been and what did we miss? On my way home, I called my mother because, for me, I need to hear my family's voices to make me feel calm. Usually I call my dad first, but I couldn't reach him so I called my mom. Right away, she said, "What's wrong?" She could tell right away, and she just listened to me for like 45 minutes and my parents are nowhere near the field of medicine so, for them, it's like, "Whatever, but I hear your distress and it's okay." I talked to my father in the morning, and he simply said just the kind of things that you want to hear. You don't want to hear an analysis; you just want to hear someone say—and this is what he said—"I'm sorry for your loss. It sounded like it was a hard day, and these things happen, and it will happen to you, but keep in mind that you do a lot of really wonderful, good things for other patients, so you should feel okay." That's all I needed to hear. I mean it was just like, "Oh-h-h, thank you, Daddy," and he goes, "Okay, have a good day," and he hung up.

19:1. For me, the difficult part is going through the death process. The closure comes when the family has accepted the fact that the patient is going to die because, often, that's the most difficult part. Once they accept it, I'm perfectly okay with that patient dying; I may not like it; I may wish things would have been different, but I'm okay as long as the parents understand that and know that there's nothing else that could have been done or there's nothing else reasonable that could have been done.

19:3. As a culture, we learn how to deal with this stuff; we study it and break it down into different things—physicians eat that up. They will go to a study session on it and break down the different areas that things could've been done better, but they're not going to talk about their own feelings. As a culture, we just say, "Deal with your own feelings and don't let that interfere with doing your job." We had an intern retreat over the weekend, and we started talking about some of the children in the hospital that we all knew, some who would pass and some who were doing really bad and at some point, somebody said, "We're outside of the hospital, let's not talk about that anymore," and suddenly the subject changed and everybody agreed. It's like, once you get out of the hospital, it's time to leave the grief that's in these walls somewhere else. I think the more seasoned attendings definitely have seen more than the younger physicians, so they have more bottled up inside. The younger physicians are bright-eyed. We see the potential for good that we can do, and the older attendings have seen the failures—the kids that they couldn't bring back. They take their feelings for a child passing and put them inside a bottle and just keep them there. You know that you're hurt by it and you want to take a minute to grieve for that child but you don't have the time, so you have to deal with only a little bit of it and then you have to move on, so it's bottled up. They don't get a chance to express their feelings or talk about how they felt when this child died. Maybe that's how they're teaching us how to deal with this— this is way they do it. I had a patient die the other day when I was post-call, and one of the other residents called and told me at night and I was glad that I was at home because I could take a minute and think about it. The kid who died had been a chronic patient of mine—he was there for months—and the next day I had to go in there and take care of another child in the exact same bed in the same spot where I'd been going in every morning for weeks seeing this other kid. That's tough.

20:8. It was more difficult for me to withdraw support for this baby than for the other two because he was awake and crying, so I had a really, really hard time doing it but I knew it was the best thing to do for the baby and for the parents. It helped that, once I pulled the tube, the baby turned blue quickly and didn't remain crying and didn't look like a well baby. He wasn't active anymore and he wasn't awake so that made it easier for me. I've been doing it for so many years, but this particular baby really upset me. I got teary-eyed and I took a deep breath and I said, "All right, you can do this. You've done this many times before, and it's okay," and I talked myself into it.

Education and Training in End-of-Life Care

Most physicians and nurses are aware of the palliative needs of their patients who are dying, but "they lack both the confidence and competence in palliative care, and have until now had little or no training in it."[3] They are inadequately trained about issues of death and dying during their preclinical and clinical years of medical school and then into their residency.[4] For example, a survey of pediatric oncologists by the American Society of Clinical Oncology (ASCO) found a serious lack of training in end-of-life care and a "strikingly high reliance on trial and error in learning to care for dying children."[5] A comprehensive review of 50 medical textbooks found that they had "little helpful information on caring for patients at the end of life."[6] Training in end-of-life care for other medical staff (e.g., nurses, social workers, psychologists) also has been found lacking.[7] For example, a review of leading textbooks in pediatric nursing reported that only 2 percent of the contents addressed end-of-life care.[8]

Knowing how to communicate "bad news" to families and promote frank discourse among patients, families, and medical staff is the cornerstone of training in end-of-life care. Training also needs to focus on self-reflection about what it is like providing end-of-life care to children and families and on strategies to help staff deal with the stresses placed on them. The Committee on Palliative and End-of-Life Care for Children and Their Families of the Institute of Medicine prescribed four general areas of training for medical staff in pediatric end-of-life care: (1) scientific and clinical knowledge and skills, (2) interpersonal skills and attitudes, (3) ethical and professional principles, and (4) organizational knowledge.[9]

A guiding principle for training in pediatric end-of-life care is that we cannot prescribe an orthodox way of dying that is appropriate for all children and families. Because there is no correct way to die, the purpose of training is to explore ways to respect and honor what patients, within the purview of family-based practice, evidence-based medicine, and patient autonomy, find is best for them.

Although strategies to train all medical staff in end-of-life care should begin early in their education, these strategies should intensify and become more focused during more specialized training. Ultimately, no amount of classroom education, reading, discussions, focus groups, or role-playing with simulated patients can ever come close to prepare staff for end-of-life care as can active and direct case-by-case clinical involvement with more experienced staff. Such involvement includes participating in staff meetings to consider options as well as being at the bedside when discussing such options with patients and families. In the words of the resident in the following narrative: "You can't just practice it outside of experiencing it." However, providing opportunities for this level of active involvement encompasses several challenges and barriers in hospital-based practice.[10]

2:3. I wish the attendings would include us more when they sit down with the family to convey the bad news. They need to grab the residents when they have these discussions with the parents. We need to go in the room and be there with the attending when they break the bad news. If we had more opportunities to learn from the people who do it often, that would be one of the most valuable experiences of your whole life. We learn esoterically in med school how to do it and then maybe have a few discussions after a lecture, but there's no way to learn how to balance the emotions without having real-life experiences. You can talk about it, you can play out scenarios about "How would you tell someone this?" but it's not the same. You can't just practice it outside of experiencing it. I don't know why attendings don't include us more, I honestly don't. Maybe our hours are such that, when it's a good time for them, it may not be a good time for us or vice versa. Maybe, when these discussions take place, we are busy doing other work, and they don't want to take us from that work. My point is that we're here to work, yet we're also here to learn, as long as there's nothing emergent. An hour that we spend here could be more valuable than 3 hours worth of lectures, so I don't know why we are not included more.

2:3. I remember, when I was a fourth-year med student, hearing a talk by one of the attendings in oncology on how to go about talking about death. She was very good at being direct; she was compassionate, but she was not going to beat around the bush to make the patients feel happier about it.

She wanted to let them know and then go from there, and I learned a lot from her. It would be great even to have a psychologist talk to us about this because death is a multidisciplinary thing, and we all need to accept that.

2:1. I don't think residents are very well prepared to deal with dying children and their families. Part of it is the way the residents rotate. It's hard to come in at the end and say, "Okay, here's a dying patient, come and take care of him," and to have that bond with the parent and the patient. It is very difficult because they don't really know them, and that's one of the reasons why it's so hard for the residents. From my standpoint, I know them in the beginning and I know them in the end, and so you build a bond, a trust. . . . Can we teach them a little bit more? We probably can, but I don't necessarily know how. I guess that's the hard question—how do you teach them to deal with that and be able to take care of the patient? Can you teach them a sort of sensitivity to the patient and the parent? How can we teach that? I don't know whether you can teach that. There are classes on death and dying, but until you're really dealing with it, it's very much in the abstract. Can we teach sensitivity? I don't think you can. I think that's going to have to be part of the intrinsic character of the person.

4:3. It's been a depressing couple of months; a lot of kids have not done well, but attendings in the ICU or the oncologists are dealing with these end-of-life issues, and they're having discussions where they'll say, "Well, it should just be me; a resident shouldn't go in there." But those are the times when the residents need to get involved because when else are we going to learn how to deal with this? It's good to have a patient like this, where you have to deal with these kinds of issues, where it faces you every day, because, in a year or in a couple of months, we're going to be making these decisions on our own. So as unpleasant as the experience was, you need to think about these things. Thinking about when is enough enough, and how do you deal with a mother who won't stop pushing, and that is the kind of experience that we need so that, when we're the ones who are making the ultimate decisions, we're not surprised. Your residency is when you want to see it all because you can see it but not be responsible for it. Some of the attendings are better than others in terms of letting residents be around for those kinds of discussions. Like when a child gets admitted and they're going to get some test done and they find that they have cancer and the oncologist's going to have to tell the parent—if you're a parent, obviously, you don't need a resident there, but it's important that the residents be there. Some attendings are a lot better about bringing you in there, plus we're the ones that are seeing these kids day in and day out and a lot of times, we'll get to know the parents better. So it's tough when you're going in and the parents are asking you these important questions, day-by-day, but you're not there when the really important decisions are being made. The best way to learn how to break the bad news is—because I don't know how you get trained to do it—to see it done. You can do all the role-playing you want, but in the end, you have to sit there while an attending is giving bad news and the mother's reacting and you get the chill down your spine and feel it. There's no real way to prepare for that. It's going to be based on what kind of person you are and how you deliver the news. In terms of how you react to the situation, you just have to be in it and watch someone else do it. It's definitely not something that you want to walk into without having seen it done before. The few times I've seen it done, I've seen parents react in a number of different ways, from outright hysterics and convulsions on the floor to stoicism and whatever. I've seen some instances where it wasn't done well at all. For example, I saw one where there was a patient who had some other kind of chronic illness and they had just found out that, in addition, this patient had leukemia. The oncology attending told the parents this in the back area, in the little workspace behind the nurses' station and not in the patient's room, not in his office, not in some private area, but in this little area. The mother became hysterical, and it was in a work area that people had to keep coming in and out of, and it was just awful. I watched it and it was painful to watch. I thought it was disgusting, so little things like that I'll put away, and, hopefully, I will never do. I've heard people say that we don't get enough training in these kinds of end-of-life issues and breaking bad news, but I don't know how you would do it, other than being present when it's being done. So it needs to be stressed to the attendings that if you see that a resident has been following this kid since he's come in and now we've got some really bad news, then that resident needs to be there. I don't think the role-playing and all the touchy-feely stuff the medical schools are doing really helps that much.

16:4. I think parents should be given the option, even if they don't think about it themselves, of organ donation. Of course, in the heat of the moment, a parent shouldn't be making that decision, but I think it's something

we, as doctors, should be taught how to approach because I didn't feel comfortable dealing with it after he had passed away. I didn't know how to go
about talking to the family about the donation that they had initially approached us about, how to bring it up. I think it's poor training on our part
as physicians that we don't know how to approach the patient who we don't
think is going to make it. Even though the parents may know that already,
we just don't know how to approach them. We don't know how to go about
getting donor consents, how it's done, when it should be done. Everyone in
the hospital kept pushing me about it; like the nursing supervisor called me
several times, and a couple of other people kept reminding me about the
organ donation. I went so far as to get the forms, but within 2 hours after
Jose had passed away, his family got up and left and I didn't have an opportunity to approach them with it; they were extremely upset still, and I didn't
think it was appropriate then. I felt that there wasn't an appropriate time,
after he had passed away, to approach that subject again.

16:2. It was helpful to have the DNR in place and go over it with the residents
because they always want to know, "Well then, what do we do? He's DNR,
so should we go in there and examine him while everybody's in there
grieving?" I don't think the residents are trained in what a DNR means.
Their mode is always to do something, and this is a time when it's okay
not to do something, but it's uncomfortable for them. They don't get
trained in residency about end-of-life care at all. Instead, they're trained
that, "Oh, there's a problem? Let's go fix it."

16:3. Do we code him if he does arrest, or do we let him pass without any
medical interventions? We would get these mandates from the ID [infectious disease] attendings literally week-to-week and his stats would
change. I felt that, as a part of a team, the residents and the interns who
were taking care of him, who saw him on a daily basis, were left out of the
loop of decision making, in terms of, if he does code, should we go all the
way in terms of aggressive intubation, giving him resuscitative medicine,
or should we just watch him die? These decisions were handed down to us,
and that was one of the most frustrating things about handling his care. So
we would just try to focus on what we can handle on a daily basis, like his
fevers or his feeding—things like that. It was the attendings talking to the
ethics committee and we weren't involved in that sort of discussion. We
were never invited to take part or listen to what was going on in terms of

what others were thinking. We only heard about the end product of the discussions.

10:5. This was the first time I had been involved in a DNR talk with parents, when it was ever certain that the patient was going to die. In medical school, we talked about it. We even had a class called "clinical practice," where we would go through case scenarios with actors having to deal with breaking bad news. However, without sounding like a cliché, there is really nothing that can prepare you for it. It's hard to take those mock situations seriously. We do, but there's just nothing that compares to being in the actual situation so, for me, this was a huge learning experience, to go through this with that family. I really don't think that medical school could have done anything differently to teach me that; you just have to actually go through it. I was fortunate enough that the team I was with was extremely competent, in my eyes, and handled the situation very well. Because the family had such different reactions at different points, I got to see how we deal with anger and sadness, and regret. They went through all of it in that DNR meeting.

A man's dying is more the
survivors' affair than his own.
— THOMAS MANN,
The Magic Mountain

As hope for a cure diminishes, the staff's disciplinary roles become more diffuse and the hierarchical relations (i.e., power differences) among the staff, in regard to families, flattens to a more level field of engagement. The staff increasingly find themselves stepping out of their professional roles to engage the family in more intimate, compassionate, and supportive ways of relating. For attendings, their roles shift from prescribing treatment protocols to clarifying remaining options and consequences. Those who are uncomfortable in this role find ways to distance themselves from the family, if not the child who is their patient. The same staff members, however, may not consistently take this stance across all cases. For example, the same resident who might distance himself from one family might, at another time, move closer to another family. Shifting patterns of relating also evolve in end-of-life care to change the valence between staff and families. For some families, a physician might be the person who becomes closest to them, while, for other families, it might be a nurse or a social worker. For children at end of life, their most intimate relationship might be with a child-life specialist. In a team approach involving different kinds of professionals and medical subspecialists, these various patterns of contingent relations are accepted and do not interfere with the primary professional responsibilities of each member. The willingness of staff to be fully present with children and families at end of life also is a matter of how families compose themselves and adjust at this time. A reciprocal interaction between families and staff naturally evolves that reflects cultural values, ways of coping, modes of expression, and levels of interpersonal comfort.

The central role of parents is to protect their children and provide for them. As end of life approaches, parents are overwhelmed at losing this role and often feel guilty for having failed their child. They are angry that more could not have been done. The hopes and aspirations that parents have for their child are part of their own identities, so parents are left with an enduring sense of not only having lost their child, but of having lost a core part of themselves, both in terms of what was and what might have been their lives.

The narratives in this chapter speak to the ways that patients and families react to end-of-life care, particularly the anguish of parents letting go of their child. The stories are told from the perspective of the medical staff; not the patients or families. Yet the range of reactions raises such questions as: What, if any, is an appropriate way to react when your child is dying before you? How do parents' reactions, such as their fear and anger, affect the staff? How does the death of a child in the hospital affect the parents of other children on the floor? How do children express their sense of their dying? When and how, in the trajectory of care and prior to the crisis, should issues about dying be explicitly raised with patients and families? How do parents' ways of relating to their child change at end of life? How likely are they to talk to their child about death? A recent study found that among 429 parents who had lost their child to cancer, 147 (34 percent) talked with their child about death, and none had regretted it. Among parents who had not talked about death with their child, 27 percent regretted not having done so; 47 percent of parents who sensed that their child was aware of his or her imminent death regretted not having talked to their child about it.[1]

1:10. They were scared. Karen was having a very tough time; it wasn't even the normal way to die; it wasn't peaceful. I think the parents realized that this was going to be ugly, and that's when I think they left her room. At that point, she no longer wanted to be in that room to see her daughter that way, with all the machines going off, and, toward the end, she started vomiting blood through her tubes. I think it would be very scary for any parent. Even though that's their child, nobody wants to see that. It's very scary. Even the doctors feel that way, even the medical staff. At the wake, mom and grandmother mentioned that Karen knew that I was nearby. But mom said that she didn't want to see Karen that way. She wanted to have another vision of Karen. So it wasn't so weird for them to leave the room; it was very appropriate.

1:10. Once her illness progressed and it was pretty evident that she was going to die, it was very emotional for the parents. No parent wants to lose a child, but their underlying personality, behavior, and coping mechanisms obviously played a big part. The dad did not have any of those skills whatsoever, so that was very difficult. Our psychiatrist had to prescribe medication for him when the death was pretty imminent. He was very erratic; he was very physical emotionally. He was in a fetal position outside of the waiting room and he wouldn't leave that position. He was lying right by the door in a fetal position. Obviously, that's not the norm, so that was difficult and that's when our psychiatrist decided to give him a prescription. Some people asked him to get up but he said, "No," and that he didn't care. When you'd approach him and wanted to talk to him to see if you could take him to a reasonable place, he didn't care. The mother was very stoic. She had her own responsibilities as a mother, and that was interesting to see. She totally understood what was happening, and she obviously could see what her husband was like during a crisis like this but it didn't really faze her because that wasn't her priority. Her priority was that she did not want to leave the bedside in case she missed anything. So mom had her own priorities and dad had his own, and we had to balance the two in between and that was very difficult.

1:10. During the week before her death, everybody came to the social worker and said, "Oh, the dad is really emotional and out of control." I would usually give them a reality check—"That's not inappropriate. It may be inappropriate to you, but it is not inappropriate for a parent who's losing a child who's intubated, who's bleeding and bloated; it's not so inappropriate." She never had a medical condition in her life, and I think that makes a big difference too, with any death. How long was that illness? This was very quick, and a lot of times, if things like that come about, usually social workers are there to remind physicians and nurses to reconsider how these parents are reacting to an unbelievable crisis, dealing with death. As long as we knew that the dad was not going to harm himself; as long as we knew he was not going to harm others—after you rule out those two things out—it's reasonable and fair to say that this is appropriate for this father who's losing a daughter. People are just going to have to know how to deal with that. That's the way I saw it, so I was very upset with the nurses because they repeatedly kept paging and paging me, wanting me to do something about this man. I finally told one nurse, "Well, how do you think you would react if this was your daughter right now?" No one had a response when you asked them that directly. Nobody's been in that position. They wanted me to somehow remove this man; they had an out-of-sight, out-of-mind type of mentality. But I understand the nurses are under a lot of stress too. They were trying to help this girl, but with the distraction of the father, I understood their point. But when it came out that way and you knew that they just wanted you to remove this man from that area so they didn't have to deal with it, then it became very difficult for me not to feel very angry at the team for treating a parent like that.

1:10. Mom, because she was very religious, talked about God and said she was very angry at God for why this was happening. This family felt also that there was medical neglect. I don't know exactly when it started, but they never understood or grasped the idea that their child had cancer and might need a liver transplant. I don't think they were able to really process that. But then, again, you had to wonder: it was a very short period—only 4 weeks—and it's difficult for any parent to process that information in such a short time. But mom was very angry with God. The day she [Karen] died, I went to see her [mom] and the doctor told me it could be hours, and at that point, believe it or not, she didn't talk about medical neglect. Instead, she just kept saying that she was just very angry with God. So like anybody who loses anybody, not even just a child, they need to place blame on somebody for the loved one's death. That's the best coping they have, at that time, and this mother was definitely very angry.

1:1. The last couple of days of her life, especially the last day, were extremely stressful both because of the complexity of the medical problems that we were facing—there had been acute and very significant deterioration—and also because of the family dynamics. This was a case of a living related liver donor, her mother, which always means that you're dealing with potentially two sick people. The mother, who was in recovery herself, had to stay with her child literally day and night at the bedside, to the point that she was physically and emotionally completely run down. It was not only a parent who potentially is losing a child, which is obviously a tremendous stress for any mother, but there was an implication that the whole transplantation was a complete failure; that they all went through this process, which potentially in the future could cause significant problems in the mother as well. So it was a double failure, although it was never articulated that way, at least to me. So this was a compounded stress. The father was extremely emotional, although a lot of times he was easier to deal with in the sense that he was happy to hear any kind of assessment, especially if it was a positive assessment. But he was also the first one to break down whenever things were getting tough—crying and being unable to stay in the room and observe whatever was going on. That became especially visible during the last few hours when he had to be removed from the unit because he could not stand everything that was going on. The mother was a very nice woman and she was very stoic most of the times, but from time to time, she had her own breakdowns and although she was not the person to scream and cry loudly, she could project her stress to everybody around in ways that, unfortunately, were very stressful for the staff. She'd say things like, "You've got to save her. You've got to find a miracle." Although she was very well aware of the severity of the situation and of the chances, at times, she was asking literally for a miracle, knowing very well that none of us has the ability to perform miracles. This was something that was perfectly understandable, as a human reaction, especially from a parent toward a dying child, but at the same time, it made it extremely difficult to work under the circumstances, because clearly you cannot meet this kind of demand.

1:1. A lot of times, being both stressed and confused about which directions things were going, they were interpreting changes or no changes in her condition as a sign that either nobody knew what to do or nobody cared. This is a very common reaction. Families of critically ill patients, when something changes, expect everybody to drop everything and run to the bedside because, for them, this clearly is the most critical thing in the world. But when you are in charge of 30 other patients, all of whom or a lot of whom are in critical condition or dying, you need to prioritize and, at any given moment, there is somebody who may need your help even more than this particular patient. I was told—I don't remember exactly which day it was—that the mother practically had a breakdown and was crying and was telling the nurse that she had a whole list of grievances about a lot of things. I talked to her and, without mentioning this piece of information, I gave her the report of the day—what we were doing and what we planned to do and she was very appreciative. So, unless there was something that I did not know about, all of these things were just natural reactions. When you cannot do something, the next best thing is to blame somebody or something for it. It was like, "I'm stressed, trying to blame it on somebody and you did not come in the room for the past 2 hours. Therefore, you don't care about me." But all of these things usually were easily recoverable. Another element was that they had a number of family members with them on a routine basis—cousins or nephews or nieces—and, for the most part, their input was positive. But there were times that they were getting as upset or even more upset than the parents themselves, and under the best possible intentions of trying to help the family, they were becoming even more inflammatory, asking, "Why did you do this?" "What are you going to do about that?" Regardless of what their intention was, this clearly was giving emotional ammunition to the parents to feel like, "Okay, it's not just me who feels this way, the entire world feels that they don't care about our child."

1:1. We had to work with the family and try to explain things to them and usually, in their defense, whenever I talked to them, no matter how upset they were with something at the beginning, they were understanding and appreciative and everything was fine but it was endless; it was a roller coaster situation. Something would happen and they would focus on that aspect, asking, "Why did we do that? or "Why don't we do that?" and "What are you going to do about this?" and "Why is this not higher?" and "What does it mean for it to be like that?" I was trying, and pretty much everybody on the staff was trying, to explain to them that you cannot isolate one finding or one number. You have to look at the global picture and make an assessment on the basis of the global not on the specific signs. But that was very difficult for them to grasp.

1:10. When the doctor did the surgery, thinking that this was just a tumor and she did not need a liver transplant, everything was okay. But the minute that they knew that she needed a transplant, the parents wanted to protect Karen. They didn't want us to talk to Karen directly and tell her what to expect if the transplant failed, so it was very hard for us to educate her and get her to know us without telling her the details. It was very hard, and that's why we tried to talk to the parents, to let them know how beneficial it would be to teach Karen, especially in that state where she's 14, that awkward age, wanting to fit into school. We tried to educate the family so they, in turn, would help Karen. But we couldn't use the word "cancer" with her, we couldn't use the word "transplant." It was not until the last minute of the transplant surgery that it was, "Okay, you can tell her about the transplant, but don't talk more about it." She trusted her family, trusted her parents to do all the work, and I think at that age most girls would. Not that they're not intelligent, it's just that many kids don't want to know. They have their priorities. She was this beautiful young girl, and all of a sudden, her parents drive her to the hospital, she has surgery, they tell her everything's going to be great afterward—I'm sure that's the way the parents presented it—but, unfortunately, it didn't work out that way. So, after Karen had the transplant, she was very depressed and very upset with the team. She had a lot of body image issues. She was a cheerleader, she was a ballerina, she was all that, and now she had a big incision and she was bloated from all the fluid overload. She was very unhappy and very angry with the team. . . . I understand, as a parent myself, that you want to protect your children, but you have to protect them in a certain sense. You still have to educate them and let children have some control over their illness. But the first control is education about your illness and about how to deal with it. . . . She was very angry, not speaking, total withdrawal, lack of eye contact, typical age-appropriate withdrawal, mouth closed, no body language, nothing. Because of her athletic background, it just impacted on a lot of things. Maybe if she wasn't such an athletic person, a body image person, maybe it wouldn't have been so bad. But it really hit her hard because she kept asking, "When am I going to lose all this fluid? When am I going to get back up? When do you think I can go back to cheerleading? Ballerina classes?"—all that stuff. . . . It was very difficult for me to balance everybody's wishes, and as an advocate for the patient, you want to educate them the most, but it's hard when they're young and have parents that you have to deal with. When it comes to kids, you're really not dealing with kids; you're ultimately dealing with the parents. That's been the most difficult hurdle working with children here.

3:10. I saw the mother becoming extremely angry, and I think that was one of her main coping mechanisms in this death. She was angry at all of us and angry at the system. She was saying, "If I wasn't Hispanic and didn't have Medicaid, I would get a private room. I wouldn't be getting pushed out of the hospital. You wouldn't be giving up on me because hospice, I think, is very American." I don't know if every culture has bought on to that so much, but she thought of hospice as killing. She said, "You know, we wouldn't give up in my culture. You're giving up on me, you're giving up on her." It was just amazing that she was so compliant with everything about Elsa's care and did everything up until the point where it had gotten to a real crisis. Then she became angry and lashed out and was resistant to a lot of our interventions. Our idea of what was good didn't match hers, and it became, like, "Who are we to say?" It became very complicated how we were telling her how her child should die. She had one version in mind, we had another, and that was the clash.

3:9. Elsa was ready to die before her mother was ready to let her. My personal beliefs are that kids know long before we know. Whether that's a concrete thought, I don't think so. Somewhere, intrinsically, they have an idea about their life course, and we wait too long to talk to children about death and dying, whether it be their own or somebody else's. They all experience it here through the relationships that they make with the other kids and with the other families here. It was Halloween, and Elsa and I were making haunted houses, which led us to talk about spirits and ghosts, and I asked her if she believed in ghosts. It was a segue into the topic, and, at this point, I knew that there was very little further treatment for her and that they were just addressing pain issues. So we were talking about spirits and ghosts and if they exist, which led us to talking about angels, and I asked her, "What do you think an angel looks like?" She threw her head back and put her arms to her side and made an image of what she perceived angels to look like. So I felt that she had already created an image of heaven for herself or where she was going to go, whatever she called that. They were a religious family, and I believe that they believed in angels and heaven and that there was an afterlife. . . . There were moments where we had some really remarkable things happen. For example, about 2 weeks before she died, she was coming in and out of consciousness, and there were many times prior to this when she was in pain and she realized that I was there because, when I entered, she said my name. She allowed me to hold her hand, and I said that I wanted to help her to feel better and to feel safe and she said, "I don't want to feel nothing anymore." I felt like this was a kid who's ready but wasn't being allowed to die; her mother was not giving her the permission that she needed. Another time we were talking about imagery and safe places and she described to me that she saw children and I said, "Do you want to go with the children? You can run with them if you want," and she threw my hand down and said, "No." The interesting thing about that was that it made me feel better, because I thought, "That's okay. She's not ready to let go, so it's okay that her mother's not ready to let go either." I started to then say to her, "You know mommy will always be with you. You will always have a connection to her. Like a kite that floats in the sky, she will always hold that string that keeps you to her and keeps you with her." This was part of the imagery that we had used before so it was something that she was familiar with, but she got upset with me again. She knew what I was getting at and what I was trying to say—she was totally aware on some level—and didn't like what she was hearing. She made me stop; she threw my hand down and would not hold my hand again and, when I started going on about her mother, she said, "No." So she was pretty clear, which was totally her prerogative and I certainly respected that. Then she went back into being delusional, so it was like I had lost her. She was with me for a little while in this image, and then she slipped back into that sort of medicated state. . . . One of the things that imagery did was to provide Elsa's mother with a language to talk with her child about dying. I tried to create that image of the kite and the string for the mother also, so as to help her find words to use and ways to communicate with her daughter without directly feeling like she's letting her child die. There's a real fine line, and people ask me all the time, "Do you ever tell a kid they're dying?" and I have never once said to a kid, "You are dying," but we certainly have talked about heaven and earth and the life process and where do people go afterward. So I can do it in a kind of euphemistic and esoteric way so that we talk around that word. Parents always think I'm going to come right out and say to their kid that they're dying, when I tell them that it's important that we talk to children about this. It's such a harsh reality. They can see it right in front of their faces but they need to have a gentler language to express what's happening, and that's partly our role in child-life. Elsa's physician and I had a lot of conversations around this, and she was very grateful to have that type of language to use with the mother and Elsa, where she could address issues because now they had a common language and image to do that and that wasn't so scary.

3:10. She was grown up in a lot of ways and yet not grown up in a lot of ways. She said, one time, that she never wanted to grow up. The day that she said that was weird for those of us who knew that she never would.

4:10. When Danny got very sick from the transplant, his mother pulled through and made such progress. It was so impressive and exciting for me, as her social worker, to watch the changes that she made. That's something that I always pointed out to her, which I think helped her and gave her a lot of confidence in herself; that she could can do this. The sicker Danny got, the more the mom pulled through. This was a great example of the human spirit. She got ornery with the staff a lot and used to blame everybody else for everything that was going on with Danny. Every time there was a problem, it was the hospital's fault, even like a little dust on the floor, she would explode and get out of control about tiny things. She couldn't control her anger or direct it in the right ways, but then, as she started to progress, she was able to sit down—she'd learned a lot of relaxation techniques from our holistic services here—kind of slow down, take a deep breath, and was able to pinpoint her anger. She knew what she was angry at and stopped displacing her anger so much on other people; and it was amazing to watch her with her son. She became an expert in his care. She knew 8,000 more things than I did about IVs and bandages and gauzes, and she knew what was what on the monitor, which I didn't know and I've been working in the hospital for 4 years. It was amazing. This woman, who I didn't think was very smart, was extremely bright in this situation. It helped her cope, to know everything that was going on all the time and be heavily involved.

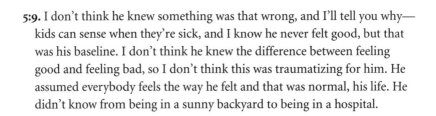

5:9. I don't think he knew something was that wrong, and I'll tell you why—kids can sense when they're sick, and I know he never felt good, but that was his baseline. I don't think he knew the difference between feeling good and feeling bad, so I don't think this was traumatizing for him. He assumed everybody feels the way he felt and that was normal, his life. He didn't know from being in a sunny backyard to being in a hospital.

5:2. They wanted to know what was going on; what we thought was going on with the lungs, with the liver, the bone marrow, and all that. You would tell them something and they would absolutely understand and maintain that. You'd tell them, "The lungs are failing. We don't know exactly why, but, at this point, there is probably hope. There are some kids who get out of this situation, but some don't. It can go up and it can go down and it usually gets worse before it gets better." Then you go back, after a couple of days, and you find that the majority of the families don't remember anything and you have to repeat the same thing but, for them, you told them something and they understood that and they maintained that. They told you, "Yeah, I know you told me. It's exactly what you told me. It's happening and it's going up and down, up and down and we know that it's very likely that he's not going to make it." That's why it was an easy family for us. You didn't have to fight with them. They would never come and say, "But you told us that this was actually good" or "You told us that if he gets better, he was probably going to survive" because we told them that, "If he gets better, he may be out of this but we are not 100 percent sure." They maintained the fact that we were saying, "I'm not 100 percent sure. I don't know what's going to happen." They never played it out like, "Oh, you're the doctor so you have to know what's going to happen." They were very, I don't know, like people should be. But, usually, it's too hard to be like that when you're in a situation like that.

5:10. The father felt so comfortable in our relationship that he collapsed on the stairwell and he just cried as I sat with him and cried too. He said, "How am I going to deal with this?" and I told him, "Day-by-day." The mother initially could not talk about it. She avoided it by putting her head underneath the pillow; that's exactly what she did. She physically put her head beneath the pillow. She could not deal with it at all. So I started working with the father because he seemed like the pillar of the relationship; he was the strength. We started to explore his feelings and his fears and his anxieties and stuff like that. They're very religious people, so I was able to bring him to a place where he was able to accept that whatever is God's will, will be. Then, because of his strength, I was able to recruit him to help me with the mom. And so his strength then became her strength. She would cry when we had these tough meetings and would just shut herself down, so I found ways to open her up. I would say to her, "Let's go get some coffee downstairs." Oftentimes, when I asked for her to come with me, I had no money, so she ended up treating me to coffee, but doing this little thing helped her to start opening up. Every time we went to get coffee and we walked to the coffee place, I did my clinical work. We started talking and she started saying, "This is really hard for me." It came to the point that when we had these meetings the past couple of days, I saw her shutting down and I would say, "You know what? You can't shut down on me. What are you feeling? What are you thinking?" She was able to cry, and she came to a place where she said, "This is hard, but you know what? I don't want my son to suffer any more." Of course parents get angry, at this point, and what I do is that I validate it. I tell them, "This is hell. This is a nightmare and there's nothing that I can say or do to take that away." So, of course, everyone is angry and everybody expresses it very differently, but the reality is that it's a very, very difficult situation. Why do innocent children have cancer? Why do a lot of them die? Why do they have to suffer? I don't have answers to that.

5:10. I helped them to feel comfortable being with their son in this condition. There's really no data showing that a child could hear, when they're under anesthesia. But what we focused on is that, while there is no data, it can't hurt. It helps parents to feel better. I also focused a lot on what great parents they were, how they've done it all, made every effort, came from another country, and told them, "Your son is a warrior; he is a champion. Let him know how much you love him." I felt that helping the mom communicate her feelings was going to help her too, at least bring them out instead of stuffing them inside. If she stuffed, stuffed, stuffed, she would deteriorate; she would get depressed. I knew they were spiritual folks, so we focused on where would Ricardo go if he died. "He would go to heaven—what does that mean?" We did a lot of work on how he's been fighting for so long, for 6 years already. And then they said, "Yes, he's in so much pain." So we built on that a little bit, and it came to the point that they were like, "We don't want him to be in pain anymore; we don't want him to suffer anymore. We want him to stop suffering." We then worked on that, "So what does that mean? That still means you're great parents. It still means what? He will be in a place where he won't be in pain."

5:10. The hardest thing for parents is when they're in the hospital room, and it's finally time to go home because the body's going to stay there. The father couldn't leave, and he wanted to wait for the body to be taken to the morgue. It was like, for him, it meant that this is really, really happening. After he left the hospital room, he was waiting outside in the area and that's when he started to collapse and he did not want the mother to see him that way. He went to another floor and then down the stairs where there was a separate room where he just collapsed; he fell on the floor and he was crying and crying. Once he went back to the mother, he stopped crying. So parents are different; it depends on what works for them. The mother was quietly crying in the corner [of the hospital room]. She was just crying. When I compare it to the father, she's more passive and he's more the patriarch of the family, but they both expressed their sorrow and they were very appropriate.

—|—

5:1. He took it one day at a time, and his not wanting to be bothered by a whole lot of medical staff and just wanting to live his own life in the hospital was admirable, especially considering what the outcome was. Why did he need to get involved with all of us? He had this indomitable spirit that was like, "Hey, leave me be. I want to watch my cartoons." If you were talking to the parents about something and blocking his TV, he'd get real pissed off at you and so, when we think about this child and reflect back on him, that was sort of neat. Some children are all too nice when they're going through therapy or all too bonded to the medical staff, but he was just still basically a kind of normal 6-year-old kid who thought this was the pits.

—|—

5:1. What made these folks easy was that they were respectful and graceful people to begin with. Just opposed to that is the other kid I had die that day, at about the same time. This family was hostile, to the point of vulgarity, and threatening, and very difficult. What made these folks easy was their general demeanor and that they were in agreement. What is difficult is when parents are not in agreement with each other, and, then, I have to do the most conservative thing [in maintaining life support]. Like mom and dad disagree or Aunt Bessie disagrees, then you are not going to turn things off. More time and more attention needs to be given to them, and that is fine, but the staff perceives that as much more difficult. The even more difficult situation is like the other one, a belligerent family who essentially are calling you a murderer, even though I had been working with them for 8 days so none of this was new information for them.

—|—

5:10. All families are different. For example, Latin families ask me a lot of questions because I am Latin and we speak the same language. Families on Medicaid, who don't often feel that they are empowered and who often feel that there is some form of institutionalized racism, come to me more readily than they would their doctor. Families that are wealthy, families that have private insurance, don't often come to me first. So what I try to do with the families that are wealthy is that I come in through the back door. Whenever doctors have meetings, I try to invite myself in so that

WHEN TREATMENT FAILS

I'm seen as being part of the team. Then I try to win them over. It's really unfortunate, but wealthy families don't understand social work. They say, "Social work is not for me. Help me set up my home care, but in terms of helping me deal with my feelings, it's not for me." So I know that already and my feelings aren't hurt. I come in the back way and, after a while, when I've gained their trust, they start saying, "You know what? Can we have a meeting about this?" That's how I coordinate meetings with the medical staff. But with Latino families, my struggle is that they want me to be their sister or their mother or their friend, which I'm not either—there has to be boundaries. They can often come to me and want to vent in a very destructive way, like, "Who's a good nurse? Who's not a good nurse? The housekeeping staff smells." I understand where they're coming from. They're angry about their child's situation. They're angry because they feel, whether it's perceived or whether it's a reality, that they are being looked down upon because they don't speak the language. Often their perceptions just don't mentally equate with reality and they just want to vent, and so I always have to draw those boundaries there with them. . . . A patient died yesterday and the social worker spent the entire day with the family, not just doing concrete services, but also helping them emotionally, providing supportive therapy. One of the attending physicians said in a meeting, "We don't always acknowledge the work that social workers do." The doctors come in to have a family meeting and then it's, "See you later. Think about what I said." Hello? There's so much more to it than that. How are parents going to make an educated decision when their emotions are all the way up here? We help them to find a balance, to think clearly, to "Let's figure this out together."

7:10. They were a dangerous family, dangerous in many ways for the people caring for them, and I always knew it and I warned people. They sucked people in. I somehow gave them the impression that I had 5 hours to spare every time I saw them, and I didn't. But I gave them an inordinate amount of time. They burnt out their first social worker. They were very angry at the first pediatrician. They were very angry at the oncologist at the other hospital where Carol had her surgery. It was very good cop/bad cop, and I knew, for Carol's sake, that I had to stay on their good side, so I did. But I always warned people that there are these two sides and you may find yourself suddenly flipped into the bad category, so don't take it personally. They just split people into good and bad, and it gave them a context to be able to deal with everything. I was squarely in the good, but, at the same time, they were very, very demanding. I couldn't walk through clinic, if they were there, and not get sucked in for an hour or more with them. At the same time, they were so decent, so decent that they would bring me food. But there were times that I would give the others short shrift when I didn't want to because they were so needy. I had very mixed emotions when she [Carol] died. I felt very sad and I really sobbed but, at the same time, relief.

7:8. When they came back from surgery, there wasn't any upbeat time. It was just at that point, "We'll see." They would say things like, "She's a gift for us to have for a short period of time." They had tried to conceive several times; they had tried and tried to conceive, and they finally did. So Carol was their "miracle baby," and they would say that too. It was hard for the grandmothers. I spoke to the father's mother just the week before Carol died. She said she was experiencing the pain bi-fold; she was experiencing it as a grandmother and as a mother and that it was so hard for her to watch her own child watch his child die.

7:10. Carol died on a Wednesday, and the Friday before she died they were still vacillating as to whether or not they wanted to consider home hospice care. They didn't know because they were trying to figure out if they wanted more chemo. If they wanted more chemo, hospice couldn't take them. So when they accepted no more chemo, they were ready to deal with hospice care. Interestingly enough, she died 3 days later, and it was all almost eerily planned perfectly. There's a theory floating around that Carol waited to die until the hospice nurse was there because her parents were so afraid of being alone with her when she died. Their biggest fear was being alone with Carol when she died at home, but at the same time, they didn't want her to die in the hospital either. The nurse was scheduled from 10:00 P.M. to 6:00 A.M. and she died at 5:20 A.M. because she knew that her parents would not have been able to handle that alone. Most parents prefer for their child to die in the hospital than at home, but they were pretty adamant and we always gave them the option of being admitted, if they changed their mind.

7:1. I said that "I know that you can do it without her, but your husband was loud and clear that he needed somebody else in the house. I think it is very difficult for him because he kept saying, 'Should I call my family?' and 'When is it going to happen? I don't want to be alone.' So, it's clear to me he needs the hospice nurse to be there. I think you could do it without her there, but he can't. He doesn't want to be alone when she dies. And he's not alone, he has you but I think it undoes him to watch you flip into efficiency mode and get X, Y, and Z done and watch you do it. He can't watch you do that. He needs you for him, so you need this person to do the pieces because your husband needs you. That's what's so remarkable about you because, while you really don't want her there, you listened to what your husband needed and you understood." The mom was very concerned about what had to be done—"Do I call 911? Do I call the coroner? Do I call the this? Do I call the that? What steps do I need to take to get the body out of my house?" kinds of things. I think this is what undid the father; that she just had the ability to flip in and out to get the job done and emote. She could just flip the switch, and he clearly couldn't do it and couldn't watch her do it.

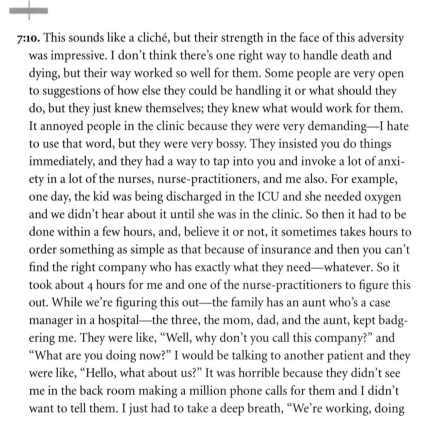

7:10. This sounds like a cliché, but their strength in the face of this adversity was impressive. I don't think there's one right way to handle death and dying, but their way worked so well for them. Some people are very open to suggestions of how else they could be handling it or what should they do, but they just knew themselves; they knew what would work for them. It annoyed people in the clinic because they were very demanding—I hate to use that word, but they were very bossy. They insisted you do things immediately, and they had a way to tap into you and invoke a lot of anxiety in a lot of the nurses, nurse-practitioners, and me also. For example, one day, the kid was being discharged in the ICU and she needed oxygen and we didn't hear about it until she was in the clinic. So then it had to be done within a few hours, and, believe it or not, it sometimes takes hours to order something as simple as that because of insurance and then you can't find the right company who has exactly what they need—whatever. So it took about 4 hours for me and one of the nurse-practitioners to figure this out. While we're figuring this out—the family has an aunt who's a case manager in a hospital—the three, the mom, dad, and the aunt, kept badgering me. They were like, "Well, why don't you call this company?" and "What are you doing now?" I would be talking to another patient and they were like, "Hello, what about us?" It was horrible because they didn't see me in the back room making a million phone calls for them and I didn't want to tell them. I just had to take a deep breath, "We're working, doing our best." Eventually, it got to the point where the mother asked me if I would like her sister to help me make phone calls, like really kind of hitting you between the eyes. I felt like I was 5 years old, and yet I knew there was this mom losing her child and she was freaking out. I just had to keep reminding myself what was happening; she wasn't mad at me—that was their bossiness. They wanted things done instantly, and I understood that. They just got to everyone. Whether they got people angry or people were in love with the family, they somehow drew everyone into them on some level. It's amazing how they could be so demanding, yet still so well liked. They had it down; it was smart, and I don't know if they realized it—I mean I don't think it was conscious; it just kind of worked that way. Everyone kind of rolled their eyes, but then 2 seconds later we'd be like, "Oh, we love them, and the baby's so cute." Clinically, I knew what was going on from the inside and I guess someone from the outside who didn't know would've been like, "That woman's a bitch!" but it was cushioned by the fact of their situation.

8:10. These parents are meshed in horror on a continuous basis and not only the horror that is happening in their lives, but the horror that is around them. Whether they want to connect to other parents or not, they hear the screams. The mom was screaming her head off on Sunday evening, screaming, screaming, screaming. Even if you wanted to close the door and not be a part of the situation, you still were indirectly a part of it. Every time a child is dying, my work with the families is processing that death; seeing where they are at and helping them through their fears that keep coming up again and again. Because we cannot give them any guarantees, the anxieties never go away. My role is that they will not be paralyzed by the fear they experienced in somebody else's child. That they will be able to look at the situation and say, "That sucks and that is painful but that is not my kid." I also try to develop their coping skills and try to help them communicate their feelings because, if they stuff this stuff up, they are just going to explode.

8:2. She started crying; she was flailing around and looking very hopeless and very despondent. The part that really got to me was that she had nobody. The father wasn't there; there was no family member. We asked her if there was anybody we could call and she said, "No, nobody." "Is there any friends we could call?" There was nobody. So we went around asking the people on the floor, the patients' moms who knew her, if they would go down and see her. I encouraged that, although medically or legally it might not have been a good thing, in terms of maintaining patient confidentiality. Are you supposed to let other parents know that William is not doing well and that his mom needs your support? I don't know if we crossed the line here. They must have heard her screaming, and it would have gotten around anyway that he wasn't doing well, so we figured, if they knew how to comfort her better than we could, then that would have been positive because she really had nobody except for the medical staff and she wasn't really that close to us because we didn't speak the language that well. So most of the Spanish moms went down, one by one, to give her support and stuff like that. That was really heart-wrenching.

8:1. It is bad enough to be here for 6 weeks, but to be here for 6 plus 6 or more begins to be interminable for the families. Especially for a family like this where the mother had another little boy as well, a little bit older, and always had to find different people to take care of him. This was a big burden for her, and the father kind of came through, at the end, but was not there a lot earlier. At the beginning of the first transplant, the mother was still trying to work. She was working at night as a waitress, and so her hours were very erratic and, if somebody didn't know that, they would assume that she was absent and inattentive to her child and not a good mom, so to speak. These kinds of judgmental-type reactions are made so quickly, out of the staff's care and concern for a child, that it got to the point where the social worker felt that she had to help out by making little signs for mom to put on the door, like, "I have to go home and wash my clothes" or "I will be back tonight" or "I am working tonight." She had to do these things because there were questions about the mom among the staff, "Where is mom anyway? We haven't seen her all morning." It is so easy to slip into that kind of bad mom category.

8:10. It was challenging to care for William and his family because the mom came here with such a wide range of social deficiencies and there was so much that she needed. She had just experienced her whole family being wiped out in Salvador a year and a half ago. The father of her 4-year-old son had died soon after that, and, soon after that, William was here for his first transplant. Then, after a couple of days of her coming to the hospital, she was mugged. Before William was born, his father left her for another woman, so she was the sole financial provider. So she had a lot going on in her life, and it was an upward hike for me to help her. But it felt like a privilege to be part of her life, and I felt satisfied that I was able to help her and that I saw my work with her come to fruition.

8:8. In the ICU, I find that what parents decide to do toward the end depends on how ready they are and how long the child has been suffering. I have had parents that have said, "That is it; enough." Even in the middle of an arrest, they say "Please, that is it, no more, no more." I have seen other cases where there is nothing left for us to do; the child has been pronounced dead and a father is doing CPR and calling us back into the room. I have had parents that said, "No, no he is not dead. I hear a heart beat," taking a stethoscope and literally listening after we had said there is nothing there. I have had parents that have said, "I don't want him to suffer anymore. I want you to give him pain medication and put him out, put him out." You get a whole range of reactions and it all depends on your own beliefs. It has nothing to do with education, nothing to do with race, color, or creed. It has to do with how much suffering can you see your child going through; that is the bottom line. I have had parents that have said, "I can't stand to see my son like that, that is not my child. I want this to end." It is the ultimate sacrifice of a parent, and it astounds me how they can see through all of this fog; rise above that fog, and land on their two feet on the other side and say, "This is what I want for my child; enough is enough." They are so brave. I don't want to say they are stoic, because they are not; you see them suffering, but they have this inner peace. They have this aura about them. You can tell from the minute you meet this family that they are going to go through hell, and they are going to be all right.

8:8. The family was asked about having an autopsy done. They did not want to permit it for the specific reason that they didn't want anything else done to him. Of course, it is possible to do an autopsy and not be able to tell, looking in the casket, that anything even happened, but they felt that that was where they had to draw the line.

8:1. We always hope that these families will stay in touch, because we anticipate that they are going to need a lot of further support. A few families actually take us up on it. The best example is a lady whose son had a transplant and he died 3 years ago and she now works here as a transporter. The way that it happened was that, at first, we stayed in touch and then she was asking about whether she could volunteer here, so we found a small amount of money, just to cover her expenses coming in to do that. I think volunteering was her way of testing out whether she was comfortable to be in this environment. She showed a certain aptitude for doing things, and so she qualified to get a job with transport. For some people, this experience, even if they lose their child, can translate into something that gives them a bridge to the future and maybe changes their thoughts about what they might do. . . . For us, especially if they have agreed to an autopsy, we are committed to stay in touch because we are going to be talking to them about the results. Otherwise, potentially it could still be helpful. For example, sometimes newly diagnosed families will ask to talk to somebody that went through this, particularly if they have a diagnosis of something really bad, like a brain stem gleomar or something. Probably the best we are going to be able to do is put them in touch with families whose child did, in fact, die but maybe he was able to go to school for a year or had some quality of life. . . . I find that, in general, the circumstances at the end go so fast that you want to slow down that clock and replay it. It is like a videotape at the wrong speed, and you feel like you want to look at it again. We do have morbidity and mortality conferences where we do that: take it apart a little bit and say, "Gee, if we had done this differently," but we probably should do the same with our relationship to the family because things were so rushed at the end that there was not really much chance for reflection about anything. We feel like we have invested so much into these complicated treatments that it would be fairly natural that somebody might stay in touch, but a lot of families don't; they just have to move on.

9:10. If I was in my office doing something, he might say, "Can I come and sit with you?" and he would sit down with me and we would just talk about anything, about movies or whatever was on his mind. I saw it as an open relationship; whenever he wanted to talk, whatever he wanted to talk about, I would talk with him about it. But every once in a while I would bring up things because, even though he didn't say it, I knew it had to be on his mind. He'd talk about going to get chemotherapy and then you're done and the next thing is getting radiation and then those radiation treatments were supposed be a certain number but then it changed to another number. So, he started to pick up on things and he would ask questions and stuff and I was trying to help him understand what was going on. . . . He didn't really say anything about dying, indirectly or directly, except that one time when he said, "Whatever happens, happens." Sometimes he would ask me, "What happened to that kid?"and I would say, "Well, that patient died" and he would go, "Oh, so he got really sick?" and I'd be like, "Yeah, he got really sick and, whatever it was, the doctors did what they could for him, but the medicine couldn't make him better"—that kind of thing. And he'd usually go, "Oh, okay" and walk away. We had our pet therapy dog who died, so that was another time when he was like, "Oh, so what happened?" I explained it to him that his owner felt like he was only going to get sicker and there was really nothing else to do so she put him to sleep because she felt it was kind to let him go. But I can't really say there ever was a time that he would say something like, "What's going to happen when I die?" I spent a lot of time talking to his sister, and she was the person that he would say things to, and she said that he'd talk to her about it, like, "When I die, I want to be buried in Puerto Rico." There was one time when the mother told me that he had made a statement that, when he died, he wanted to be cremated and he wanted his ashes spread in the jungle in Puerto Rico and his mother was joking, "How am I going to get to the jungle? I can't pray in the jungle. It has to be somewhere else." I say this because, although he didn't necessarily have those conversations with me, I know he had them with his mom and his sister. . . . It's tough for me to have to tell a kid that one of their friends or someone they knew died, but at the same time, it's important to be honest with the kids. If I didn't tell them the truth, I'd be doing more of a disservice by just pretending like it didn't happen because that is the reality of what happens here. It is hard. You take a deep breath and then you say it, and I feel that I'm doing something to help by saying it. . . . We had a really nice relationship, and it was good that I was able to be there with him and to sit with him and not even necessarily even say anything, but just to sit there together. That said a lot; that he had someone who wanted to sit with him. Even the time when his attending was talking to his parents about how his prognosis was that last week, his mother asked me, "Can you sit with him for a little while?" I wanted to go to the meeting, but I said, "Okay, I'll sit with him," and I think that was important because I could tell that his mind was racing "They're having another meeting, what's going on here?" I said, "Do you know what they're talking about?" and he goes, "Well, I know they're talking about me."

9:8. I didn't get the sense at all, on Thursday, that he thought he might not make it because he'd come in not feeling well before and we've always been able to fix the problem and send him home. But the next day he was a lot more tachypnek [breathing fast] and having difficulty breathing so I think, by that afternoon, he knew that something was not right. We were with him until probably 7:00 that night and then he went home and died 24 hours later. When he left, the mother and I said, "Goodbye," and she thanked me and I said, "Well, what's your plan here?" She said, "We don't have a plan. We're probably never coming back." The mother knew and I think that John knew because he's smart. I hugged him goodbye, and I kissed him, and I told him I loved him, and I told him, "Do what your mother says." He said to me, "Yeah, I will because she bugs out if I don't." So although we didn't exchange words, I think he knew.

9:10. The last Friday that he was here, I had a lot of conversations with the mom because she wanted to know, "How can I tell him this?" She didn't want to tell him he was going to die and said, "I wish you could tell him, but I don't want you to tell him until that time," but she knew that that wasn't possible because I wasn't going to be with him at home. She wanted me to give her ways of talking about it with him. I told her that you don't have to directly say, "You're dying," but you can say that you're dying in other ways. I told her that he's old enough to understand concretely and that he knew that he had a tumor in his lung and that it had gotten bigger. I explained that one way you could tell him is to say that we've decided that chemotherapy will not help anymore and that we didn't want to put him through that anymore; the nausea, the vomiting, and hair loss, if it wasn't going to make him better. I told her that "If you can't say that, maybe that's too hard to say—which I can understand, I couldn't imagine having to tell my kid that—then you can let him know that, if his body is getting tired, he can rest now." I thought the most important thing was for her to tell him that she was going to be okay because he was always worried about his mother and how she would be when he was gone. So that was kind of what I told her to do. I spent some time with his sister as well because she's the kind of kid who just holds everything inside. She said, "I cry in the shower, but I don't let anyone know how I'm really feeling. I tell everyone that we have to think positive, but I know that I'm going to lose my baby brother. I don't want to think that, but I know that." It was nice to go to the wake because I spent a little time talking to her, because everyone would ask her how she's doing and she would say, "I don't want to talk about it," but then she just started to tell me the whole story about how John died: "Well, do you know what happened?" and "This is what he did," and "This is how I feel. I don't really see him as dead yet but I know tomorrow, when they bury him, that's when it's really going to hit me." She talked about that day that he died and how she was at his bedside and her interpretation of what happened—him saying that he didn't want to go yet and how hard it was for her mother.

9:1. On a personal level, he certainly taught me about courage. He was a kid, a young man, whose father was incredibly ill with cancer. His father would come often, but his father had something called a tracheotomy, which is a tube in the throat because he'd had a tumor that was obstructing his airway. So, for a big part of the time, his father could only talk in a gruff way. His father had always been a really active, vital, healthy, runner kind of guy, and he had to put on all this weight because he'd been on steroids and he'd had heart problems and he'd been in and out of the hospital multiple times. John adored his father and always had this positive outlook, not in denial but just this faith that "My dad's tough. He's going to make it. It's going to be okay." So that's how he dealt with it. The hospital really is, no matter how nice we try to make it with child-life and activities, not a nice place to be. It's not your home, there's no privacy, it's noisy, the food is awful, and he was in and out of the hospital, and in and out of the hospital, yet he never complained. This was a kid who never complained. Once, twice, maybe, during the whole year or so that I knew him he said something about wishing he didn't have to go through this, but he just was a very brave kid. A lot of it was about protecting his parents. He just didn't want to show weakness, because his father had shown a lot of strength and he wanted to be there for his dad. He didn't want his dad to be worrying about him, and he knew that his mother was already worrying about his dad, so he didn't want her to worry about him. He just was a really brave kid, but not in a sickly-sweet way. He'd occasionally make little sarcastic jokes about the food or the hospital, so it's not like he was oblivious or such a goody-two-shoes you couldn't stand it.

10:1. Families look for help trying to understand what's going on. They take in what we say, and then they bounce it off other families here that are going through similar situations. This family certainly knew other families of kids with brain tumors that were having problems with reoc-currences, and most people dealing with them felt that, at least at the end, they were accepting it.

—————

10:1. The day before she died, the parents asked me—they didn't come out and say sedative—if there was some medication they could have to lessen their stress. So we sat down and talked about how to go about doing that, and they were perfectly fine. We didn't get to it because she died before we could get that in place, but I was more than willing to give them a pre-scription for something, if needed, and we talked about the first step pos-sibly being sitting and talking with somebody and then moving on to a prescription for something. But having to think about medicating the par-ents is really uncommon, and, in this case, they were the ones who initi-ated the request. One of the things we don't do well in medicine is to pharmacologically take care of the family because, when we talk about controlled substances, we all have this fear of giving somebody something who is not under our direct care, but these people may need something and we don't have the resources to take care of this issue. Knowing what it's like to be in the emergency room, I just don't understand having the parents go through probably the most stressful situation in their life and to have to send them to the adult ER only to be seen by somebody who has never seen them before in their life just for them to then get a psychiatric consult. This is something that we should have thought about or done a long time ago, especially with the number of bone marrow transplant pa-tients that we are taking care of and knowing that they're as high risk as they are.

—————

11:2. I've sent families to go talk to the mom and go stay with the mom be-cause "She needs you right now." The families are very close and they al-ways end up talking to each other and they all know what's going on with each other. You're not supposed to release any information—tell some-body who is not a direct parent or guardian of a patient what's wrong with somebody or what's happening, aside from what they pick up just by being there—so you really have to distract them from asking questions that you cannot answer. Sometimes I say, "Mom needs you right now," or "Why don't you go pray for the little baby." I turn it around and give them something else to do to take their minds off asking the direct question. When a child dies, you have to say the child died because they're going to hear about it anyway. If they ask you, "Is she gone?" you say "Yes," but while it's happening, you cannot say whether she's doing better or not. When they question why a child has died, we mostly evade the question, especially in a situation like this when we didn't even know. Most of the time, the kids are very sick, and we tell them, "She was very sick, and we tried all we could and we couldn't bring her back." That kind of thing but not more specific than that.

13:10. There were times when her mother would come in and say to me, "Rebecca has a question, and maybe you are the person we can ask that of." Rebecca would ask me about going back to school. When the standard therapy ended and she was going on more experimental stuff and, after the transplant had not worked, Rebecca's questions were, "How do I tell my friends when they say, 'So, are you cured? Are you better now?' How do I say, 'No' without leading into a whole lot of other questions?" Rebecca understood what was going on. She knew what her prognosis was, she knew what her disease was, but she did not want to talk about it and involve her friends in all this, and you had to respect that; that was fine. . . . Her mom told me that they have always been honest with her. They told her that her cancer came back, and she read the assent for more treatment. But, if you went down a path that she didn't want to go down, she would divert the conversation. So, you got to take your cues from what she wanted to know and Rebecca's way of coping was, "You can tell me once, but I don't want to talk about it anymore. I'm ready to move on from that." She would hear it and then say, "Okay, it's not going so well. I have to take this medicine, okay, but here's what I also want to do. I want to take my SATs; I want to get my driver's license; I want to be in my Shakespeare club; I want to read this book; and I want to go to school." She went to school up until the very last day practically. This was a kid who was living to the last possible moment. She just said, "This is something that is going on but it's not my life—it doesn't define me."

13:8. I'll never forget Rebecca because she was an incredible person. The therapy she received and the side effects she had would have floored anybody, and this girl dragged herself to school everyday. She took every single one of her medicines; a lot of teenagers will hide them or throw them away. Six weeks before she died, she went to Paris. She did everything she wanted to, and that's amazing because a lot of people can't just pick themselves up from this. It got to a point when she knew she had an illness that was going to kill her, but she just kept on. Rebecca didn't act like she was dying, ever.

13:10. There definitely was a shift in her thinking that things were getting worse. The family had their hopes hung on this [bone marrow] transplant; that it was going to be the cure-all. When it wasn't, she started reading assent forms and hearing about things that say "Phase I Studies" and "experimental." She was reading and signing assents that said, "This may or may not be curative." She was reading that stuff because she was required to look at it and give assent, and that is when that shift occurred. As difficult as it is to get assents, I think it's important to do that, but you need to have somebody there and not just hand them a piece of paper. You need to have somebody there that goes over the information with them. One time, when she was signing the assent, I asked her, "What's it like to read this information? She said, "Sometimes it's scary to read it." And I said, "What do you think about having these experimental medications?" and she's like, "Well, I know that they write on them anything that can possibly happen, and I know that these aren't the things that always happen." You have to be careful about what information is given and how it is given. Maybe different assents need to be signed by different-aged children. The same assents sometimes need to be geared toward a 7-year-old and sometimes geared toward a 13-year-old and written differently at different ages. Despite all this information she was getting from the assent forms, Rebecca chose not to sit in on the meetings with her parents to discuss treatment options with the staff. She didn't want to be involved in that, even when it became end-of-life kinds of meetings.

15:6. I couldn't even comprehend what the mom was going through. The only thing she kept saying was, "This is all my fault. My husband has two healthy daughters from a previous marriage, so this is all my fault." That was mom's first thing. She said, "My two children have cancer and they are both going to die and this is my fault." She never elaborated to me about it, and I never pursued the matter because I got the sense from her that she didn't want to talk about the way things were going and the horror of the situation. That first night, I just tried to comfort her and said, "Look, we are going to get through this and we'll do everything we can for Justine." But that night, I almost lost it. She was the most incredible woman. She cared for George the whole time that he was sick with just amazing strength. And then the same thing when it came time for Justine. She had all this experience in the hospital that made it so she could just go get stuff and do stuff. She wouldn't refuse help but very much didn't want help with taking care of her kids. It really became her life. She was immensely strong. But that night, when she was saying that they're both going to die, there was some part of her that was saying it and knowing it. It was shortly before that that George's disease came back with a vengeance and no matter what we were going to do—we were going to try a few more things—the likelihood of him surviving had dropped and then, suddenly, she was hit with the news that her other child, who had been this beautiful, healthy, articulate, incredibly intelligent 4-year-old now had a brain tumor. There aren't even words to say, at that point. All I felt like I could do was just be there and do the best that I could for Justine and try and comfort mom through the night; just give her every consideration possible.

15:10. All the families get to know each other on the floor, and they really stand by for each other. Like, when George died yesterday, Mrs. Givanni, Anthony's mother, took the time out, left Anthony with the nurses' aide, and spent the entire morning in George's room with mom and dad and other family members. She just sat there, just to be with them through this whole thing. And Mr. Kapelli came into the room to offer support, and so did Mrs. Moldorno, who spent the last 2 months in and out of the hospital. All these families have children who are in bad shape, yet they rallied yesterday to be there for George's family. Everybody on the floor knew that he was dying. I don't know who specifically told them, but the parents all talk with each other. I know that Mr. Kapelli was closest to George's mother because when his daughter was diagnosed, they shared the same room. So they were talking and all the parents talk among each other. They serve as a kind of an informal support group. A lot of the rooms here are double rooms, so these kids are often in the same room with each other and their families are talking. And then parents come out and wander the halls, especially when they are here at night, and the nurses' station is a congregation place where people talk and people walk from room to room. They also meet in the clinic because, when children are diagnosed around the same time, the parents are hanging out in the same area in the clinic. They get to talking and get to know each other and then they get to know each other on the inpatient side of things. People will actively look for each other, like, when some parents come in, they ask who else is here so they can go visit. While we don't display a list of names of patients on the floor, for patient confidentiality reasons, we are not going to not tell them, because it's a wonderful source of support for the parents. It creates some problems for our social workers when parents hear that some people are getting some things that other people aren't, usually for eligibility reasons and insurance things. But, for the most part, it is a positive thing to have parents talking with each other.

15:10. Knowing that Justine was 4, even though she talked like a 12-year-old, she didn't have the full capability or grasp of death. From what I remember from my developmental pediatrics, it's more like going to sleep and the person is gone, but kids her age don't have the ability to abstract and equate the sense of loss. It is more like a lost toy or a friend that moved away kind of a thing. But she did have some comprehension of it. There was a day earlier this week when she asked her mother, who was crying, "Mommy, are you crying for George, are you crying for me, or are you crying for us both?" So there was a degree of comprehension there but, because of her disease, she was having these waxing and waning periods of lucidity—some days she could barely be aroused and, other days she was articulate to that level of understanding and articulation. . . . We tried to do whatever was best for the family, and it was best for them to have their two children there where they could see them both. I am not totally against children being around for the passing of their siblings. I've seen many siblings here when their brothers or sisters died. When George died, his mother picked him up and brought him to Justine in the next bed and said, "I want you to give George a goodbye kiss. He is going to sleep now." And she [Justine] gave him a kiss and patted him on the head, and everybody in the room basically just lost it. Mom was such a stoic person that all she did was cry. There was no screaming, there was no gnashing of teeth, or wailing, or prostrating, or anything like that. It was just very somber, and so, for Justine, it wasn't a huge upheaval. It was just that mommy was sad, but mommy's been sad. So I don't think that her being there, for whatever short life she had left, was going to be destructive to her psyche. She saw her mommy sad, and she got to say goodbye to her brother. . . . This raises the issue about how old a child should be to be there when a brother or sister is dying. I don't know. I think that any self-respecting pediatrician would look at the situation, look at the child, look at the family, and do what is best for the child and the family. I think that, in an intact family where there aren't issues and where the child is capable of dealing with it and has been dealing with it, it's perfectly acceptable if you make the judgment that this child can handle it and the best thing is for them to be there with their family and to say goodbye. I think that offers a degree of closure for a child at any age. I don't know if people would agree with me, but from my experience, that's my take on the situation. If the child was dying at home, it would be the parents' call on whether or not siblings should be there, so maybe the hospital should try to replicate the support of home conditions and allow parents to make the decision. It's the parents' call, and that's what we did having Justine and George in the same room. It was mom's call, and she made the call and we went with it. I don't think that it's our place to dictate what parents allow or don't allow their children to see. We can recommend, we can offer advice, but when it comes down to it, I feel it's their decision.

15:7. When George was really sick, we tried to do things with Justine to keep Justine busy and, when Justine was really sick, we tried to do things with George to keep him busy, so that mom could focus on the one child. I tried to do whatever I physically or emotionally could do to be supportive. We'd play with Justine. We would put her in a wheelchair and bring her to the nurses' station because if they were in the room together, they were both competing for mom's attention. We would take George down to the candy store, those sorts of things. I think that helped a little, so that she had some free time to focus on one child at a time. But, in the end, George couldn't leave his room, and Justine didn't want to leave. She wanted to be a part of what was going on. She was really scared. At first I didn't know if it was a good idea having them both in the same room, but they were separated when George had to go to the ICU. Mom initially had wanted them in separate rooms but when she had to go back and forth between the two, she realized it was just going to be way too difficult, so when he came back from the ICU, they were in the room together. I wasn't sure how Justine would react, but in the end it was best because, when we tried to close the curtain and keep her separate, she kept opening it. She really wanted to know what was going on. She got mad at the people who tried to close her off. So I think keeping her informed and keeping her a part of it, even though she was so young, really was the right decision. Even though she was sad, at least she knew what happened and

she got to say good-bye to him. As horrible as it was, she held him and
kissed him goodbye.

16:1. In the beginning, I never had chances to speak with Jose alone because
his mother didn't want me to. She didn't want me to have conversations
with him because I might tell him bad news. So we had a long discussion,
and I finally convinced her to let me tell him that he had a tumor. I don't
think he knew he had cancer until months later. But I could deal with
telling him he had a malignancy, explaining what cancer was like, from a
mechanistic perspective. But he really wasn't that interested in hearing
about it. When we would start having more medical discussions, he would
just walk off; he wanted to go play. That's kind of unusual in 14-year-olds,
but it's variable. Some of them want to know everything, and I see that
more in the boys. Girls have different ways of coping. That's not completely true, but that's my knee-jerk reaction. But yes; I've seen other kids
his age not wanting to know about their disease.

16:11. As late as 7 days before he passed away, his mom was refusing to
come to a family meeting to discuss his medical situation and get permission from her to discuss it with him. She said, "No, absolutely not. I don't
want to talk about death, death, death. I want to enjoy the time that we
have. If we say death, death, death, it's going to make him say it and then
he'll think it'll bring it on sooner." I asked her, "Do you think that he
knows?" and she said, "No." "But really, in his heart of hearts, do you
think he knows?" and she said, "Maybe in his heart of hearts. But I don't
want to talk about death. I'm just tired of talking about death." In her
eyes, she was trying to protect him, and that was sad because children,
especially adolescents, are very aware of what's going on. They can read
nonverbal signs, people's facial expressions, to know what's going on. The
idea of trying to protect their child is understandable, but it's ineffective
and counterproductive. It creates more anxiety, there's more ambiguity
for the child or adolescent who's unclear about what's going on. At least if
they knew what was going on, they could talk about it; talk about treatment. They could say, "I'm scared," or, "I don't want to die." I've also
come to appreciate that, while the parents are trying to protect their child,
the child is often an active participant in trying to protect the parents by
not bringing it up because they see they can't handle it. Jose was involved
in that dance. He was very astute; he was a quiet boy but very astute. He'd

say, when mom went out of the room, "She was crying." She'd come back, her eyes were all red and he realized that.

18:10. When he originally got diagnosed, his parents didn't want to tell him what he had. It took a while for his parents to come around and realize that it was important for him to be involved in his own care and to understand more about what was happening to him and then being able to figure out ways to face it and to deal with it. So, at first this put me in a tough position because at 14, you can have a very good understanding of what's happening to your body, and you should be able to have some say about what's happening to you. So it was difficult and we worked with mom. She was like, "You can tell him that he has a tumor, but you can't tell him he has cancer because, if you tell him that he has cancer, he's not going to fight it and he's not strong enough." So we didn't focus on that. We didn't tell him he had cancer, but we talked about chemotherapy and we explained to him what's going to happen. So we kind of went along with what mom said we could talk about and the other things, we just left it as is. But he figured it out, and then, once he was able to find out who he could trust, he would ask questions. I was always honest with the mother and told her that, if he came up and point blank asked me a question, I wasn't going to lie about it. And she said, "Okay, that's fair, but I don't want you telling him." I explained that even if I don't use the word "cancer," other kids are going to say things like, "I have cancer, what are you here for?" But it was still like, "No, no, no, don't tell him." We go through this, at first, with a lot of parents. Often, parents say, "Don't tell them they have cancer," or, "Don't use that word," but then they're totally fine with the rest of it. But the words "cancer center" are right on the entrance to this building.

16:11. His sister, who was about 10 years old, came to the unit but didn't want to set foot in the room. I wanted to make sure that she knew this was one of her last opportunities to say goodbye. So one of the child-life specialists took her to the child-life room and helped her make a memory box. Some time later, the psychiatry fellow met with her and said, "She's appropriately upset." So, in the end, it was okay that she didn't want to go in the room; she wanted to remember him as he used to be. That's all you can do, is to offer an opportunity.

16:4. The thing that came up the night that he was dying was that he came
from a large Dominican family and there must have been about 40 relatives here that night. They were all over. There were relatives in this conference room, in the back conference room, they were spilling out into the
hallways. They brought everyone, like little kids aged 5, 6 to grandparents.
It was very difficult dealing with so many family members because we're
on an oncology floor where all the kids are on the brink of life or death.
We talked to the different groups of relatives and explained that they
couldn't be in the hallway, they had to be in his room, but there couldn't
be a gigantic number of people in his room because that was disruptive to
him as well. We had to put a limit on how many people were allowed in
his room at one time. It was hard, because if he had been at home, that
wouldn't have been so much an issue. It's horrible to have to say, "You
can't disturb and upset the other children and families on the floor," but
it's true. I think that was really the hardest thing surrounding Jose's
death. . . . All the parents on the floor knew what was happening. A couple
of the parents asked me questions, "What's happening? "What's going
on?" "He's dying, isn't he?" One of the moms of another patient had been
in Jose's room the whole night, the night before—and her son's pretty sick
too—and about an hour before Jose passed away she lost control and
started screaming. We went to see her and she said, "I'm tired. I can't take
it anymore. I want to kill myself," while poor Jose is dying in the room. I
wound up having to send this other mother to psychiatry and then send
her to the Psych ER. On her way to the Psych ER, she ran into some of
Jose's family members who said, "He's dying. He's dying." So she wound
up back in his room and I had to tell her, "I need you to go to the Psych
ER. You can either come out of Jose's room and go down peacefully and
not disturb his family, or I'll have to have security come." It was a mess
and about 15 minutes later Jose died. She had said these things before, and
we had psychiatry involved. She was extremely tearful, at that point, and I
felt like I had to take a stand with her because I knew that Jose was going
to pass away that night and I was worried that Jose's mother, who had her
own psychiatric problems, would get hysterical and feed into this. I didn't
want to have two hysterical moms on the floor. When I called psychiatry, I
explained the situation and said, "I have to take her threat seriously," and
they said, "Absolutely. We think you did the right thing," and they came to
see her. We had a psych plan in place for Jose's mother because she had
been hysterical two or three times in the past—same sort of thing that this
mom did, threatening to kill herself—but she turned out to be completely
appropriate. Unfortunately, this other mom was hospitalized overnight in

psychiatry and, as far as I know, she's still hospitalized, which is unfortunate because her child's doing so much better now.

16:10. I remember once, when I asked him, "What you most afraid of? Are you scared? Are you in pain?" he said, "I'm in pain, but I'm not afraid." Over the last 2 years, as he felt more comfortable with me, he would ask me more questions, like a lot of kids do, like, "What's heaven like? What do you think it's like?" I'd say, "Well, what do you think it's like?" and he'd say, "I think it's a place like whatever you want it to be, it is," and then kind of left it like that. Because Jose was a jokester, he liked talking about ghosts and stuff, and I said, "Yeah, when you go to heaven, you'll probably go around joking with people because that's what you like to do," and he said, "Yeah, I would be really good at that—spooking people out." I learned that, with him, you couldn't push the issue; he had to bring it up and then you kind of went with it and then you kind of knew when he was at a point where he didn't want to take it further. He would have this kind of look, this grin on his face, and that's when you knew he was done with that and didn't want to talk about it anymore. . . . Every once in a while you would get a sense of what he was thinking. A lot of times, he would say things to me like, "One thing I see is that life isn't promised to you forever and I don't make plans because I realize that I'm sick and I'm happy for what I'm able to do. Three years ago they told me that I was going to die of this and I'm still here." That was how he figured it all out, and he knew eventually it would happen but he didn't know when. He just learned to deal with whatever he had and make the best of it, and that's incredible for someone his age to come up with that.

16:10. Jose wrote a letter to his family telling them, "I'm going to be okay. You don't have to worry about me." I don't know if he was able to say it to them when he was alive, but, at least, he was able to write it. I was happy knowing that he was able to do this so, at least, he left his family with something to know how he felt and that he was okay with it.

17:2. In the beginning, Christianna knew that she had disease in her lungs and in her leg, and then when she had the surgery, we told her, "Right now it looks like all the disease is gone, but it could come back so we want to keep you on the therapy because the chances of it coming back are very high." After that piece of information, they didn't want us to give her any more than absolutely necessary information. It wasn't so much the father as the aunt, the dad's younger sister. She had no children so when the mother died, she raised the children and she was very, very protective of Christianna—emotionally, spiritually, and physically. She was a very pleasant woman, and everything was fine until the relapse. She had so much faith that she was going to get better, and that faith was shattered when she [Christianna] came back with the disease. Part of it may be that she really didn't understand as much as the father did because she wasn't there at the very beginning during the prognosis talks we had about what we expected and how she presented. And when you look at Christianna, you think she looks great, so it's hard to relate that with death and dying. In the aunt's mind, that was not compatible with her reality, and she didn't want to face that part at all.

17:10. The aunt was under a lot of pressure, and she kept complaining to different people that "This hasn't happened. Why hasn't that happened?" She was splitting the people. Like, if she were told, "You have to speak with this one nurse; this is your nurse and she will relay the information to me," she'd tell the nurse, the resident, the fellow, the attending, the kitchen person—anybody who would listen to her, because she was so desperate to have some human contact. Then I would get a phone call from every single one of those people. I understood what she went through, up to a certain level. I probably will never fully go through that or understand it, but I imagine that if I had to be with a relative in the hospital for months and that person was dying and I didn't have anybody to help me, then, you know what? I would look pretty psychotic. So I felt terrible for her. I'm sure I'll come up against another patient like that, so I have to prepare myself to deal with things like that in the future. I learned that in the future, with a case like this, I need to keep everyone more in the loop; the fellows, the attendings, the residents, and the nurse-practitioner about what's going on. My experience with this family was very difficult and I felt attacked on many occasions, but I have to move beyond that because I have to work with these people day in and day out. I kept telling myself that she was just reacting naturally and, for me, it's a job. This was not my best case. I don't think I've ever had such a difficult experience as I did here.

19:3. It was the fellow who started to talk to the mother to explain what had happened, and when he got to the point of telling her, "We were unsuccessful," she just put her head down because she couldn't face him; that's when the mom figured it out. I didn't realize that they had walked out and were going to talk to the mom, so I didn't follow them and, by the time I realized they were down the hallway, I decided not to go in and interrupt. I knew when mom realized what happened because there was this awful cry coming from the end of the hallway. . . . This mother's 15½ years old. She came out and was like, "Why? Why? It was my baby, why?" and then she had a classic teenage comment, "I bought all these clothes for her and we were going to chill in the summertime, oh God." Eventually, the father and the whole family came. It was a two-patient room, so they moved the other patient to a different room; he was a 5-year-old, so he was somewhat traumatized by all this happening as well. We cleared out the room, except for the crib and the baby, and we took all of the monitors out of the room. Certain things had to stay, like the nasogastric tube that had been used and her NG tube, and she'd been intubated, so that was in and then, of course, her IV. There were certain pieces that could not be taken off of her because mom had requested an autopsy and, for autopsy purposes, that stuff has to stay in because they want to know what foreign bodies were there so that, when they're actually doing the procedure, they know what lesions came from external objects. We let the family stay for a long, long time and the mom was basically just torn apart and her mom, the grandmother, was grieving but also very angry. She kept making comments like, "This baby should never have been on this floor. Why was this baby on this floor? She should have been in the ICU."

20:8. This was kind of easy, considering that they're a together couple and very supportive of each other and they both knew this is what they wanted to do [withdraw care]. But sometimes you have parents that, one wants it, the other one doesn't, and then you're stuck in the middle, and that's really hard because you have to have both of them agreeing to this or you just can't do it. So you just hold it off and you watch the baby get sicker and sicker and sicker, until eventually either the baby dies or both parents come to an agreement. Sometimes, when a baby's been here for a long time, for months and months, we see marriages start to break up and sometimes you see parents that are really together and remain very close and very supportive of each other. But the longer the child is in the hospital, the greater the burden on the marriage. Over time, you see some parents not talking to each other as much as they were, or they start visiting at different times and not together.

20:8. We encourage parents to bring siblings with them except when they're really young, like maybe under 5 when they don't really know what's going on and they don't really get it. But I think, if you have a 5-year-old that's pretty intelligent, it can be important for them to be a part of it because, a lot of times, they just feel like they're not part of that family. Some families absolutely don't want their children to have anything to do with it, and a lot of parents say, "Yeah, I want my other children here."

20:1. We [Neonatal Intensive Care Unit] have a memorial service once a year for children who have died in our unit. It's nondenominational and all parents of children who expire here are invited and about 10 to 15 percent of the families come. In the last few years we've been attempting to in-clude more readings that parents send in or read poems, make tributes. There's a board so if they would like, they can put up a picture of the child. We light a candle for each child. As their name is called out, the parents come up and light a candle. They move to the garden afterward and plant bulbs near a rather lopsided tree that's growing in the garden that has a plaque by it. The people who come are clearly the ones who would like to have that one day that they can openly remember their child and everyone else who had a child who died. It's becoming increasingly noisy, because they bring subsequent children or siblings so that there is this element of the ever-turning cycle of life. People come back pregnant and there is this optimism, but they don't forget the child or children that have been lost. I think it's important that we be there for them and say, "Yes, we weren't able to cure him, but we can stand as physicians and care team members and remember these children." Most of the time, these babies never went home, so the only people who really knew their baby were us; so it's very important for them to come back so that we can remember their baby.

Conclusions | 8

Gracious dying is a huge,
macabre and expensive joke on
the American public.
— JESSICA MITFORD
The American Way of Death

How likely is it that those working in pediatric end-of-life care would see a mother who, soon after learning that one of her two children will likely die from cancer, learns that her other child also will soon die from a different kind of cancer (Story 15); see a mother care for a child who has terminal cancer at the same time his father (her husband) does (Story 9); see a mother who, soon after her child dies from complications of a bone marrow transplant, has to decide if she wants her second and only surviving child to have a bone marrow transplant, for the same reason because, if he doesn't, he will certainly die prematurely (Story 4); be a nurse who has to withdraw life support from a newborn who is awake and active and then watch him die (Story 20); learn about a mother, a nurse, who has to withhold CPR from her child so that he can die peacefully at home, despite her child's ardent pleas for her to give him CPR (Story 9); care for a child whose parents had her (their only child) after six miscarriages and then had to watch her die when she was 5 years old (Story 12); decide whether to use radiation, in place of failed chemotherapy and surgeries, to eradicate a brain tumor in a baby even though it might cause mental retardation or to wait until the baby is older to reduce the risk of retardation but also risk the chance that she might die (Story 10); question if a 5-year-old boy, in intractable pain, is asking to die when he screams, "I can't take this anymore" (Story 2)? These are dramatic and poignant cases, but they are not necessarily unusual for those involved in pediatric end-of-life care—these are the things that happen.

The most compelling part of these narratives is the diverse ways in which they capture the vicissitudes of end-of-life issues in pediatrics. In most of the narratives, it is difficult to recognize which discipline is being voiced, in terms of the issues being raised and ways of speaking about them. Residents don't sound that much different than attendings or nurses or social workers. The one exception is the nurses: as a group, they were more inclined to withdraw life support sooner than later, compared to physicians (e.g., Story 7). Physicians' narratives generally are more concerned with medical issues; child-life specialists' and social workers' with psychosocial issues; and nurses' narratives fall somewhere in between. Yet all of the disciplines convey the gamut of issues (medical and psychosocial) that all members of a treatment team share in any given case.

The narratives also are diverse across cases. Each case is demanding in its own particular way and argues against the idea that we can prescribe standardized guidelines that have universal application. Pediatric end-of-life care is highly particularized and, therefore, cannot easily be generalized. As medicine moves along the trajectory of a child dying, a pattern of interacting forces emerges which involves the child's disease status along with the beliefs, values, desires, strengths, resources, vulnerabilities, expectations, hopes, and limitations of a particular family at a particular time. These forces come to constitute, for the staff, a context of empathic care that is highly individualized for every child and family.

Withdrawing Care

As new scientific findings, technologies, and medications lead to ever more complicated diagnostic and treatment procedures with more uncertain outcomes, questions about when to withhold or withdraw end-of-life care for children escalate. When considering decisions about when to withhold or withdraw care, it is important to remember that, in each narrative where decisions were made to either withhold or withdraw care or to push more aggressively for cure, the child died and, often, died in pain because care for curative intent was not withheld or withdrawn sooner. Missing here are narratives in which aggressive approaches to push the limits sometimes result in children surviving and going on to have healthy and productive lives. Aggressive care in pediatric oncology, for example, accounts, in part, for a cure rate of 75 to 80 percent today. I am reminded of the attending physician who questioned the "go for broke" approach of one of her colleagues but then said, "When looking out in the clinic, I see a couple of saves that I would have written off, from my perspective, who have made it and are alive and healthy, so I'm glad that there are these people" (Story 2).

Who should decide when and how to continue seeking ever more aggressive kinds of medical interventions and diagnostic studies? This is an ethical issue because the question rests on a series of risk/benefit ratios that have to be considered (i.e., the ratio of benefit to burden of treatment as judged by patients, families, institutional resources, scientific evidence, etc.).[1] The principled reply is that it is a collaborative decision, rationally and systematically negotiated, and arrived at through consensus of the various subspecialty teams involved in caring for a child as well as the child's family. In practice, however, it very different.

Aggressive and experimental treatments test the evidence-based (i.e., scientific) limits of a single subspecalty, so that it is not reasonable to expect all of the medical teams to be on board at this level of end-of-life decision making. In the narratives, this often is seen in regard to how an ICU team relates to an oncology team. How their differences in perspective and knowledge are conveyed to the families is of paramount importance. Ideally, according to the principle of patient autonomy, the family and the patient are partners with the staff in decision making, but the narratives show us how difficult it is to involve children or parents.

Many children simply don't want this burden and walk away from it when approached. Perhaps the fault lives in how they are approached and how options are communicated to them, but the adolescents in the narratives consistently avoided this issue even when it was sensitively and carefully communicated (Stories 13 and 16). It is more likely that children react this way because they have qualitatively different ways of reasoning about time (i.e., more concrete than abstract) and, consequently, are less reflective than we are about the need to justify the meaning or purpose of their lives.[2] In at least one other story, the child chose to defer to the parents' wishes regarding symptom management, even when it was detrimental to the child's own comfort and quality of life and against medical advice (Story 1). Nevertheless, we need to continually question the extent to which dying children participate in a conspiracy of silence with adults who love, care, and want to "protect" them[3] and monitor what they want to know. The narratives provide ample evidence of how this occurs.

Without the child's participation, the burden of end-of-life decisions falls on the parents, and here we see many illustrations of how difficult it is for parents to ever give up hope and face the likelihood of losing their child. This is dramatically illustrated in Stories 3 and 4, but denial that their child is dying is a recurring theme in most of the narratives. In only two stories do we find that parents were ready to withdraw support before the medical team (Stories 5 and 12). Is the parents' reluctance to face the realities of their children dying due, in part, to the staff's hesitancy to communicate with them about it openly and honestly? The narratives present ample evidence that the staff generally is disinclined to convey bad news and generally waits to the end to initiate DNR discussions with parents. Discussing a DNR order was the usual means by which staff initiated discussions with parents that were explicitly focused on the likelihood of death (e.g., Story 7). Would it have been preferable for them to have discussed the DNR order earlier? How does the staff know when it is appropriate to break down the patients' or parents' denial? In cases of chronic deterioration, it could be done at the first signs that standard treatment is failing. But this is difficult because, from the narratives, we see how circuitous the trajectory of death is; the emotional roller coaster is difficult enough for children and parents (and staff) without discussing DNR before it appears inevitable. Most parents fervently cling to hope, and the stories present no evidence that earlier, more frank, and less optimistic discussions by physicians with patients and families might lessen their extent of denial.

Are pediatricians overly optimistic when they are conveying information about end-of-life options?[4] Yes, most of them are, as are most physicians, but what is the cost of their reluctance to abandon hope? From the narratives do we get any sense that a false sense of hope will compromise the child's quality of life? Was any child lied to, either directly or indirectly, about his or her chances of survival? We often speak of the need to be honest with adults who might be dying because they have a need to put their lives in order (whatever that might mean). Do we see any evidence that children have similar needs? What comes across so forcefully in the narratives is that principles of honesty and patient autonomy are not cut-and-dried in the press of end-of-life care. If there is one principle that can be derived from the narratives, with regard to communicating with children and families about end-of-life care, it is to always leave the door open so that the patient or family can open it further if they so choose and with whom. As we have seen, alliances and bonds between staff and families become stronger at end of life and may also shift. At the start of care, the patient's primary attending physician usually has the strongest alliance, but, as conditions worsen, we see in the stories how patients and families turn to others for guidance and support. One patient, for example, never talked about dying with anyone except the child-life specialist (Story 16); in other stories, parents turned to a social worker as their advocate, while others aligned themselves with a nurse.

The narratives also show that the varieties of pain and suffering at end of life are not due to the indifference, ignorance, or unwillingness of the staff to do all that they could, within the parameters of curative intent and parental concerns, to manage a child's pain and suffering. This picture contradicts the one that is so often presented depicting physicians, particularly pediatricians, as reluctant to use adequate doses of opioids and nonopioid analgesics to manage pain.[5] Frequently, too, parents will interfere with adequate pain management because of fears that it will hasten their child's death (Stories 1, 3, 4, and 15). Textbooks about palliative care promote the idea that pain management can always be achieved. In contrast, the scenarios captured in these narratives show that, under the best of circumstances, under the direction of well-trained and compassionate medical staff, including members of a specially trained pain team, adequate pain control, for all patients, is rarely realized. Sometimes this is because the focus is on cure rather than comfort. Some pain syndromes and symptoms are profoundly difficult to control even when pain management specialists are not afraid of using high doses of narcotics.

Good communication between the staff and the children and their families is the hallmark of excellence in end-of-life care, and yet it is the most difficult aspect of care to prescribe. In no other aspect of medicine is the staff and family more subtly and reciprocally entwined. The staff's ability to listen in order to first discern the emotional, cultural, and psychological context of the family is paramount and goes against the sense that physicians are the ultimate sources of authority. Instead, listening promotes a more collaborative and negotiated way for physicians and families to interact in the child's best interest.[6] Although some staff are more adept at listening than others, the narratives provide numerous opportunities to understand how physician/patient relations are negotiated in contexts of empathy and benevolence. Such negotiations require a set of skills that are difficult to define and teach, but staying abreast of the families' changing perspectives and beliefs is critical. The narratives illustrate different ways of communicating and, more significantly, convey how the staff's ways of communicating, on a case-by-case basis, reflect how they reciprocally interact with children and families.

About 20 percent of families enter the system of hospital-based care in pediatrics with preexisting psychological problems.[7] The stresses on parents caring for their children and dealing with the medical system, particularly when care moves from curative intent to end-of-life palliative care, can exacerbate already fragile relations and can create enormous problems for the staff; it helps if they are prepared for such possibilities. Questions arise about appropriate and inappropriate ways of adapting to a child's end of life. For example, the father who assumed a fetal position on the floor outside the waiting room was seen as behaving pathologically by some of the nurses but not by the social worker (Story 1; see also Story 16).

Ethical Concerns

Ethics always is more a matter of case-based questions than of principled or standardized guidelines of practice. In addition to the ethics of withdrawing care and symptom management, the narratives provide a stockpile of ethical challenges for clinical case analysis in pediatric end-of-life care. Consider, for example, the two siblings who had Wiskott-Aldrich Syndrome (Story 4), a genetic disease for which there is no cure except bone marrow transplant (BMT). Without it, children will die, even with continuing supportive care, by the time they are 11 or 12 years old. The mother in Story 4, after considerable deliberation, finally agreed with the attending physician's advice to consent to BMT for her older child. This child then died from complications of the transplant, and the mother was subsequently asked to consider BMT for her other child. The attending physician no longer felt able to advocate as strongly for the second child, and so the mother decided to refuse the procedure for him. But if just the second child had been presented, the attending would unequivocally have advocated the transplant (just as he had for the mother's first child). The ethical issue, in this regard, is whose agent is the physician—the mother's, who suffered terribly from the prolonged dying and complicated death of one of her two children, or the child's? Is the physician ethically obligated to act in the best interests of the second child to advocate (perhaps to the extent of seeking a court order) for another BMT, which will again run the risk of death (and further suffering for this mother) but also the possibility of cure and the promise of a full life?[8]

In many of the narratives, interns and residents issue a clarion call to become more involved in decision making in end-of-life care. Accordingly, ways need to be found to free them from the immediacies of patient care so that they can take part in the decision-making process, and ways need to be explored for them to learn to convey bad news to patients and families. They can't be expected simply to follow directives at this level of patient care or to acquire difficult and demanding interpersonal skills outside the context of practice.

The staff can do this kind of work, day-after-day because they are a self-selected group who knowingly chose their jobs. Hence, they are resilient and competent in finding their own ways of coping and moving on. There is no single way of coping, and the different roads to resilience for the staff have to be protected and preserved. Just as recent studies have questioned the value of bereavement counseling for all parents who have lost a child,[9] so we have to be careful not to impose counseling on the staff. Routine institutionalized interventions to help staff grieve, whether in groups or individually, are unwarranted. Staff members don't want such interventions, although they often speak of seeking opportunities to talk to colleagues about the challenges they face each day. Having the staff meet outside the hospital to reinvigorate their collegiality and to develop and maintain interpersonal relations in roles other than strictly hospital care is an appealing idea (see Story 15).

As a reflection of hospital-based pediatric care, these narratives are skewed and biased because for every death the staff faces, there are hundreds of cures and successful recoveries; for every hostile and angry family that has lost a child, there are hundreds of families happy to be taking their child home. Unlike those who provide hospice care, hospital-based pediatrics never is focused solely on end of life, and, for most pediatric specialists in this country, a dying patient is very rare.

End-of-Life Care Is Idiographic

This book began with the compelling idea that end-of-life care in pediatrics always is idiographic and inductive. Accordingly,

> it works by passing the existing principles of the philosophical and religious moral traditions through the grid of particular personal and clinical histories to learn gradually what these principles command, prohibit, or tolerate [in each individual case]. This knowledge is not all worked out in advance, completed, and awaiting to be applied. The clinical ethical order within these principles . . . cannot be made explicit as a whole. It is manifested slowly and only partially as it is worked out in the case-by-case practical judgments reached at the bedsides of utterly unique persons as their disease advances and their biographies come to a close.[10]

To the extent that these narratives capture the "particular personal and clinical histories" of medical staff involved in this demanding and challenging work, they will help us to better appreciate and come to terms with the difficult and frustrating issues associated with the end-of-life care of children and their families. They render greater depth and breadth of understanding than the usual dry, uninstantiated, abstract approaches to end-of-life care in pediatrics.

Notes

PREFACE

1. Bearison, D. J. (1991). *"They never want to tell you": Children talk about cancer.* Cambridge, MA: Harvard University Press (1993). Translated as *"Keiner spricht mit mir darüber"—Krebskranke kinder erzählen von ihren efrahrungen.* Munich, Germany: Droemer Knaur Verlag.

2. Saunders, C. M. (2004). Foreword. In D. Doyle, G. Hanks, N. I. Cherny, & K. Calman (Eds.)., *Oxford textbook of palliative medicine,* 3rd ed. (pp. xvii–xx). Oxford: Oxford University Press.

3. Groopman, J. (2004). *The anatomy of hope.* New York: Random House (p. 59).

4. Sontag, S. (1977). *Illness as metaphor.* New York: Farrar, Straus & Giroux; Sontag, S. (1988). *AIDS and its metaphors.* New York: Farrar, Straus & Giroux.

5. Lakoff, G., & Johnson, M. (1980). *Metaphors we live by.* Chicago: University of Chicago Press; Kovecses, Z. (2002). *Metaphor: A practical introduction.* New York: Oxford University Press.

6. Examples include passed away, one's loss, down under, gone, kicked the bucket, bought the farm, 6 feet under, gone to his maker, answered the last call, bit the big one, bit the dust, bought the box, croaked, checked out, faded away, in the sweet hereafter. A formidable alphabetical list of euphemisms for dying is available at: http://phrontistery.50megs.com/longpig/dead.html (December 12, 2003).

7. Richard Neuhaus speaks of inextricable links in the ways we conceptualize and practice sex and death, including procreation as a drive toward immortality. Neuhaus, R. J. (2002). *As I lay dying.* New York: Basic Books. See also Gorer, G. (1986). *Death, grief and mourning in contemporary Britain.* London: Cresset Press.

8. It is interesting to note that the study of sex, like death and dying, is constrained by limits on what can be reasonably measured in a quantitative and standardized form in laboratory-type experiments. Hence, essential aspects often are subject to interpretive and qualitative kinds of inquiries. Wiederman, M. W., & Whitley, B. E., Jr. (2002). *Handbook for conducting research on human sexuality.* Mahwah, NJ: Erlbaum.

9. Haynes, R. B., Davis, D. A., McKibbon, A., & Tugwell, P. (1984). A critical appraisal of the efficacy of continuing medical education. *Journal of the American Medical Association, 251,* 61–64; Cabana, M. D., Rand, C. S., Powe, N. R., Wu, A. W., Wilson, M. H., Abboud, P., & Rubin, H. R. (1999). Why don't physicians follow clinical practice guidelines? A framework for improvement. *Journal of the American Medical Association, 282,* 1458–1465; Greco, P. J., & Eisenberg, J. M. (1993). Changing physicians' practices. *New England Journal of Medicine, 329,* 1271–1274.

10. William James believed, for example, that if you want to understand religion you must find the most religious person at his or her most religious moment (James, W. [1902/1982]. *The varieties of religious experience: A study in human nature.* New York: Penguin Books). The Roman poet and Epicurean philosopher Lucretius expressed similar sentiments: "If you would like to know what men really are, the time to learn comes when they stand in danger or in doubt. For then at last words of truth are drawn from the depths of the heart, and the mask is torn off, reality remains" (Lucretius [1924]. *On the nature of the universe,* Transl. by W. H. D. Rouse. Cambridge, MA: Harvard University Press.

CHAPTER 1: PEDIATRIC END-OF-LIFE CARE

1. Some examples of this kind of qualitative research about end-of-life care are: Sourkes, B. (1995). *Armfuls of time: The psychological experience of the child with a life-threatening illness.* Pittsburgh: University of Pittsburgh Press; Bluebond-Langner, M. (1978). *The private worlds of dying children.* Princeton, NJ: Princeton University Press; Finkbeiner, A. K. (1996). *After the death of a child: Living with loss through the years.* New York: Free Press; Diamond, J. C. (1998). *". . . because cowards get cancer too."* London: Vermilion; Picardie, R. (1998). *Before I say good-bye.* Middlesex, England: Penguin Books; Epstein, F. (2003). *If I get to five: What children can teach us about courage and character.* New York: Henry Holt; Talbot, K. (2002). *What forever means after the death of a child: Transcending the trauma, living with the loss.* New York: Brunner-Routledge; Barnard, D., Towers, A., Boston, P., & Lambrinidou, Y. (2000). *Crossing over: Narratives of palliative care.* New York: Oxford University Press.

There is, of course, a venerable tradition of physicians writing about medicine. Some recent and notable examples are: Gawande, A. (2002). *Complications: A surgeon's notes on an imperfect science.* New York: Henry Holt & Co.; Candib, L. M. (1995). *Medicine and the family: A feminist perspective.* New York: Basic Books; Verghese, A. (1994). *My own country: A doctor's story of a small town and its people in the age of AIDS.* New York: Simon & Schuster; Borkan, J., Reis, S., Steinmetz, D., & Medalie, J. H. (Eds.) (1999). *Patients and doctors: Life changing stories from primary care.* Madison: University of Wisconsin Press; Nuland, S. B. (1994). *How we die: Life's final chapter.* New York: Knopf; Groopman, J. (2004). *The anatomy of hope.* New York: Random House; Sacks, O. (1995). *An anthropologist on Mars.* New York: Vintage Books; Campo, R. (1997). *The poetry of healing: A doctor's education in empathy, identification and desire.* New York: Norton; Alvord, L. A., & Cohen Van Pelt, E. (1999). *The scalpel and the silver bear: The first Navaho woman surgeon combines Western medicine and traditional healing.* New York: Bantam.

2. Ferrell, B. (2003, November). *End of Life Nursing Education Consortium (ELNEC): National efforts to improve pediatric palliative care.* Paper presented at the meeting of the Initiative for Pediatric Palliative Care, New York, New York.

3. Rabow, M. W., Hardie, G. E., Fair, J. M., & McPhee, S. J. (2000). End-of-life case content in 50 textbooks from multiple specialities. *Journal of the American Medical Association, 283,* 771–778.

4. Field, M. J., & Behrman, R. (Eds.). (2003). *When children die: Improving palliative and end-of-life care for children and their families.* Washington, DC: National Academies Press (p. 355).

5. American Psychological Association Working Group on Assisted Suicide and End-of-Life Decisions. (2000, May). *Report to the Board of Directors of the American Psychological Association.* Washington, DC: American Psychological Association.

6. Contro, N., Larson, J., Scofield, S., Sourkes, B., & Cohen, H. (2002). Family perspectives on the quality of pediatric palliative care. *Archives of Pediatric and Adolescent Medicine, 156,* 14–19.

7. Virani, R., & Sofer, D. (2003). Improving the quality of end-of-life care. *American Journal of Nursing, 103,* 52–60.

8. Nuland, S. (1994). *How we die: Reflections on life's final chapter.* New York: Knopf. Nuland describes cancer, for example, in the following way: "Cancer, far from being a clandestine foe, is in fact berserk with the malicious exuberance of killing. The disease pursues a continuous, uninhibited circumferential, barn-burning expedition of destructiveness, in which it heeds no rules, follows no commands, and explores all resistance in a homicidal riot of devastation. Its cells behave like members of a barbarian horde run amok . . . to plunder everything within reach" (p. 207). See also Gawande, A. (2002). *Complications: A surgeon's notes on an imperfect science.* New York: Henry Holt.

9. Goldman, A. (1998). Life threatening illnesses and symptom control in children. In D. Doyle, G. W. C. Hanks, & N. MacDonald (Eds.), *Oxford textbook of palliative medicine,* 2nd ed. (pp. 1032–1043). Oxford: Oxford University Press.

10. Collins, J. J. (2004). Paediatric palliative medicine: Symptom control in life-threatening illness. In D. Doyle, G. Hanks, N. I. Cherny, & K. Calman (Eds.), *Oxford textbook of palliative medicine,* 3rd ed. (pp. 789–798). Oxford: Oxford University Press; Collins, J. J. (2003). Current status of symptom measurement in children. In R. K. Portenoy & E. Breweri, *Issues in palliative care research.* New York: Oxford University Press.

11. Pitorak, E. F. (2003). Care at the time of death. *American Journal of Nursing, 103,* 45–52.

12. Goldman, A. (1998). Life threatening illnesses and symptom control in children. In D. Doyle, G. W. C. Hanks, & N. MacDonald (Eds.), *Oxford textbook of palliative medicine,* 2nd ed. (pp. 1032–1043). Oxford: Oxford University Press.

13. Timmins, J. G. (1985). Pharmaceutical problems in children. *British Journal of Pharmaceutical Practice, 7,* 242–246.

14. Levetown, M., & Carter, M. A. (1998). Child-centered care in terminal illness: An ethical framework. In D. Doyle, G. W. C. Hanks, & N. MacDonald (Eds.), *Oxford*

textbook of palliative medicine, 2nd ed. (pp. 1107–1117). Oxford: Oxford University Press; Dominica. F (1987). Reflections on death in childhood. *British Medical Journal, 294,* 108–110.

15. Vernick, J., & Karon, M. (1965). Who's afraid of death on a leukemia ward? *American Journal of Diseases of Children, 109,* 393–397; Waechter, E. H. (1971). Children's awareness of fatal illness. *American Journal of Nursing, 71,* 1168–1172; Spinetta, J. J., Rigler, D., & Karon, M. (1973). Anxiety in the dying child. *Pediatrics, 52,* 841–845; Spinetta, J. J., Rigler, D., & Karon, M. (1974). Personal space as a measure of a dying child's sense of isolation. *Journal of Consulting and Clinical Psychology, 42,* 751–756; Hilden, J. M., Watterson, J., & Charastek, J.(2000). Tell the children. *Journal of Clinical Oncology, 18,* 3193–3195.

16. Bearison, D. J. (1991). *"They never want to tell you": Children talk about cancer.* Cambridge, MA: Harvard University Press.

17. Such a conspiracy, however, remains the norm in many developed countries. For example, a survey in 1992 found that only 18.2 percent of adult patients in Japan who died of cancer had been told their diagnosis while 98 percent of their families were told. Patients would have been told if they had asked, but that was not considered culturally appropriate. Ishikawa, Y., et al. (1992). *Cancer death in middle age. Report of the Statistics Bureau of the Ministry of Health and Welfare of Japan.* See also Charlton, R., & Dovey, S. (1995). Attitudes to death and drying in the UK, New Zealand, and Japan. *Journal of Palliative Care, 11,* 42–47; Kimura, R. (1986).

In Japan, parents participate but doctors decide. *Hastings Center Report, 16,* 22–23; Kashiwagi, T. (1998). Palliative care in Japan. In D. Doyle, G. W. C. Hanks, & N. Mac-Donald (Eds.). *Oxford textbook of palliative medicine,* 2nd ed. (pp. 796–814). Oxford: Oxford University Press. In this country, 45 years ago, 90 percent of physicians reported that they preferred not to reveal a cancer diagnosis to an adult patient, consequently denying the patient any opportunity to participate in health care decisions; see Oken, D. (1961). What to tell cancer patients. *Journal of the American Medical Association, 175,* 1120–1128. This is no longer the case in the United States.

18. McCallum, D. E., Byrne, P., & Breweri, E. (2000). How children die in hospitals. *Journal of Pain Symptom Management, 20,* 417–423.

19. Bluebond-Langner, M. (1978). *The private worlds of dying children.* Princeton, NJ: Princeton University Press; Lansdown, R., & Benjamin, G. (1985). The development of the concept of death in children aged 5–9 years. *Child Care Health and Development, 11,* 13–20; Faulkner, K. W. (2001). Children's understanding of death. In A. Armstrong-Dailey & S. Zarbock (Eds.), *Hospice care for children,* 2nd ed. New York: Oxford University Press; Sourkes, B. (1996). The broken heart: Anticipatory grief in the child facing death. *Journal of Palliative Care, 12,* 56–59; Spinetta, J. J., & Maloney, L. (1975). Death anxiety in the outpatient leukemic child. *Pediatrics, 56,* 1034–1037; Spinetta, J. J. (1974). The dying child's awareness of death: A review. *Psychological Bulletin, 81,* 256–260; Kubler-Ross, E. (1983). *On children and death.* New York: Macmillan; Goldman, A., & Christie, D. (1993). Children with cancer talk about their own death with their families. *Pediatric Hematology Oncology, 10,* 223–231; Stevens, M. M. (2004). Paediatric palliative medicine: Psychological adaptation of the dying child. In D. Doyle, G. Hanks, N. I.

Cherny, & Calman (Eds.), *Oxford textbook of palliative medicine,* 3rd ed. (pp. 798–806). Oxford: Oxford University Press.

20. Levetown, M., & Carter, M. A. (1998). Child-centered care in terminal illness: an ethical framework. In D. Doyle, G. W. C. Hanks, & N. MacDonald (Eds.), *Oxford textbook of palliative medicine,* 2nd ed. (pp. 1107–1117). Oxford: Oxford University Press (p. 1107).

21. King, N. M. P., & Cross, A. W. (1989). Children as decision makers: Guidelines for pediatricians. *Journal of Pediatrics, 115,* 10–16; Doyal, L., & Henning, P. (1994). Stopping treatment for end-stage renal failure: The rights of children and adolescents. *Journal of Pediatric Nephrology, 8,* 768–791; Grant, V. J. (1991). Consent in pediatrics: A complex teaching assignment. *Journal of Medical Ethics, 17,* 199–204; Grisso, T., & Vierling, L. (1978). Minors' consent to treatment: A developmental perspective. *Professional Psychology, 9,* 412–427; Leikin, S. (1993). The role of adolescents in decisions concerning their cancer therapy. *Cancer* (suppl.), *71,* 3342–3346; American Academy of Pediatrics, Committee on Bioethics (1995). Informed consent, parental permission and assent in pediatric practice. *Pediatrics, 95,* 314–317; American Academy of Pediatrics, Committee on Bioethics. (1996). Ethics and the care of critically ill infants and children. *Pediatrics, 93,* 149–152.

22. American Academy of Pediatrics (1994). Guidelines on forgoing life-sustaining medical treatment. *Pediatrics, 93,* 532–536; Hilden, J. M., Watterson, J., & Chrastek, J. (2000). Tell the children. *Journal of Clinical Oncology, 18,* 3193–3195.

23. Ways of helping parents cope with end-of-life care for their child are discussed in Hilden, J., & Tobin, D. R. (2003). *Shelter from the storm.* Cambridge, MA: Perseus; Moldow, D. G., & Martinson, I. (1991). *Home care for seriously ill children: A manual for parents.* Alexandria, VA: Children's Hospice Intl.

24. Bowlby, J. (1977). The making and breaking of affectional bonds I & II. *British Journal of Psychiatry, 130,* 201–210, 421–431; Ainsworth, M., Blehar, M., Waters, E., & Wall, S. (1978). *Patterns of attachment: A psychological study of the strange situation.* Hillsdale, NJ: Erlbaum.

25. Field, M. J. & Behrman, R. (Eds.). *When children die: Improving palliative and end-of-life care for children and their families.* Washington, DC: National Academies Press (p. xv).

26. Klass, D. (1988). *Parental grief: Solace and resolution.* New York: Springer; Miles, M. S., & Demi, A. S. (1986). Guilt in bereaved parents. In T. A. Rando (Ed.), *Parental loss of a child* (pp. 97–118). Champaign, IL: Research Press; Rubin, S. (1993). The death of a child is forever: The life course impact of child loss. In M. S. Stroebe, W. Stroebe, & R. O. Hansson (Eds.), *Handbook of bereavement* (pp. 285–299). Cambridge: Cambridge University Press; Rosof, B. (1994). *The worst loss: How families heal from the death of a child.* New York: Henry Holt.

27. Whittam, E. H. (1993). Terminal care of the ding child: Psychosocial implications of care. *Cancer, 71,* Suppl., 3450–3462; Morgan, R., & Murphy, S. B. (2001). Care of children who are dying of cancer. *The New England Journal of Medicine, 342,* 347–348.

28. Himelstein, B. P., Hilden, J. M., Boldt, A. M., & Weissman, D. (2004) Pediatric palliative care. *New England Journal of Medicine, 350,* 1752–1762 (p. 1758).

29. Saunders, C. M. (2004). Foreword. In D. Doyle, G. Hanks, N. I. Cherny, & K. Calman (Eds.). *Oxford textbook of palliative medicine,* 3rd ed. (pp. xvii–xx). Oxford: Oxford University Press (p. xvii).

30. Wolfe, J., Klar, N., Grier, H. E., Duncan, J., Salem-Schatz, S., Emanuel, E. J., & Weeks, J. C. (2000). Understanding of prognosis among parents of children who died of cancer: Impact on treatment goals and integration of palliative care. *Journal of the American Medical Association, 284,* 2469–2475 (p. 2473).

31. Carter, B. (2003, November). *Pediatric pain and symptom management: A first step toward pediatric palliative care.* Paper presented at the meeting of the Initiative for Pediatric Palliative Care National Symposium, New York; Carter, B. S., Howenstein, M., Gilmer, M. J., Throop, P., France, D., & Whitlock, J. A. (2004). Circumstances surrounding the death of hospitalized children: Opportunities for Pediatric palliative care. *Pediatrics, 114,* 361–366. Another study reported a median length of terminal hospitalization of 4 days and a mean of 16.3 days. Feudtner, C., Christakas, D. A., Zimmerman, F. G., Muldoon, J. H., Neff, J. M., & Koepsell, T. D. (2002). *Pediatrics, 109,* 887–893.

32. Kissane, D. W. (2004). Bereavement. In D. Doyle, G. Hanks, N. I. Cherny, & K. Calman (Eds.). *Oxford textbook of palliative medicine,* 3rd ed. (pp. 1137–1151). Oxford: Oxford University Press.

33. In *"They never want to tell you": Children talk about cancer,* I discussed eight narrative themes that prevailed in almost all of the children's stories about having cancer. Among them was the theme of spirituality. Whether or not they came from religious families, children, in a variety of different ways, found solace by putting themselves in the hands of God. See also Bohannon, J. (1991). Religiosity related to grief levels of bereaved mothers and fathers. *Omega, 23,* 153–159; Miller, W. R., & Thoresen, C. E. (2003). Spirituality, religion, and health: An emerging research field. *American Psychologist, 58,* 24–35.

34. Khaneja and Milrod found that a majority of attending physicians, but not residents or fellows, often considered a patient's death as a personal failure. Despite their sense of failure, they were more prepared to deal with issues of death and dying than residents or fellows (71 percent vs. 13 percent and 56 percent, respectively). Khaneja, S., & Milrod, B. (1998). Educational needs among pediatricians regarding caring for terminally ill children. *Archives of Pediatric and Adolescent Medicine, 152,* 909–914.

See also Meier, D. E., Back, A. L., & Morrison, R. S. (2001). The inner life of physicians and care of the seriously ill. *Journal of the American Medical Association, 286,* 3007–3015, for a fuller account of physicians' emotions regarding the death of their patients. Along with a sense of failure, physicians caring for patients at the end of life can develop a sense of helplessness, frustration, and guilt, as a result of which these physicians often withdraw from patients.

See also Feifel, H. (1986). Foreword. In F. Wald (Ed.), *In the quest of the spiritual component of care for the terminally ill: Proceedings of a colloquium* (pp. 15–22). New Haven, CT: Yale School of Nursing.

35. The idea that end-of-life care without curative intent is beyond the pale of medicine—and hence its failure—is reflected in the way medicine is defined: "The science or practice of the diagnosis and treatment of illness and injury and the preservation of

health; *spec.* the science or practice of restoring and preserving health"—*The Oxford English Dictionary.*

36. Nuland, S. (1994). *How we die: Reflections on life's final chapter.* New York: Knopf.

37. Saunders, C. M. (2004). Foreword. In D. Doyle, G. Hanks, N. I. Cherny, & K. Calman (Eds.), *Oxford textbook of palliative medicine,* 3rd ed. (pp. xvii–xx). Oxford: Oxford University Press.

38. Feudtner, C., Silveira, M. J., & Christakis, D. A. (2002). Where do children with complex chronic conditions die? Patterns in Washington State, 1980–1998. *Pediatrics, 109,* 6576–6660.

39. NHPCO facts and figures. Alexandria, VA: National Hospice and Palliative Care Organization, July 2003. (Accessed April 26, 2004 at http://www.nhpco.org/templates/1/homepage.cfm); Carter, B. S., Howenstein, M., Gilmer, M. J., Throop, P., France, D., & Whitlock, J. A. (2004). Circumstances surrounding the death of hospitalized children: Opportunities for pediatric palliative care. *Pediatrics, 114,* 361–366.

40. Quill, T. E. (2004). Dying and decision making: Evolution of end-of-life options. *New England Journal of Medicine, 350,* 2029–2032.

41. Huijier, H. A. (2003, November). Cultural challenges in family centered care. Paper presented at the Initiative for Pediatric Palliative Care National Symposium, New York, NY.

42. Dominica, F. (1998). Development in the United Kingdom. In D. Doyle, G. W. C. Hanks, & N. MacDonald (Eds.), *Oxford textbook of palliative medicine,* 2nd ed. (pp. 1098–1100). Oxford: Oxford University Press.

43. Levetown, M. (1996). Ethical aspects of pediatric palliative care. *Journal of Palliative Care, 12,* 35–39; American Academy of Pediatrics Committee on Bioethics and Committee on Hospital Care (2000). Palliative care for children. *Pediatrics, 106,* 351–357.

44. A bill was recently introduced in the U.S. Congress (September 17, 2003) titled the Children's Compassionate Care Act and the Pediatric Palliative Care Act in the Senate (S 1629) and House (HR 3127), respectively. The purpose of this legislation is to improve palliative and end-of-life care provided to children with life-threatening medical conditions.

45. McCallum, D. E., Byrne, P., & Breweri, E. (2000). How children die in hospital. *Journal of Pain Symptom Management, 20,* 417–423. One study found that parental adaptation following home care of their dying child was more favorable than allowing their child to die in the hospital. Lauer, M. E., Mulhern, R. K., Wallskog, J. M., & Camitta, B. M. (1983). A comparison study of parental adaptation following a child's death at home or in the hospital. *Pediatrics, 71,* 107–112.

46. Field, M. J., & Behrman, R., (Eds.). (2003). *When children die: Improving palliative and end-of-life care for children and their families.* Washington, DC: National Academies Press.

47. Field, M. J., & Behrman, R. (Eds.). (2003). *When children die: Improving palliative and end-of-life care for children and their families.* Washington, DC: National Academies Press.

48. Aside from cancer, other illnesses that account for the death of children are neurodegenerative and metabolic diseases, cystic fibrosis, muscle disorders (e.g., muscular dystrophy), cardiac diseases, and liver and renal disease. Goldman, A. (1998). Life threatening illnesses and symptom control in children. In D. Doyle, G. W. C. Hanks, & N. MacDonald (Eds.), *Oxford textbook of palliative medicine,* 2nd ed. (pp. 1032–1043). Oxford: Oxford University Press.

49. Robinson, L. L. (1993). General principles of the epidemiology of childhood cancer. In P. A. Pizzo, & D. G. Poplack (Eds.), *Principles and practice of pediatric oncology,* 2nd ed. (pp. 3–10). Philadelphia: J. P. Lippincott; Parkin, D. M., Stiller, C. A., Draper, G. S., Bieber, C. A., Terracini, B., & Young, J. L. (Eds.). *International incidence of childhood cancer,* International Agency for Research on Cancer. Geneva: World Health Organization.

50. Hilden, J. M., Emmanuel, E. J., Fairclough, D. L., Link, M. P., Foley, K. M., Clarridge, B. C., Schnipper, L. E., & Mayer, R. J. (2001). Attitudes and practices among pediatric oncologists regarding end-of-life care: Results of the 1998 American Society of Clinical Oncology Survey. *Journal of Clinical Oncology, 19,* 205–212 (p. 207).

51. Meyer, E. C., Burns, J. P., Griffith, J., & Truog, R. D. (2002). Parental perspectives on end-of-life care in the pediatric intensive care unit. *Critical Care Medicine, 30,* 226–231.

52. Feudtner, C., Hays, R. M., Haynes, G., Geyer, J. R., Neff, J. M., & Koepsell, T. D. (2001). Deaths attributed to pediatric complex chronic conditions: National trends and implications for supportive care services. *Pediatrics, 107,* e99.

53. Martinson, I. M. (1993). Hospice care for children: past, present, and future. *Journal of Pediatric Oncology Nursing, 10,* 93–98; Liben, S. (1996). Pediatric palliative medicine: obstacles to overcome. *Journal of Palliative Care, 12,* 24–28; Sahler, O. J., Frager, G., Levetown, M., Cohn, F. G., & Lipson, M. A. (2000). Medical education about end-of-life care in the pediatric setting: principles, challenges, and opportunities. *Pediatrics, 105,* 575–584.

54. Phase I studies test investigational treatments that offer only a slight chance of cure and often cause significant increases in pain and morbidity. However, at the point where it is offered to patients and families, it is the only option that offers any chance at all of cure.

55. Children's Oncology Group, Task Force on End-of-Life Care, Semi-annual Meeting, San Antonio, TX (October 2001).

56. Hoy, A. M. (2004). Training specialists in palliative medicine. In D. Doyle, G. Hanks, N. I. Cherny, & K. Calman (Eds.), *Oxford textbook of palliative medicine,* 3rd ed. (pp. 1166–1175). Oxford: Oxford University Press. According to Hoy, "Palliative medicine was first recognized as a medical speciality by the Royal College of Physicians in the United Kingdom in 1987" (p. 1166). In the United States, certification in Pain and Palliative Care has been available since 1995.

57. In the next 50 years, there will be a fourfold increase worldwide among those aged 65 and older (from 0.4 to 1.5 billion). United Nations (1998). *United Nations population database: The sex and age distribution of the world populations.* New York: United Nations.

58. Field, M. J., & Cassel, C. K. (Eds). (1997). *Approaching death: Improving care at the end of life*. Washington, DC: National Academies Press.

59. APA Working Group on Assisted Suicide and End-of-Life Decisions (2000, May). *Report to the Board of Directors of the American Psychological Association*. Washington, DC: American Psychological Association; New York State Task Force on Life and Law. (2000). *When death is sought: Assisted suicide and euthanasia in the medical context*, 2nd ed. Albany: New York State Department of Health; Roy, D. J. (2004). Ethical issues: Euthanasia and withholding treatment. In D. Doyle, G. Hanks, N. I. Cherny, & K. Calman (Eds.), *Oxford textbook of palliative medicine*, 3rd ed. (pp. 84–97). Oxford: Oxford University Press.

60. Mello. M. M., Burns, J. P., Truog, R. D., Studdert, D. M., Puopolo, A. L., & Brennan, T. A. (2004). Decision making and satisfaction with care in the pediatric intensive care unit: Findings from a controlled clinical trial. *Pediatric Critical Care Medicine, 5*, 40–47 (p. 44).

61. Steinhauser, K. E., Christakis, N. A., Clipp, E. C., McNeilly, M., McIntyre, L., & Tulsky, J. A. (2000). Factors considered important at the end of life by patients, family, physicians, and other care providers. *Journal of the American Medical Association, 284*, 2476–2482; Steinhauser, K. E., Clipp, E. C., McNeilly, M., Christatkis, N. A., McIntyre, L. M., & Tulsky, J. A. (2000). In search of a good death: Observations of patients, families, and providers. *Annals of Internal Medicine, 132*, 825–832; Fried, T. R., Bradley, E. H., Towle, V. R., & Allore, H. (2002). Understanding the treatment preferences of seriously ill patients. *New England Journal of Medicine, 346*, 1061–1066; Bradley, E. H., Hallemeier, A. G., Fried, T. R., et al. (2001). Documentation of discussions about prognosis with terminally ill patients. *American Journal of Medicine, 111*, 218–223.

62. Field, M. J., & Behrman, R. (Eds.). (2003). *When children die: Improving palliative and end-of-life care for children and their families*. Washington, DC: National Academies Press (p. 30).

63. World Health Organization. (1990). *Cancer pain relief and palliative care*. WHO Technical Report Series 804. Geneva: WHO (p. 11).

64. American Academy of Pediatrics, Committee on Bioethics and Committee on Hospital Care (2000). Palliative care for children. *Pediatrics, 1067*, 351–357 (p. 352).

65. Collins, J. J., Devine, T. D., Dick, G. S., et al. (2002). The measurement of symptoms in young children with cancer: The validation of the Memorial Symptom Assessment Scare in children aged 7–12. *Journal of Pain and Symptom Management, 23*, 10–16; Varni, J. W., Burwinkle, T. M., Katz, E. R., Meeske, K., & Dickinson, P. (2002). The PedsQL in pediatric cancer: Reliability and validity of the Pediatric Quality of Life Inventory Generic Core Scales, multi-dimensional fatigue scale, and cancer module. *Cancer, 94*, 2090–2106.

66. Frank, A. W. (2004). *The renewal of generosity: Illness, medicine and how to live*. Chicago: University of Chicago Press.

67. Doyle, D., Hanks, G., Cherny, N. I., & Calman, K. (2004). Introduction. In D. Doyle, G. Hanks, N. I. Cherny, & K. Calman (Eds.), *Oxford textbook of palliative medicine*, 3rd ed. (pp. 1–4). Oxford: Oxford University Press.

68. Portenoy, R. K., & Breweri, E. (Eds.) (2003). *Issues in palliative care research*. New York: Oxford University Press; Lloyd-Williams, M. (Ed.) (2003). *Psychosocial issues in palliative care*. New York: Oxford University Press.

69. McCallum, D. E., Byrne, P., & Breweri, E. (2000). How children die in hospital. *Journal of Pain Symptom Management, 20*, 417–423. See also Lantos, J. D., Berger, A. C., Zucker, & A. R. (1993). Do-not-resuscitate orders in a children's hospital. *Critical Care Medicine, 21*, 52–55.

70. Council on Ethical Judicial Affairs of the American Medical Association. (1991). Pediatrics and the patient self-determination act. *Pediatrics, 1265*, 1868–1871.

71. Sussman, E. J., Hersch, S. P., Nannis, E. D. et al. (1982). Conceptions of cancer: The perspectives of child and adolescent patients and their families. *Journal of Pediatric Psychiatry, 7*, 253–261; Leikin, S. (1993). The role of adolescents in decisions concerning their cancer therapy. *Cancer* (suppl.), *71*, 3342–3346; Freyer, D. R. (1992). Children with cancer: Special considerations in the discontinuation of life sustaining treatment. *Journal of Medical and Pediatric Oncology, 20*, 136–142.

72. Foley, K. M., & Gelband, H. (Eds.). (2001). *Improving palliative care for cancer*. Washington, DC: National Academies Press.

CHAPTER 2: NARRATIVE THEORY, MEDICINE, AND METHODS

1. Kristjanson, L. J., & Coyle, N. (2004). Research in palliative medicine: Qualitative research. In D. Doyle, G. Hanks, N. Cherny, & K. Calman (Eds.), *Oxford textbook of palliative medicine*, 3rd ed. (pp. 138–144). Oxford: Oxford University Press.

2. Bruner, J. (2002). *Making stories: Law, literature, life*. New York: Farrar, Straus & Giroux (p. 5).

3. Angel, S. (2004). *The tale of the scale: An odyssey of invention*. New York: Oxford University Press.

4. Burke, K. (1945). *Grammar of motives*. New York: Prentice-Hall.

5. Bruner, J. (2002). *Making stories: Law, literature, life*. New York: Farrar, Straus & Giroux (p. 31).

6. Clandenin, D. J., & Connelly, F. M. (1994). Personal experience methods. In H. K., Denzin & Y. S. Lincoln (Eds.), *Handbook of qualitative research* (pp. 413–427). Thousand Oaks, CA: Sage (p. 416); Murray, M. (2003). Narrative psychology and narrative analysis. In P. M. Camic, J. E. Rhodes, & L. Yardley, *Qualitative research in psychology: Expanding perspectives in methodology and design*. Washington, DC: American Psychological Association.

7. Nelson, K. (1966). *Language in cognitive development: The emergence of the mediated mind*. New York: Cambridge University Press; Danto, A. C. (1965). *Analytical philosophy of history*. Cambridge: Cambridge University Press; Harre, R., & Gillet, G. (1994). *The discursive mind*. Thousand Oaks, CA: Sage; Shotter, J., & Gergen, K. (Eds.) (1989). *Texts of identity*. Newbury Park, CA: Sage; Schafer, R. (1982). Narration in the psychoanalytic dialogue. In Spence, D. (Ed.), *Narrative truth and historical truth: Meaning and interpretation in psychoanalysis*. New York: Norton; White, H. (1987). *The content of form: Narrative discourse and historical representation*. Baltimore, MD: Johns Hopkins University Press.

8. Day, J. D., & Tappan, M. B. (1996). The narrative approach to moral development: From the epistemic subject to dialogical selves. *Human Development, 39*, 67–82;

Wertsch, J. V. (Ed.) (1985). *Culture communication and cognition: Vygotskian perspectives.* New York: Cambridge University Press; Vygotsky, L. S. (1978). *Mind in society: The development of higher psychological processes.* Cambridge, MA: Harvard University Press.

9. Riessman, C. K. (1993). *Narrative analysis.* Thousand Oaks, CA: Sage.

10. Hunter, M. K. (1991). *Doctors' stories: The narrative structure of medical knowledge.* Princeton, NJ: Princeton University Press; Greenhalgh, T. (1998). Narrative-based medicine. London: BMJ Publishing; Kleinman, A. (1988). *The illness narratives: Suffering, healing, and the human condition.* New York: Basic Books; Verghese, A. (2001). The physician as storyteller. *Annals of Internal Medicine, 135,* 1012–1017; Charon, R. (2004). Narrative and medicine. *New England Journal of Medicine, 350,* 862–864; Frank, A. (2004). *The renewal of generosity.* Chicago: University of Chicago Press; Campo, R. (2004). Just the facts. *New England Journal of Medicine, 351,* 1167–1169.

11. Flood, D. H., & Soricelli, R. L. (1992). Development of the physician's narrative voice in the medical case history. *Literature and Medicine, 11,* 64–83.

12. For example, one study found value in having veterans of the Normandy invasion tell their stories, another found value in having women tell stories about having had an abortion, and yet another in having victims talk about terrorist attacks in Israel. Harvey, J. H., Stein, S. K., & Scott, P. K. (1995). Fifty years of grief: Accounts and reported psychological reactions of Normandy invasion veterans. *Journal of Narrative and Life History, 5,* 315–332; Ellis, C., & Bochner, A. P. (1992). Telling and performing personal stories: The constraints of choice in abortion. In C. Ellis, & M. Flaherty (Eds.), *Investigating subjectivity* (pp. 79–101). Newbury Park, CA: Sage; Tuval-Mashiach, R. (2004, May). The narrative approach on coping with trauma: Implications for the treatment of adolescents. Paper presented at the second bi-national conference on treating traumatized children and adolescents. Jerusalem, Israel; Tuval-Mashiach, R., Freedman, S., Bargai, N., Boker, M., Hadar, H, & Shalev, A. Y. (2004). Coping with trauma: Narrative and cognitive perspectives. *Psychiatry, 67,* 280–294.

13. Piaget, J. (1923). La pensée symbolique et la pensée de l'enfant. *Archives de Psychologies, 18,* 273–304; Freud, S. (1963). *Therapy and technique.* New York: Collier; Kvale, S. (2003). The psychoanalytical interview as inspiration for qualitative research. In P. M. Camic, J. E. Rhodes, & L. Yardley (Eds.), *Qualitative research in psychology: Expanding perspectives in methodology and design.* Washington, DC: American Psychological Association.

14. Gilbert, K. R. (2002). Taking a narrative approach to grief research: Finding meaning in stories. *Death Studies, 26,* 223–239.

15. Narratives were audiotaped and transcribed verbatim by specially trained doctoral students in psychology. Informed consent was obtained from participants according to the standards of the medical center's Institutional Review Board, and a Certificate of Confidentiality was obtained from the U.S. Department of Health and Human Resources to further insure the confidentiality of participants. All names cited in the narratives are fictitious.

Narratives were elicited from 30 attending physicians, 12 fellows, 2 house physicians, 9 residents, 4 interns, 2 medical students, 9 nurse practitioners, 19 registered nurses, 13 social workers, 1 psychologist, and 8 child-life specialists. Some of the participants were involved in more than one case. Narratives ranged from approximately half an hour to an hour and a half. Four people (2 physicians and 2 nurses) declined to participate.

16. The narratives are verbatim transcriptions, with the following editorial guidelines taken to render them easier to read: (1) repetitions were deleted, (2) colloquial kinds of typical and repetitive oral speech (e.g., "you know," "hmm," "like," "uh") were deleted, and (3) grammatical inconsistencies (mostly in verb tenses) were corrected to fit the syntax of the sentence. The names of patients and their families were changed, and the names of staff were substituted with their professional titles. Occasionally, words in parentheses were added for clarifying or explaining (in place of a glossary) what participants were saying. Breaks in narratives are indicated by three periods (four when it is at the end of a sentence). As is always the case when transcribing oral speech, determination of how to indicate clauses, sentences, and paragraphs was made at the discretion of the author with the intent to convey the contextual meaning of the narrator.

CHAPTER 3: TWENTY STORIES ABOUT HOW CHILDREN DIE

1. Arias, E., MacDorman, M. F., Strobino, D. M., & Guyer, B. (2003). Annual summary of vital statistics–2002. *Pediatrics, 112,* 1215–1230.

2. Feudtner, C., Hays, R. M., Haynes, G., Geyer, J. R., Neff, J. M., & Koepsell, T. D. (2001). Deaths attributed to pediatric complex chronic conditions: National trends and implications for supportive care services. *Pediatrics, 107,* e99.

3. Nuland, S. B. (1993). *How we die: Reflections on life's final chapter.* New York: Random House (pp. xvi & xvii, respectively).

4. Nuland, S. B. (1993). *How we die: Reflections on life's final chapter.* New York: Random House (p. xvii).

5. Centers for Disease Control and Prevention (1999, July 30). Control of infectious diseases. *Morbidity and Mortality Weekly Report, 48,* 621–629.

6. For a discussion of the many conflicting legal standards that have been used to define death, see Kolata, G. (1997, April 27). When death begins. *New York Times;* Veatch, R. M. (1989). *Death, dying and the biological revolution: Our last quest for responsibility,* rev. ed. New Haven, CT: Yale University Press.

7. Meyer, E. C., Burns, J. P., Griffith, J., Truog, R. D. (2002). Parental perspectives on end-of-life care in the pediatric intensive care unit. *Critical Care Medicine, 30,* 226–231.

8. Atul Gawande, in a book about the limits of modern medicine, cites some remarkable findings about autopsies. He reports that 40 percent of autopsies reveal a "major misdiagnosis" in the cause of death and that in about a third of these cases, the patients would have survived if treatment, appropriate to the diagnosis, had been administered. He also states that the rate of misdiagnosis found by autopsies has not changed since 1938. Such an alarming finding needs to be qualified, however, by further findings that today less then 10 percent of autopsies are performed in hospitals compared to the end of the World War II, when autopsies were considered a routine procedure in the death of any patient in a hospital. This is not because families of the

deceased are more reluctant to consent to autopsies (80 percent do consent when asked), but that physicians are more reluctant to request it because advanced technologies such as CT, ultrasound, and nuclear scanning allow them to feel less uncertain about their patients' causes of death. Gawande then claims that because "physicians did not consider the correct diagnosis in the first place" (p. 198), they never made use of advanced technologies by ordering the appropriate diagnostic tests. His point, worth considering, is that we don't always know why a patient dies in a hospital because we don't always know the appropriate diagnosis and therefore the appropriate medical intervention to cure and restore health. See Gawande, A. (2002). *Complications: A surgeon's notes on an imperfect science.* New York: Henry Holt.

9. A code is a call for nursing, physician, and respiratory therapy staff to come immediately to a patient's bedside to resuscitate or otherwise provide emergency care for a patient who has had a sudden event resulting in inadequate cardiac and/or respiratory function.

CHAPTER 4: WITHHOLDING AND WITHDRAWING CURATIVE TREATMENTS

1. Morgan, E. R., & Murphy, S. B. (2001). Care of children who are dying of cancer. *The New England Journal of Medicine, 342,* 347–348. According to J. Hilden & D. R. Tobin *(Shelter from the storm: Caring for a child with a life-threatening condition,* Cambridge, MA: Perseus, 2003), "Medical culture currently tilts toward the philosophy that no condition is truly hopeless, that there is always some therapy worth trying. Such a philosophy can make parents who don't choose high-tech therapy feel that they are wrong, or bad parents" (p. 39).

2. Whittam, E. H. (1993). Terminal care of the dying child: Psychosocial implications of care. *Cancer, 71,* Suppl., 3450–3462; Wiener, J. M. (1970) Attitudes of pediatricians toward the care of fatally ill children. *Journal of Pediatrics, 76,* 700–705.

3. Cantagrel, S., Ducrocq, S., Chedeville, G., & Marchand, S. (2000). Mortality in a pediatric hospital: Six-year retrospective study. *Archives Pediatrique, 7,* 725–731; McCallum, D. E., Byrne, P., & Breweri, E. (2000). How children die in hospital. *Journal of Pain and Symptom Management, 20,* 417–423; van der Wal, M. E., Renfurm, L. N., van Vught, A. J., & Gemke, R. J. (1999). Circumstances of dying in hospitalized children. *European Journal of Pediatrics, 158,* 560–565.

4. President's Commission for the Study of Ethical Problems in Medicine and Biomedical and Behavioral Research (1983). *Deciding to forgo life-sustaining treatment. A report on the ethical, medical and legal issues in treatment decisions.* Washington, DC: U.S. Government Printing Office; Council on Ethical and Judicial Affairs of the American Medical Association (1986). *Withholding or withdrawing life-prolonging treatment.* Chicago: American Medical Association.

5. Freyer, D. R. (1992). Children with cancer: Special considerations in the discontinuation of life-sustaining treatment. *Medical and Pediatric Oncology, 28,* 136–142 (p. 136)

6. Freyer, D. R. (1992). Children with cancer: Special considerations in the discontinuation of life-sustaining treatment. *Medical and Pediatric Oncology, 28,* 136–142.

7. Wolfe, J., Klar, N., Grier, H. E., Duncan, J., Salem-Schatz, S., Emanuel, E. J., & Weeks, J. C. (2000). Understanding of prognosis among parents of children who died of cancer: Impact on treatment goals and integration of palliative care. *Journal of the American Medical Association, 284*, 2469–2475.

8. Tulsky, J. A., Fischer, G. S., Rose, M. R., & Arnold, R. M. (1998). How do physicians communicate about advance directives. *Annals of Internal Medicine, 129*, 441–449.

9. The range of time from DNR to death was between 1 hour and 30 days. McCallum, D. E., Byrne, P., & Breweri, E. (2000). How children die in hospital. *Journal of Pain and Symptom Management, 20*, 417–423.

10. Hilden, J. M., Emmanuel, E. J., Fairclough, D. L., Link, M. P., Foley, K. M., Clarridge, B. C., Schnipper, L. E., & Mayer, R. J. (2001). Attitudes and practices among pediatric oncologists regarding end-of-life care: Results of the 1998 American Society of Clinical Oncology Survey. *Journal of Clinical Oncology, 19*, 205–212.

11. Treatment in pediatric oncology almost always involves enrolling patients on experimental treatment protocols and clinical trials. The National Department of Health and Human Services (Title 45, Part 46), mandates that, in such cases, pediatricians must elicit the assent of children. "Assent means a child's affirmative agreement to participate in research. Mere failure to object should not, absent affirmative agreement, be construed as assent" (NIH, 1996; p. 15). Furthermore, it is the pediatrician's responsibility to determine when children are capable of providing assent relative to the age, maturity, and psychological state of a given child (National Department of Health and Human Services [DHHS] 1996). Additional protection for children involved as subjects in research is provided in the *Federal Register* [45 DFR 46]. Pp. 4–17.

12. Leikin, S. (1989). A proposal concerning decisions to forgo life-sustaining treatment for young people. *Journal of Pediatrics, 115*, 17–22.

13. Schneider, C. E. (1998). *The practice of autonomy: Patients, doctors, and medical decisions.* New York: Oxford University Press.

14. Nitschke, R., Humphrey, G. B., Sexauer, C. L., Catron, B., Wunder, S., & Jay, S. (1982). Therapeutic choices made by patients with end-stage cancer. *Behavioral Pediatrics, 101*, 471–476 (p. 475).

15. Leikin, S. (1989). A proposal concerning decisions to forgo life-sustaining treatment for young people. *Journal of Pediatrics, 115*, 17–22 (p. 21).

16. Schneider, C. E. (1998). *The practice of autonomy: Patients, doctors, and medical decisions.* New York: Oxford University Press; Zussman, R. (1995). Reflections on field work in a medical setting: Medicine, medical ethics, and the sociological voice. Paper presented at the Conference on the Sociology of Medical Ethics. Ann Arbor, MI, September 1995.

17. Fleischman, A. R., Nolan, K., Dubler, N. N., Epstein, M. F., Gerben, M. A., Jellinek, M. S., Litt, I. R., Miles, M. S., Oppenheimer, S., Shaw, A., van Eys, J., & Baughan, V. C. (1994). Caring for gravely ill children. *Pediatrics, 94*, 433–439; Hinds, P. S., Oakes, L., Furman, W., Quargnenti, A. Olson, M. S., Foppiano, P., & Srivastava, D. K. (2001). End-of-life decision making by adolescents, parents, and healthcare providers in pediatric oncology: Research to evidence-based practice guidelines. *Cancer Nursing, 24*, 122–136.

18. The American Academy of Pediatrics, Committee on Bioethics. (1995). Informed consent, parental permission and assent in pediatric practice. *Pediatrics, 95,* 314–317; American Academy of Pediatrics, Committee on Bioethics. (1996). Ethics and the care of critically ill infants and children. *Pediatrics, 93,*149–152.

19. Meyer, E. C., Burns, J. P., Griffith, J., & Truog, R. D. (2002). Parental perspectives on end-of-life care in the pediatric intensive care unit. *Critical Care Medicine, 30,* 226–231.

20. Slevin, M. L., Stubbs, L., Plant, H. J., Wilson, P., Gregory, W. M., Ames, P. J., & Downer, S. M. (1990). Attitudes to chemotherapy: Comparing views of patients with cancer with those of doctors, nurses, and general public. *British Medical Journal, 300,* 1458–1460; Rayson, D. (2003). Sweet time unafflicted. *Supplement to Journal of Clinical Oncology, The art of oncology: When the tumor is not the target, 21,* 46–47s.

21. Ashwal, S., Perkin, R. M., & Orr, R. (1992). When too much is not enough. *Pediatric Annals, 21,* 311–314, 316–317; Cassell, E. J. (1982). The nature of suffering and the goals of medicine. *New England Journal of Medicine, 306,* 639–645; Orlowski, J. P. (1992). How much resuscitation is enough resuscitation?*Pediatrics, 90,* 997–998.

22. Epstein, F. (2003). *If I get to five: What children can teach us about courage and character.* New York: H. Holt (p. 54).

CHAPTER 5: PAIN AND SUFFERING

1. Hilden, J., & Tobin, D. R. (2003). *Shelter from the storm: Caring for a child with a life-threatening condition.* Cambridge, MA: Perseus (p. 3).

2. National Institutes of Health. (2002). NIH State-of-the-science statement on symptom management in cancer: Pain, depression, and fatigue. *NIH State Science Statements, 19,* 1–29.

3. Portenoy, R. K., & Bruera, E. (Eds.) (2003). *Issues in palliative care research.* New York: Oxford University Press; Nuland, S. (1994). *How we die: Reflections on life final chapter.* New York: Knopf; Gawande, A. (2002). *Complications: A surgeon's notes on an imperfect science.* New York: Henry Holt.

4. Collins, J. J., Byrnes, M. E., Dunkel, I. J., Lapin, J., Nadel, T., Thaler, H. T., Polyak, T., Rapkin, B., & Portenoy, R. K. (2000). The measurement of symptoms in children with cancer. *Journal of Pain and Symptom Management, 19,* 363–377; Collins, J. J., Devine, T. D., Dick, G. S., Johnson, E. A., Kilham, H. A., Pinkerton, C. R., Stevens, M. M., Thaler, H. T., & Portenoy, R. K. (2002). The measurement of symptoms in young children with cancer: the validation of the Memorial Symptom Assessment Scale in children aged 7–12. *Journal of Pain and Symptom Management, 23,* 10–16.

5. Wolfe, J., Grier, H. E., Klar, N., Levin, S. B., Ellenbogen, J. M., Salem-Schatz, S., Emanuel, E. J., & Weeks, J. C. (2000). Symptoms and suffering at the end of life in children with cancer. *New England Journal of Medicine, 342,* 326–333.

Another survey, however, found that "81 per cent of parents reported that the amount of pain medication their children received at the end of life was usually or always enough." Meyer, E. C., Burns, J. P., Griffith, J., & Truog, R. D. (2002). Parental perspectives on end-of-life care in the pediatric intensive care unit. *Critical Care Medicine, 30,* 226–231 (p. 227).

6. Foley, K. M. (1995). Pain, physician assisted dying and euthanasia. *Pain, 4,* 163–178.

7. Fossa, S. D., et al. (1990). Quality of life and treatment of hormone resistant prostatic cancer. *European Journal of Cancer, 26,* 1133–1136.

8. Waco, G. A., Cassidy, R. C., & Schechter, N. L. (1994). Pain, hurt, and harm: The ethics of pain control in infants and children. *New England Journal of Medicine, 331,* 541–544; Zeltzer, L. (1994). Pain and symptom management. In D. J. Bearison & R. K. Mulhern (Eds.), *Pediatric psychooncology: Psychological perspectives on children with cancer* (pp. 61–83). New York: Oxford University Press; Sirkia, K., Saarinen, U. M., Ahlgren, B., & Hovi, L. (1997). Terminal care of the child with cancer at home. *Acta Pediatrics, 86,* 1125–1130; Field, M. J., & Behrman, R. (Eds.). (2003). *When children die: Improving palliative and end-of-life care for children and their families.* Washington, DC: National Academies Press.

9. Walco, G. A., Cassidy, R. C., & Schechter, N. L. (1994). Pain, hurt, and harm: The ethics of pain control in infants and children. *New England Journal of Medicine, 331,* 541–544.

10. Foley, K. M. (1995). Pain, physician assisted dying and euthanasia. *Pain, 4,* 163–178.

11. McGrath, P. A. (1990). *Pain in children: Nature, assessment and treatment.* New York: Guilford.

12. McGrath, P. A., & Brown, S. C. (2004). Paediatric palliative medicine: Pain control. In D. Doyle, G. Hanks, N. Cherny, & K. Calman (Eds.), *Oxford textbook of palliative medicine,* 3rd ed. (pp. 775–789). Oxford: Oxford University Press (p. 775).

13. Freyer, D. R. (1992). Children with cancer: Special considerations in the discontinuation of life-sustaining treatment. *Medical and Pediatric Oncology, 20,* 136–142 (p. 141); Tadmor, C. S., Postovsky, S., Elhasid, R., Barak, A. B., & Arush, M. W. (2003). Policies designed to enhance the quality of life of children with cancer at the end-of-life. *Pediatric Hematology and Oncology, 20,* 43–54.

14. Conte, P. M., & Walco, G. A. (2006). Pain and procedure management. In R. T. Brown (Ed.), *Comprehensive Handbook of Childhood Cancer and Sickle Cell Disease.* New York: Oxford University Press.

15. Howard, R. F. (2003). Current status of pain management in children. *Journal of the American Medical Association, 290,* 2464–2469 (p. 2464).

16. Meyer, E. C., Burns, J. P., Griffith, J., & Truog, R. D. (2002). Parental perspectives on end-of-life care in the pediatric intensive care unit. *Critical Care Medicine, 30,* 226–231.

17. Enskar, K., Carlsson, M., Golsater, M., Hamrin, E., & Kreuger, A. (1997). Life situation and problems as reported by children with cancer and their parents. *Journal of Pediatric Oncology Nursing, 14,* 18–26.

18. PCA is a system that allows patients to self-administer controlled doses of opioids in response to pain at frequent intervals. It has been successfully used with children as young as 5 years of age. See Berde, C. B., Lehn, B. M., Yee, J. D., Sethna, N. F., & Russo, D. (1991). Patient-controlled analgesia in children and adolescents: A randomized,

prospective comparison with intramuscular administration of morphine for postoperative analgesia. *Journal of Pediatrics, 118,* 460–466.

CHAPTER 6: STAFF REACTING

1. Heaven, C. M., & Maquire, P. (2003). Communication issues. In M. Lloyd-Williams (Ed.). *Psychosocial issues in palliative care.* New York: Oxford University Press; Von Gunten, C. F., Ferris, F. D., & Emanuel, L. L. (2000). Ensuring competency in end-of-life care: Communication and relational skills. *Journal of the American Medical Association, 284,* 3051–3057; Ptacek, J. T., & Eberhardt, T. L. (1996). Breaking bad news: A review of the literature. *Journal of the American Medical Association, 276,* 496–502.

2. Davies, B., & Orloff, S. (2004). Paediatric palliative medicine: Bereavement issues and staff support. In D. Doyle, G. Hanks, N. Cherny, & K. Calman (Eds.), *Oxford textbook of palliative medicine,* 3rd ed. (pp. 831–839). Oxford: Oxford University Press.

3. Doyle, D., Hanks, G., Cherny, N. I., & Calman, K. (2004). Introduction. In D. Doyle, G. Hanks, N. I. Cherny, & K. Calman (Eds.), *Oxford textbook of palliative medicine,* 3rd ed. (pp. 1–4). Oxford: Oxford University Press (p. 3).

4. Khaneja, S., & Milrod, B. (1998). Educational needs among pediatricians regarding caring for terminally ill children. *Archives of Pediatric and Adolescent Medicine, 152,* 909–914; Mermann, A. C., Gunn, D. B., & Dickinson, G. E. (1991). Learning to care for the dying: A survey of medical schools and a model course. *Academy of Medicine, 66,* 35–38; Rappaport, W., & Witzke, D. (1993). Education about death and dying during the clinical years of medical school. *Surgery, 113,* 163–165; Sahler, O. J., Z., Frager, G., Levetown, M., Cohn, F. G., & Lipson, M. A. (2000). Medical education about end-of-life care in the pediatric setting: Principles, challenges, and opportunities. *Pediatrics, 105,* 575–584; Von Gunten, C. F., Ferris, F. D., & Emanuel, L. L. (2000). Ensuring competency in end-of-life care: Communication and relational skills. *Journal of the American Medical Association, 284,* 3051–3057.

5. Hilden, J. M., Emmanuel, E. J., Fairclough, D. L., Link, M. P., Foley, K. M., Clarridge, B. C., Schnipper, L. E., & Mayer, R. J. (2001). Attitudes and practices among pediatric oncologists regarding end-of-life care: Results of the 1998 American Society of Clinical Oncology Survey. *Journal of Clinical Oncology, 19,* 205–212 (p. 206).

6. Rabow, M. W., Hardie, G. E., Fair, J. M., & McPhee, S. J. (2000). End-of-life case content in 50 textbooks from multiple specialities. *Journal of the American Medical Association, 283,* 771–778.

7. Field, M. J., & Behrman, R. (Eds.). (2003). *When children die: Improving palliative and end-of-life care for children and their families.* Washington, DC: National Academies Press.

8. Field, M. J., & Behrman, R. (Eds.). (2003). *When children die: Improving palliative and end-of-life care for children and their families.* Washington, DC: National Academies Press.

9. Ferrell, B. (2003, November). *End of Life Nursing Education Consortium (ELNEC): National efforts to improve pediatric palliative care.* Paper presented at the meeting of the Initiative for Pediatric Palliative Care, New York, New York.

10. Field, M. J., & Cassel, C. K. (Eds). (1997). *Approaching death: Improving care at the end of life*. Washington, DC: National Academies Press.

CHAPTER 7: PATIENTS AND FAMILIES REACTING

1. Kreicbergs, U., Valdimarsdottir, U.; Onelov, E., Henter, J., & Steineck, G. (2004). Talking about death with children who have severe malignant disease. *New England Journal of Medicine, 351,* 1175–1186. See also Wolfe, L. (2004). Should parents speak with a dying child about impending death? *New England Journal of Medicine, 351,* 1251–1253; and Nitschke, R. (2000). Regarding guidelines for assistance to terminally ill children with cancer: Report of the SIOP Working Committee on psychosocial issues in pediatric oncology. *Medical and Pediatric Oncology, 34,* 271–273.

CHAPTER 8: CONCLUSIONS

1. Doyal, L., Goldman, A., Larcher, V., & Chantler, C. (2004). Ethical issues: Palliative medicine and children: Ethical and legal issues. In D. Doyle, G. Hanks, N. I. Cherny, & K. Calman (Eds.), *Oxford textbook of palliative medicine,* 3rd ed. (pp. 70–75). Oxford: Oxford University Press (p. 71).

2. Piaget, J. (1981). *Intelligence and affectivity*. Palo Alto, CA: Annual Reviews; Vygotsky, L. (1978). *Mind in society*. Cambridge, MA: Harvard University Press.

3. Children quickly come to perceive that many adults simply are not able to talk to them about death, dying, and end-of-life decisions. Despite their own fears, children's hesitancies to spontaneously talk about issues about their dying in such situations often are more a reflection of the fears and anxieties they discern among others around them than their own. See Bearison, D. J. (1991). *"They never want to tell you": Children talk about cancer*. Cambridge, MA: Harvard University Press.

4. Fallowfield, L. (2004). Communication and palliative care: Communication with the patient and family in palliative medicine. In D. Doyle, G. Hanks, N. I. Cherny, & K. Calman (Eds.), *Oxford textbook of palliative medicine,* 3rd ed. (pp. 101–107). Oxford: Oxford University Press.

5. Walco, G. A., Cassidy, R. C., & Schechter, N. L. (1994). Pain, hurt, and harm: The ethics of pain control in infants and children. *New England Journal of Medicine, 331,* 541–544; Schechter, N. L. (1989). The undertreatment of pain in children: An overview. *Pediatric Clinics of North America, 36,* 781–794.

6. Bearison, D. J., Minian, N., & Granowetter, L. F. (2002). Medical management of asthma and folk medicine in an Hispanic community. *Journal of Pediatric Psychology, 27,* 385–392.

7. Kazak, A., Rourke, M., & Crump, T. (2003). Families and other systems in pediatric psychology. In M. Roberts (Ed.), *Handbook of pediatric psychology,* 3rd ed. (pp. 159–175). New York: Guilford.

8. King, N.M.P., & Cross, A.W. (1989). Children as decision makers: Guidelines for pediatricians. Journal of Pediatrics, 115, 17–22; Leikin, S. (1989). A proposal concerning decisions to forgo life-sustaining treatment for young people. *Journal of Pediatrics, 115,*

17–22; Fletcher, J. C., van Eys, J., & Dorn, L. D. (1993). Ethical considerations in pediatric oncology. In P. A. Pizzo & D. G. Poplack (Eds.), *Principles and practices of pediatric oncology* (pp. 1179–1201). Philadelphia: Lippincott; American Academy of Pediatrics, Committee on Bioethics. (1996). Ethics and the care of critically ill infants and children. *Pediatrics, 93*, 149–152; Kleespies, P. M. (2004). *Life and death decisions: Psychological and ethical considerations in end-of-life care.* Washington, DC: American Psychological Association.

9. Murphy, S. A., Johnson, C., Cain, K. C., Gupta, A. D., Diamond, M., Lohan, J., & Baugher, R. (1998). Broad-spectrum group treatment for parents bereaved by the violent death of their 12 to 28 year-old children: A randomized controlled trial. *Death Studies, 22*, 209–235; Allumbaugh, D. L., & Hoyt, W. T. (1999). Effectiveness of grief therapy: A meta-analysis. *Journal of Consulting Psychology, 46*, 370–380; Kato, P. M., & Mann, T. (1999). A synthesis of psychological interventions for the bereaved. *Clinical Psychology Review, 19*, 275–296.

10. Roy, D. J. (2004). Ethical issues: Euthanasia and withholding treatment. In D. Doyle, G. Hanks, N. I. Cherny, & K. Calman (Eds.), *Oxford textbook of palliative medicine,* 3rd ed. (pp. 84–97). Oxford: Oxford University Press (p. 84).

Index

Page numbers followed by t indicate tables.

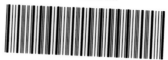